www.harcourt-international.com

Bringing you products from all Harcourt He~~alth~~ companies including Baillière Tindall, Chur~~chill~~ Mosby and W.B. Saunders

- **Browse** for latest information on new books, journals and electronic products

- **Search** for information on over 20 000 published titles with full product information including tables of contents and sample chapters

- **Keep up to date** with our extensive publishing programme in your field by registering with eAlert or requesting postal updates

- **Secure online ordering** with prompt delivery, as well as full contact details to order by phone, fax or post

- **News** of special features and promotions

If you are based in the following countries, please visit the country-specific site to receive full details of product availability and local ordering information

USA: www.harcourthealth.com

Canada: www.harcourtcanada.com

Australia: www.harcourt.com.au

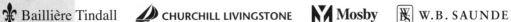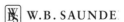

Baillière Tindall   CHURCHILL LIVINGSTONE   Mosby   W.B. SAUNDE~~RS~~

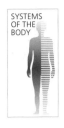

SYSTEMS
OF THE
BODY

SELF-ASSESSMENT
IN
ME

0027643

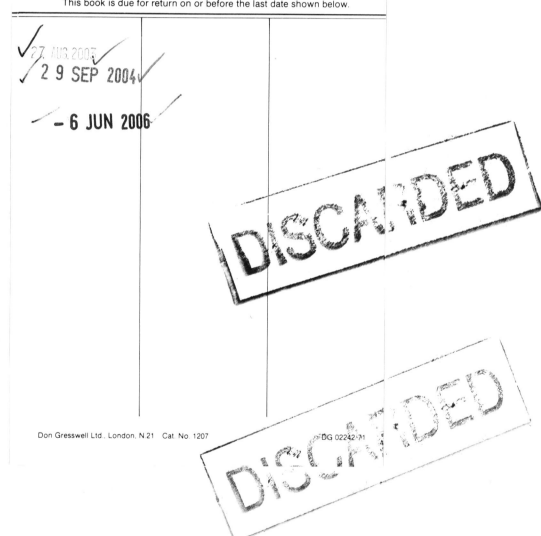

£17.20
pm

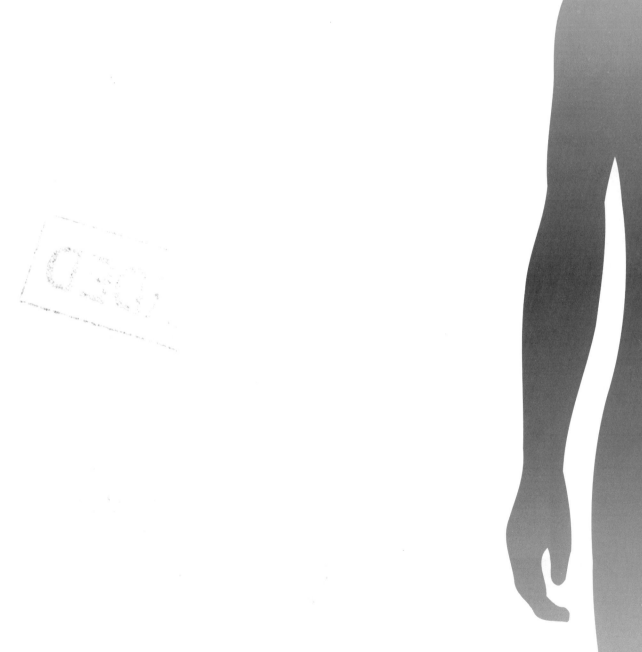

SYSTEMS OF THE BODY

Commissioning Editor: Michael Parkinson
Project Development Manager: Lynn Watt
Project Manager: Frances Affleck
Designer: Erik Bigland
Illustrator: MTG

SELF-ASSESSMENT IN INTEGRATED MEDICAL SCIENCES

Wai-Ching Leung

MA MRCP(UK) MRCPCH MRCGP MRCPsych DCH DO DRCOG PGCE AdvDipEd

Lecturer in Public Health Medicine,
Health Policy and Practice,
University of East Anglia,
Norwich,
UK

With a contribution from

Katharine E.A. Darling

BSc(Hons) MB BS BSs MRCP(UK)

Wellcome Research Fellow,
Department of Infectious Diseases,
Hammersmith Hospital,
London,
UK

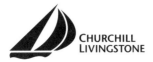

CHURCHILL
LIVINGSTONE

EDINBURGH LONDON NEW YORK PHILADELPHIA ST LOUIS SYDNEY TORONTO 2002

CONTENTS

PART 1
GENERAL BASIC MEDICAL SCIENCES 1

1. The cell   3

2. General principles of pharmacology   15

3. Nutrition and energy   30

4. General principles of pathological processes   41

5. General principles of infectious diseases   54
   K. Darling

6. General principles of histology and embryology   70

7. General principles of genetics   74

PART 2
SYSTEM-BASED BASIC MEDICAL SCIENCES 87

8. Blood and bone marrow   89

9. The cardiovascular system   105

10. The respiratory system   133

11. The gastrointestinal system   154

12. The liver and biliary system   170

13. The endocrine system   175

14. The reproductive system   197

15. The renal and urinary system   215

16. The nervous system   231

17. The musculoskeletal system   262

Index   269

PART 1
GENERAL BASIC MEDICAL SCIENCES

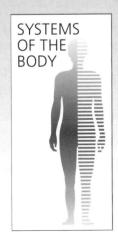

SYSTEMS
OF THE
BODY

The Cwith 1

1.1 The following organelles may contain DNA:
   A The nucleus
   B Lysosomes
   C Rough endoplasmic reticulum
   D Mitochondria
   E Golgi apparatus

1.2 The cytoskeleton:
   A Is only present in muscle cells
   B Allows the cell to change shape
   C Allows the cell to move
   D Facilitates movement of organelles from one part of the cell to another
   E Plays an important role in mitosis

1.3 The following have an important role in the process of translation in protein synthesis:
   A Double-stranded DNA
   B Transfer RNA
   C Ribosomes
   D Lysosomes
   E Cilia

1.4 The following statements about the human cell membrane are true:
   A It consists of a phospholipid molecule bilayer
   B The non-polar hydrophobic tails of the molecules are exposed to the outside
   C Cholesterol molecules regulate the fluidity of the cell membrane
   D The outside of the cell is electronegative compared to the inside
   E It is freely permeable to organic ions

1.5 Given that there are more negatively charged non-diffusible proteins inside cells than in interstitial fluids, the following statements are true:
   A Cells would swell and rupture if active transport of ions out of cells ceases
   B The concentrations of diffusible ions on the inside and the outside of the cell membrane are equal
   C The product of the concentrations of sodium and chloride inside the cell is equal to the product outside the cell
   D An electrical gradient exists across the cell membrane at equilibrium
   E The Na^+,K^+-ATPase generates a negative electrical potential inside the cell

1.6 The following statements about membrane potentials across cell membranes are true:
   A The equilibrium potential for chloride ions is the membrane potential at which the rates of influx and efflux of chloride ions are equal

   B The equilibrium potential for chloride ions increases if the chloride ion concentration is doubled both inside and outside the cell
   C The resting membrane potential in a motor neurone normally closely approximates the equilibrium potential for sodium ions
   D The resting membrane potential for sodium ions is about −90 mV
   E The resting membrane potential for potassium ions is about +60 mV

1.7 The following statements about protein synthesis in human are true:
   A Translation is the process for the synthesis of mRNA
   B The mRNA manufactured in the nucleus is shorter than the final mRNA which enters the cytoplasm
   C Amino acids are coded by a group of three bases (codon)
   D All codons specify particular amino acids
   E All amino acids are coded for by unique codons

1.8 The types of protein embedded in the cell membrane include:
   A Carriers
   B Ion channels
   C Hormone receptors
   D ATP
   E Enzymes

1.9 Energy is needed for the following mode of transport across the cell membrane:
   A Diffusion
   B Facilitated diffusion
   C By a carrier against a chemical gradient
   D By a carrier against an electrical gradient
   E Osmosis

1.10 The following statements about Na^+,K^+-ATPase are true:
   A Energy is absorbed when the enzyme catalyses the hydrolysis of an ATP molecule
   B It is absent in the brain
   C It transports one sodium ion out of the cell for each potassium ion transported in
   D Inhibition results in an increase in intracellular calcium concentration
   E Inhibition may result in improved contraction of the cardiac muscle

1.11 Common examples of the mechanisms for chemical messengers outside the cell to exert intracellular effects include:

1 **Q** GENERAL BASIC MEDICAL SCIENCES

The Cell

A Acting via cytoplasmic or nuclear receptors to start transcription of specific mRNA
B Opening ion channels in the cell membrane
C Direct entry into the nucleus to start transcription of specific mRNA
D Inducing altered electrical potential inside the cell
E Binding to membrane receptors to initiate release of intracellular messengers

1.12 Recognised second messengers include:
A Calmodulin
B G protein
C Cyclic AMP
D Inositol triphosphate
E Noradrenaline (norepinephrine)

1.13 Gap (communicating) junctions:
A Allow small molecules to pass from the inside to the outside of a cell
B Allow small molecules to pass from the inside of one cell to another
C Are impermeable to ions
D Are important in synchronising the contraction of heart muscle
E Are essential in tissues lacking in blood supply

1.14 Proteins:
A Are only found outside cells
B May be synthesised outside cells
C May be able to bind hormones
D Are often linear in shape
E May catalyse chemical reactions

1.15 The following statements about enzymes are true:
A They catalyse chemical reactions
B They cannot act on more than one substrate
C They act by increasing the activation energy
D Only one enzyme can catalyse a given chemical reaction
E A given enzyme can only catalyse one chemical reaction

1.16 The following statements about the concentration of enzymes are true:
A Measurement may be useful in detecting liver diseases
B It may be measured by the initial rate of disappearance of substrates
C It may be measured by the initial rate of appearance of products
D It may be measured by the average rate of disappearance of substrates over a day
E It may be measured by the average rate of appearance of products over a day

1.17 The following statements about the genetic code are true:
A The code in humans differs significantly from that in other mammals
B One codon may code for more than one amino acid
C Chain termination occurs in translation when a codon codes for 'glycine'
D Frameshift mutation by one nucleotide is often silent
E Mutation of the third nucleotide in the codon is often silent

1.18 Mitosis:
A Results in two daughter haploid cells
B Occurs in cancer cells
C Occurs in neurones
D Occurs in fully formed red blood cells
E Occurs in skin cells

1.19 Isoenzymes:
A Are enzymes which catalyse different biochemical reactions
B Are physically identical
C Are chemically identical
D Are often present in different cell types
E Are usually produced by genes on different chromosomes

1.20 The following statements about the rate of enzyme-catalysed reactions in vivo are true:
A It approximately doubles for every 10°C rise in temperature between 0°C and 100°C
B It approximately doubles for every 10-fold increase in hydrogen concentration between pH 2 and pH 10
C An increase in enzyme concentration usually results in a significant increase in reaction rate
D An increase in substrate concentration always results in a significant increase in reaction rate
E It can be predicted from the value of ΔG^0 (change in free energy) of the reaction

1.21 The following statements are consistent with the Michaelis–Menten equation on enzyme reactions:
A The Michaelis constant K_m is the enzyme concentration which produces half-maximal velocity
B When the substrate concentration is very much less than K_m, the initial rate of reaction is directly proportional to the substrate concentration

C When the substrate concentration is very much more than K_m, the initial rate of reaction is inversely proportional to the substrate concentration

D When the substrate concentration is equal to K_m, the initial rate of reaction is half maximal

E The value of K_m can be easily determined by the intercepts of a plot of substrate concentration against initial velocity

1.22 The following statements about the effects of enzyme inhibitors are true:

A A non-competitive inhibitor combines with an enzyme at the same site as the substrate

B A competitive inhibitor increases the apparent Michaelis constant K_m of the enzyme

C A competitive inhibitor reduces the maximal velocity V_{max} of the reaction

D A non-competitive inhibitor increases the maximal velocity V_{max} of the reaction

E A non-competitive inhibitor increases the apparent Michaelis constant K_m of the enzyme

1.23 Mechanisms for regulating enzyme activities in vivo include:

A Secretion of inactive precursors of enzymes

B Feedback inhibition by end products

C Compartmentalisation of enzymes in different cellular organelles

D Hormonal entry from outside the cell

E Feedback regulation at allosteric sites by metabolites

1.24 Allosteric enzymes:

A Often contain a single binding site for both the substrate and the allosteric effector

B Characteristically obey the Michaelis–Menton equation

C Often result in a sigmoid substrate saturation curve

D May affect the apparent K_m of the reaction

E May affect the V_{max} of the reaction

1.25 An athlete took part in a marathon race. There was a net flow of oxygen, carbon dioxide, water and glucose across the cell membrane of the muscle cells. This was essential for the production of energy.

A Is the net flow of oxygen, carbon dioxide and glucose in or out of the cell?

B What are the two components of the cell membrane across which substances may pass from one side of it to the other?

C Across which component of the cell membrane does oxygen pass? Describe the structure of this component.

D Explain, by completing Table 1.1, how the four substances pass through the cell membrane.

1.26 Table 1.2 shows the concentration of sodium, potassium and chloride ions inside and outside human nerve cells. The equilibrium potentials for the specific ions are also shown.

A What are the mechanisms by which sodium ions can pass through the cell membrane? Indicate whether energy is required for each mechanism you mentioned.

B i Calculate the total intracellular concentration of (a) cations and (b) anions.

ii What other major substances make up for the difference? Can these substances pass through the cell membrane freely?

C i From your answer in (B) above, what effects do these intracellular substances have on the osmotic pressure?

ii How might such osmotic pressure adversely affect human cell function? Explain.

iii What mechanism is available to prevent such adverse effects on cell function?

Table 1.1

Passage through cell membrane	Oxygen	Carbon dioxide	Glucose	Water
Through which component of the cell membrane?				
Transport process?				
Property of the substance that facilitates this mode of transport?				
Is energy required for the process?				

Table 1.2

Ion	Concentration (mmol/l of water)		Equilibrium potential (mV)
	Inside cell	Outside cell	
Sodium	18	150	+60
Potassium	150	5	−90
Chloride	9	125	−70

Resting membrane potential = −70 mV.

1

Q

GENERAL BASIC MEDICAL SCIENCES

The Cell

D Consider the forces acting on a chloride ion across the cell membrane.
  i In which direction does the concentration (chemical) gradient drive the chloride ion? Explain.
  ii In which direction does the electrical gradient drive the chloride ion?
  iii Explain what is meant by 'equilibrium potential for chloride ion'.
  iv Take the numerical value for RT/FZ_{Cl} to be −26.71, where R = gas constant, T = absolute temperature, F = the faraday (number of coulombs per mole of charge), Z_{Cl} is the valence of chloride ion (−1). Show the calculation for the equilibrium potential for chloride ion in the table (to the nearest mV).
  v Are forces other than the chemical and electrical gradient required to explain the distribution of Cl^- across the membrane? Explain.

E Consider the forces acting on a potassium ion across the cell membrane.
  i In which direction does the concentration (chemical) gradient drive the potassium ion? Explain.
  ii In which direction does the electrical gradient drive the potassium ion?
  iii Are forces other than the chemical and electrical gradient required to explain the distribution of K^+ across the membrane? Explain.

F Consider the forces acting on a sodium ion across the cell membrane.

  i In which direction does the concentration (chemical) gradient drive the sodium ion? Explain.
  ii In which direction does the electrical gradient drive the sodium ion?
  iii Are forces other than the chemical and electrical gradient required to explain the distribution of Na^+ across the membrane? Explain.

G What is the mechanism that may explain your answers to (Eiii) and (Fiii) above?

1.27 The cell encounters exogenous substances (e.g. bacteria). Describe how the cell usually eliminates such substances, highlighting the functions of the cell organelles involved.

1.28 In protein synthesis, organelles need to be transported from one part of the cell to another.
  A What cell structures are responsible for this transport?
  B What other functions do these structures have?
  C Name one drug that inhibits this function.
  D What therapeutic use do such drugs have?

1.29 Complete Table 1.3 regarding the different processes in protein synthesis – from the double-stranded DNA to the secretion of synthesised protein. In the last column, consider an initial DNA segment containing the sequence ATA-GCG, which codes for part of a polypeptide of the synthesised protein. (*Note* The DNA triplet ATA codes for Tyr (tyrosine) and GCG codes for Arg (arginine)).

Table 1.3

Transformed from:	Transformed to:	Part of cell where process takes place	Process	Resulting information represented by initial DNA segment ATA-GCG
Double-stranded DNA	Single-stranded DNA			
Single-stranded DNA	Pre-mRNA			
Pre-mRNA	mRNA			
mRNA	Peptide chain			
Peptide chain	Final peptide chain			
Final peptide chain	Final protein			
Final protein	Secreted protein			

Table 1.4

	Source and destination of message	Are effects local or general?	How fast are the effects?	Are second messengers involved?
Acetylcholine				
Noradrenaline (norepinephrine)				
Levothyroxine (thyroxine)				

Table 1.5

Concentration of S (mmol/l)	Initial rate of reaction (units)
10.0	0.29
5.0	0.25
3.3	0.22
2.5	0.20
2.0	0.18
1.7	0.17
1.4	0.15
1.3	0.14
1.1	0.13

1.30 For each of the following examples, describe the mechanisms by which chemical messengers outside cells may affect cell function:
  A Acetylcholine acting on the motor end-plate
  B Noradrenaline (norepinephrine) acting on heart muscle (via β_1 receptors)
  C Levothyroxine (thyroxine)
  D Further compare these mechanisms by completing Table 1.4

1.31 An experiment was performed to investigate the rate of reaction catalysed by a recently discovered enzyme X, at different concentrations of the substrate S. S can be measured using optical methods. The initial rate of reaction was estimated by measuring the rate of disappearance of S within the first 20 s. The results obtained are given in Table 1.5.
  A What kind of chemical is an enzyme?
  B In this experiment, is it preferable to measure the average rate of reaction over, say, 10 min, rather than the initial rate of reaction in the first 20 s? Explain.
  C What factors must be controlled in this experiment?
  D How would the concentration of X vary with time if it were measured?
  E For a particular concentration of S, how would you expect the rate of reaction to vary over a range of temperature (say, from 5°C to 90°C)? Explain.
  F What is meant by an 'allosteric enzyme'? Give one example.
  G By plotting an appropriate graph, determine whether there is any evidence that enzyme X is an allosteric enzyme. Explain.
  H Can you determine how many binding sites there are for substrate S for each molecule of X? Explain.
  I Calculate the Michaelis constant K_m and the maximum velocity (V_{max}) for X.

GENERAL BASIC MEDICAL SCIENCES

The Cell

1.1 A D

The nucleus consists mostly of chromosomes which carry the genetic message of the cell. The chromosomes are made up of DNA. Without the nucleus, the cell cannot divide and eventually dies (e.g. red blood cells). However, the mitochondria contains a small amount of DNA which codes for a small number (13) of the proteins in the ATP generating system in the mitochondria. This may be clinically important, as mutation in the mitochondrial DNA may result in rare muscular disorders with a special pattern of inheritance. Mitochondria may have been independent microorganisms which became incorporated into the cell in the course of evolution.

1.2 B C D E

The cytoskeleton is a system of fibres which maintains the shape of the cell, allows the cell to change shape and move, and facilitates movement of organelles from one part of the cell to another. The fibres vary in diameter, and include microtubules (the largest), intermediate filaments and microfilaments. The microtubules are constantly assembled and disassembled, and help to form tracks for the transport of organelles such as mitochondria and secretory granules to move to the part of the cell where they are needed. Microfilaments consist of actins, and are responsible for the movement of organelles, as well as the contraction of muscles.

1.3 B C

Translation is the process by which a polypeptide chain of a protein is formed from the processed messenger RNA, and occurs in the ribosomes. The amino acids in the cytoplasm are activated by adenosine monophosphate and an enzyme, and each activated amino acid is attached to a transfer RNA. The tRNA–amino acid complex is then attached to the processed mRNA in the ribosomes. Double-stranded DNA is only found in the nucleus. Lysosomes contain enzymes which would destroy most cellular components, and act as a digestive system for the cell. Cilia are projections from the cells.

1.4 A C

Human cell membrane basically consists of a phospholipid bilayer. Each phospholipid molecule consists of a polar hydrophilic phosphate head and two non-polar hydrophobic tails. The polar heads are exposed to the outside and the cytoplasm of the cell, whilst the non-polar tails are buried within the cell membrane. Cholesterol molecules are present to stabilise the cell membrane and regulate its fluidity by filling the gaps between the tails of phospholipid fatty acid tails whilst simultaneously preventing too close placing. The inside of the cell is almost invariably electronegative relative to the outside, although the magnitude of this resting potential varies amongst tissues. The membrane is impermeable to intracellular organic anions, and this results in an asymmetry of the distribution of permeant anions at equilibrium. This is the Donnan effect, and is the cause of the membrane potential.

1.5 A C D E

Since there are more negatively charged non-diffusible proteins inside cells, there are more osmotically active particles inside than outside cells. Hence, cells would swell and rupture if there were no active transport of ions out of cells. This active transport is carried out by Na^+,K^+-ATPase. The concentration of the diffusible ions is governed by the Gibbs–Donnan equation. For any pair of cation and anion with the same valency, the outside to inside concentration ratio of the cation is the same as the inside to outside concentration ratio of the anion. In other words, the product of the concentrations of the cation and anion inside the cell is equal to the corresponding product outside the cell. Since the distribution of positive and negative charged ions across the membrane is asymmetrical, there is an electrical gradient across the membrane at equilibrium. Furthermore, the Na^+,K^+-ATPase pumps three Na^+ out of the cells in exchange for every two K^+ into the cells. This also contributes to the electrical gradient across cell membranes.

1.6 A

The equilibrium potential for any diffusible ion is the membrane potential at which the rates of influx and efflux of the ions are equal. The magnitude of the membrane potential can be determined by the Nernst equation:

$$E_x = \frac{RT}{F} \ln \frac{[X_o]}{[X_i]}$$

Hence, doubling the concentrations of the relevant ions both inside and outside the cells would not alter its equilibrium potential. The resting membrane potential differs slightly amongst tissues. In the motor neurone, the resting membrane potential is about −70 mV, which is entirely accounted for by the chloride equilibrium potential. The equilibrium potential for sodium ions is about +60 mV, and accounts for the membrane potential of neurones at depolarisation during an action potential. The electrical potential for potassium ions is about −90 mV, and is important when tissues are hyperpolarised.

1.7 C

The process of synthesis of mRNA in the nucleus is known as transcription, whilst the synthesis of protein from mRNA in the ribosomes is known as translation. In eukaryotic cells, segments of DNA which code for protein synthesis (exons) are separated from segments which do not

GENERAL BASIC MEDICAL SCIENCES

(introns). The mRNA molecules synthesised in the nucleus are spliced to eliminate the introns before entering the cytoplasm. Hence the final mRNA is shorter than the mRNA synthesised in the nucleus. In translation, each amino acid is coded for by a group of three bases (codon). Out of the 64 codons, only 61 code for particular amino acids, whilst the other three code for chain termination. As there are only 20 amino acids, most are coded for by more than one codon.

1.8 A B C E
There are different proteins embedded in the cell membranes, with a variety of functions. They include (a) structural proteins, (b) ion channels (which allow ions to pass in and out of the cell when activated), (c) carriers (which facilitate diffusion of substances across the membrane down an electrochemical gradient), (d) pumps (which actively transport substances across the membrane), (e) receptors (which cause physiological changes inside the cells when bound to a hormone or a neurotransmitter), (f) enzymes (which catalyse biochemical reactions at the surface of the membrane). ATP is a high-energy phosphate compound and not a protein.

1.9 C D
Diffusion is the movement of a substance from an area of higher to lower concentration (chemical gradient). Ions may also move down an electrical gradient. Osmosis is the diffusion of solvent (e.g. water) molecules from areas with a lower to a higher solute concentration. All these processes do not require energy. Diffusion down a chemical or electrical gradient may be facilitated by a protein (carrier), and no energy is required. However, transport of substances against a chemical or electrical gradient require energy, which is usually provided by the hydrolysis of ATP by Na^+,K^+-ATPase.

1.10 D E
The enzyme Na^+,K^+-ATPase is present throughout all the cells in the body, and is responsible for a large part of the basal metabolism. It catalyses the hydrolysis of ATP to ADP, and energy is released in the process. This energy is used to transport three Na^+ out of the cell for every two K^+ transported in, and results in a net positive charge outside the cell. It may be linked to a second active transport system (e.g. for transport of glucose across the intestinal mucosa). Digoxin inhibits the enzyme. This results in a decrease in intracellular sodium concentration and hence a decrease in the sodium gradient across the cell membrane. The normal exchange of an inflow of sodium ions for an outflow of calcium ions is reduced, and the intracellular calcium level increases. This facilitates the contraction of cardiac muscle (positively inotropic effect).

1.11 A B E
The commonest mechanism for chemical messengers to exert intracellular effects is binding to a membrane receptor to initiate the release of intracellular mediators (second messengers). Other mechanisms include acting via cytoplasmic or nuclear receptors to initiate transcription of certain mRNAs (e.g. thyroid hormone), and opening of specific ion channels in the membrane (e.g. acetylcholine acting on the nicotinic receptors to open the sodium channels).

1.12 A B C D
Second messengers are intracellular mediators the release of which is triggered by extracellular chemicals (first messenger) binding to membrane receptors. An example is noradrenaline (first messenger) binding to β_1-adrenergic membrane receptors, which triggers the increase of intracellular cyclic AMP (second messenger). Many second messengers have been identified in recent years, and include cyclic AMP, cyclic GMP, calcium-binding proteins (e.g. calmodulin), G proteins, inositol triphosphate and diacylglycerol.

1.13 B D E
Gap (communicating) junctions are channels which connect one cell to another, and are composed of polypeptides called connexin. They allow passage of small polar molecules such as metabolites and amino acids, and ions. They are essential to allow nutrients to travel from one cell to another in tissues lacking in blood supply (e.g. cornea, bone). They are also important in synchronising the contraction of cardiac or uterine muscle by allowing rapid transfer of calcium ions.

1.14 C E
Proteins may be found outside cells (e.g. immunoglobulins), in the plasma membrane (e.g. hormone receptors) and inside cells (e.g. haemoglobin). However, they are all synthesised inside cells in ribosomes. Whilst polypeptides are linear, the shape of proteins is determined by the exact nature of their folding (i.e. the tertiary structure). Most non-structural proteins are globular in shape (e.g. haemoglobin). They are capable of binding to other molecules (ligands) at specific regions (binding sites). Enzymes are proteins, or rarely RNA molecules, capable of binding to ligands and initiate the catalysis of a chemical reaction involving the ligands.

1.15 A
Although most chemical reactions are catalysed by enzymes (which are proteins), it was discovered in the mid-1980s that some RNA molecules (ribozymes) may also catalyse reactions. Most enzymes can act on more than one substrate. Different enzymes may catalyse the same

1 **A**

The Cell

GENERAL BASIC MEDICAL SCIENCES

chemical reaction, and different enzymes may catalyse the same reaction. Enzymes speed up reaction by lowering the activation energy barrier, but do not change the final equilibrium.

1.16 A B C

Measurement of the concentration of enzymes is often useful in the diagnosis of diseases. For example, in liver or heart diseases, specific enzymes are often released from the damaged liver or cardiac cells. Enzyme concentration is most commonly measured by the initial rate of disappearance of substrates or the appearance of products. The initial rate must be measured, as the rate of reaction decreases with time as the concentration of substrates falls. Enzyme concentration may sometimes be measured by immunological methods using antibodies to the enzyme.

1.17 E

There are three nucleotides in a codon. Hence, a trinucleotide codon codes for 64 amino acids. As there are only 20 amino acids, an amino acid may be coded for by more than one codon. Of the different codons which code for a particular amino acid, the first two nucleotides are often the same, but the third nucleotide may differ. Hence, mutation of the third nucleotide is often silent and has no effect on the functioning of the resulting protein. On the other hand, one codon only codes for one amino acid. There is one codon (AUG) which codes for 'start', and three codons which code for 'stop'. Chain termination occurs with the 'stop' codon. Frameshift mutation by one nucleotide usually results in a wholly incorrect amino acid sequence, and hence a non-functional protein.

1.18 B E

Mitosis is a type of cell division in somatic cells, and is essential for growth, tissue formation and repair. It starts with a parent diploid cell (consisting of two sets of chromosomes) and ends with two diploid daughter cells. In contrast, meiosis is the other type of cell division, which is responsible for the production of gametes. It starts with a diploid cell and ends with two haploid daughter cells. Mitosis occurs in all embryonic tissues. It also occurs in all tissues throughout life apart from fully specialised end cells such as neurones. Fully formed red blood cells do not have a nucleus and are therefore unable to undergo mitosis. Cancer cells undergo mitosis at a faster rate than normal cells. This is important in the treatment of cancer, as several cytotoxic drugs and radiotherapy act by inhibiting mitosis via different mechanisms.

1.19 D

Isoenzymes are enzymes which catalyse the same biochemical reactions, but are of physically and chemically distinct forms. They are often present in different cell types (e.g. isoenzymes of lactate dehydrogenase are present in the heart, skeletal muscle and the liver). Isoenzymes are products of genes which are closely related. Often, they are made up of the same subunits combined in different ways. Clinically, identification of the specific form of isoenzymes may pinpoint where an abnormal enzyme is produced, and hence the likely diagnosis in the patient.

1.20 C

Increase in temperature results in increase in the kinetic energy and the frequency of collision between molecules of the reactants. Hence, the rate of reaction increases with temperature below a certain threshold. However, when the temperature reaches a certain level, the energy in the enzyme molecule may exceed that needed to break the chemical bonds that maintain the secondary and tertiary structure of the molecule. As a result, denaturation occurs. Hence, the relationship between the rate of reaction and temperature is bell-shaped, and there is an optimum temperature which gives rise to a maximum rate of reaction. Similarly, there is an optimum pH for a given enzymatic reaction, and this optimum pH depends on the particular biochemical reaction and the enzyme. For most biochemical reactions in vivo, there is an excess of substrates over enzymes. Hence, the rate of reaction increases with the concentration of enzymes. However, an increase in the concentration of substrates will not increase the rate of reaction unless there are sufficient free enzymes around to react. Whilst the value of ΔG^0 (change in the free energy of the reaction) will dictate the direction of the reaction for which it will be spontaneous, it does not predict the rate of reaction. The rate of reaction depends on the magnitude of the energy barrier.

1.21 B D

The Michaelis–Menten equation describes how the initial rate of reaction varies with substrate concentration whilst keeping other factors constant. The Michaelis constant K_m is defined as the substrate concentration that produces half-maximal velocity. The Michaelis–Menten equation is as follows:

$$V_i = \frac{V_{max}[S]}{k_m + [S]}$$

where V_i is the initial rate of reaction, V_{max} is the maximal velocity, K_m is the Michaelis constant, and $[S]$ is the substrate concentration. It can be easily shown that when $[S] \ll K_m$, V is approximately directly proportional to $[S]$. When $[S] = K_m$, V_i is approximately equal to V_{max}. When $[S] > K_m$, V_i is approximately equal to $1/2\ V_{max}$.

From the equation, it can be seen that a direct plot of V_i and $[S]$ would be difficult to interpret. However, rearranging the equation to

$$\frac{1}{V_i} = \frac{K_m}{V_{max}} \frac{1}{[S]} + \frac{1}{V_{max}}$$

It can be seen if we perform a double reciprocal plot of $1/V_i$ and $1/[S]$, K_m and V_{max} can be calculated.

1.22 B
A competitive enzyme inhibitor usually binds to the substrate binding site of the enzyme, whereas a non-competitive inhibitor usually binds to another site of the enzyme. In the presence of a competitive enzyme inhibitor, increase of substrate concentration will eventually overcome the inhibition. Hence, the maximal velocity is unchanged, but the Michaelis constant K_m (the substrate concentration that produces half-maximal velocity) is increased. On the other hand, for non-competitive inhibitors, the maximal velocity is reduced as increase in substrate cannot overcome the inhibition, but the K_m is unchanged as the substrate binding site of the enzyme is unaffected.

1.23 A B C E
There are many ways of regulating enzyme activities in vivo. The enzymes may be kept separate in different cellular organelles (e.g. enzymes involved in the citric acid cycle are kept in the mitochondria); enzymes may be secreted in an inactive form so that they may be activated rapidly if necessary (e.g. chemotrypsin is secreted in an inactive form), there may be direct feedback inhibition from the end products, or there may be allosteric inhibition at an allosteric site different from the substrate site.

1.24 C D E
Allosteric enzymes are enzymes whose activity is affected by effectors at allosteric sites separate from the catalytic sites. It is an important mechanism for regulating enzyme activities. It does not obey the Michalelis–Menten equation, which predicts a hyperbolic substrate saturation curve. The substrate saturation curve is often sigmoid in shape, similar to the oxygen dissociation curve of haemoglobin. It indicates the phenomenon of cooperativity between different substrate binding sites, and that the presence of a substrate molecule at a catalytic site increases the chance of a second substrate binding at a second catalytic site. Allosteric enzymes may affect either K_m or V_{max}.

1.25
A
Muscle cells consume oxygen and glucose and produce carbon dioxide. Hence, oxygen and glucose enter the cells and carbon dioxide leaves them.

B
Substances may pass from one side of the cell membrane to the other through the lipid bilayer or via transmembrane proteins (proteins that span the cell membrane).

C
Oxygen passes across the lipid bilayer. The lipid bilayer consists of two layers of phospholipid molecules which have a hydrophilic (polar) head end and a hydrophobic (non-polar) tail end. The head ends are exposed to either the cytoplasm or the outside of the cells; the tail ends are buried inside the membrane.

D
See Table 1.6.

1.26
A
The major mechanisms by which sodium ions can pass through the cell membrane are:
- diffusion through the lipid bilayer (slow) – no energy required

Table 1.6

	Oxygen	Carbon dioxide	Glucose	Water
Through which component of the cell membrane?	Lipid bilayer	Lipid bilayer	Transport proteins	Lipid bilayer and water channels
Transport process?	Diffusion	Diffusion	Facilitated diffusion	Diffusion
Property of the substance that facilitates this mode of transport?	Non-polar molecules	Small uncharged molecules	Presence of glucose transporters	Small uncharged molecules, presence of water channels
Is energy required for the process?	No	No	No	No

11

The Cell

- facilitated diffusion through voltage-gated channel – no energy required
- facilitated diffusion through ligand-gated (e.g. acetylcholine receptor) channels – no energy required
- active transport via Na^+,K^+-ATPase – energy required.

B

i Intracellular concentration of (a) cations (Na^+ and K^+) = 18 + 150 = 168 mmol/l of water, and (b) anions (Cl^-) = 9 mmol/l of water.

ii Phosphates, non-diffusible protein anions and bicarbonate ions make up the rest of the anions. Non-diffusible protein anions cannot pass through the membrane.

C

i Osmotically active particles can exert osmotic pressure only when they are in contact with another solution across a membrane permeable to the solvent but not to the solute. Since there are non-diffusible protein anions inside the cells, the osmotic pressure inside the cell is increased.

ii Since human cells have flexible cell walls, the osmotic pressure may cause the cells to swell and rupture.

iii Swelling and rupture of the cell is prevented by Na^+,K^+-ATPase pumping sodium ions out of the cells (3 Na^+ out of cells for every 2 K^+ into cells).

D

i Since the concentration of Cl^- is higher outside than inside the cell, the chemical gradient drives the ion into the cell.

ii Since the resting membrane potential is negative inside the cell, the electrical gradient drives the negative Cl^- out of the cell.

iii 'Equilibrium potential for Cl^-' is the membrane potential at which the number of chloride ions entering the cell equals the number of chloride ions leaving the cell.

iv By the Nernst equation, $E_{Cl} = (RT/FZ_{Cl})\ln([Cl_o^-]/[Cl_i^-])$; hence, $E_{Cl} = -26.71\ln(125/9) = -70$ mV.

v Since the resting membrane potential (–70 mV) is the same as the equilibrium potential for Cl^-, no other forces are required to explain the distribution of the ion across the membrane.

E

i Since the concentration of K^+ is higher inside than outside the cell, the chemical gradient drives the ion out of the cell.

ii Since the resting membrane potential is negative inside the cell, the electrical gradient drives the positive K^+ into the cell.

iii Since the equilibrium potential for K^+ (–90 mV) is more negative than the resting membrane potential

(–70 mV), another force tending to drive K^+ inside cells is required to explain the distribution of K^+ across the membrane.

F

i Since the concentration of Na^+ is higher outside than inside the cell, the chemical gradient drives the ion into the cell.

ii Since the resting membrane potential is negative inside the cell, the electrical gradient also drives the positive Na^+ into the cell.

iii Since both chemical and electrical forces drive Na^+ into the cell, there must be another mechanism driving the Na^+ out of the cell.

G

The mechanism which drives Na^+ out of the cell and K^+ into the cell is active transport by Na^+,K^+-ATPase.

1.27

The cell eliminates exogenous substances by the following steps:

1. The cell engulfs the exogenous substances by phagocytosis (a form of endocytosis): the substance makes contact with the cell membrane which then invaginates, leaving the engulfed substances in a membrane-lined vacuole.

2. The vacuole merges with a lysosome to form a phagocytic vacuole. A lysosome is a large irregular structure, surrounded by a membrane, which contains acids and lysosomal enzymes.

3. The exogenous substances are 'digested' inside the phagocytic vacuole by acids and enzymes. The products are absorbed through the wall of the vacuole or discharged outside the cell by exocytosis.

1.28

A

Microtubules are responsible for the transport of organelles from one part of the cell to another.

B

Microtubules are often responsible for the formation of spindles in mitosis during cell division.

C

Colchicine (and vinblastine) inhibits the assembly of microtubules. Paclitaxel binds tightly to microtubules so that they become totally immobilised.

D

Such drugs may be used in the treatment of malignancy as they preferentially affect dividing cells. Immobilisation of microtubules leads to cell death as the organelles cannot move and cell division is impossible.

1.29
See Table 1.7.

1.30
A
Acetylcholine is released in vesicles by terminal buttons of neurones and transmitted across the synaptic cleft to the motor end-plate. It acts by opening sodium channels in the cell membrane.

B
Noradrenaline (norepinephrine) is released by adrenergic post-ganganglionic nerve fibres or the adrenal medulla and acts by binding to β_1 receptors of heart muscle. This activates adenyl cylase and causes an increase in the intracellular production of cyclic AMP. cAMP activates

protein kinase A, which phosphorylates proteins to produce physiological effects.

C
Levothyroxine is released by the thyroid gland. It acts by binding to receptors in the nucleus or cytoplasm. This increases the transcription of selected mRNA to produce the required physiological effects.

D
See Table 1.8.

1.31
A
An enzyme is a stereospecific protein that catalyses a chemical reaction in the body.

B
The initial rate of reaction should be measured because the rate of reaction decreases with time as the substrate is depleted.

Table 1.7

Transformed from:	Transformed to:	Part of cell where process take place	Process	Resulting information represented by initial DNA segment ATA-GCG
Double-stranded DNA	Single-stranded DNA	Nucleus (nucleolus)	Splicing	ATA-GCG
Single-stranded DNA	Pre-mRNA	Nucleus (nucleolus)	Transcription	UAU-CGC
Pre-mRNA	mRNA	Nucleus	Post-transcriptional processing	UAU-CGC
mRNA	Peptide chain	Cytoplasm (ribosomes)	Translation	Tyr-Arg
Peptide chain	Final peptide chain	Cytoplasm (endoplasmic reticulum)	Post-translational modification	Tyr-Arg
Final peptide chain	Final protein	Cytoplasm (endoplasmic reticulum)	Protein folding	Tyr-Arg
Final protein	Secreted protein	Golgi apparatus	Secretion (exocytosis)	Tyr-Arg

Table 1.8

	Source and destination of message	Are effects local or general?	How fast are the effects?	Are second messengers involved?
Acetylcholine	Across the synaptic cleft	Local	Fast	No
Noradrenaline (norepinephrine)	From sympathetic nervous tissue to heart muscle	General	Moderate	Yes – cAMP
Levothyroxine	From thyroid gland to target tissue	General	Slow	No

GENERAL BASIC MEDICAL SCIENCES

SYSTEMS OF THE BODY

The Cell

C

Factors that must be controlled in the experiment include:
- concentration of all substrates
- pH
- temperature
- any cofactors
- (enzyme concentration – although we do not expect the rate of reaction to differ).

D

The enzyme concentration would remain constant with time.

E

For the biological range of temperature (e.g. from 5°C to 40°C), the rate of reaction should increase with temperature (roughly doubling for every 10°C rise in temperature); however, the rate of reaction decreases drastically above this temperature owing to denaturation of the enzyme.

F

An allosteric enzyme is an enzyme with regulatory sites to which an allosteric effector (usually a product of the reaction) can bind and alter enzyme activity. Examples are phosphofructokinase and hexokinase. The interaction between haemoglobin and oxygen is another example.

G

The interaction of enzyme and substrate can be described in a non-allosteric enzyme by the Michaelis–Menten equation:

$$V = V_{max}[S]/([S] + K_m)$$

Rearranging this equation gives:

$$1/V = 1/V_{max} + [(K_m/V_{max}) \times (1/[S])]$$

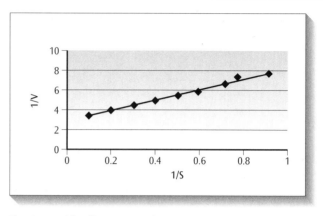

Fig. 1.1 Michaelis–Menten plot.

Hence, a plot of $1/V$ against $1/[S]$ should be linear (Fig. 1.1). It can be seen the plot is almost linear; thus, there is no evidence that enzyme X is an allosteric enzyme. However, the presence of allosteric sites for substances other than the substrate and products of the reaction cannot be ruled out.

H

There is no evidence of co-operative effects. It is likely that there is only one binding site for S.

I

From Fig. 1.1, the intercept is at 2.9 on the $1/V$ axis and with a slope of 5.5.

Hence, $1/[V_{max}] = 2.9$,

$V_{max} = 1/2.9 = 0.34$ units

$K_m/V_{max} = 5.5$

Hence, $K_m = 5.5 \times 0.34 = 1.87$

14

General principles of pharmacology

2.1 The relationship between pharmacological effect and log dose for drugs A and B is shown in Fig. 2.1. The following conclusions can be drawn from the figure:
A The dose–response curve for drug A is linear
B Drug B produces a higher maximal response than drug A
C Drug B is more potent than drug A
D The EC_{50} is lower for drug B than drug A. (The EC_{50} value is the concentration of drug which gives rise to 50% of the maximal response)
E Both drugs produce the pharmacological effect by the same mechanism

2.2 The following are the results of loss of sensitivity of target tissues to a drug:
A A reduction in the concentration of the drug
B A reduction in the maximal response of the drug
C A reduction in the EC_{50} value
D A shift of the log dose–response curve to the right
E A shift of the log dose–response curve downwards

2.3 An antidepressant highly selective for its antidepressant effect:
A Achieves a higher antidepressant effect than other drugs
B Has a lower EC_{50} value than for other effects such as sedation
C Has a higher potency for depression than other drugs
D Has a higher potency than for other effects such as sedation
E Has a higher therapeutic index

2.4 The following statements about enzyme inhibitors are true:
A The therapeutic effect may be due to an increase in substrate concentration
B The therapeutic effect may be due to a decrease in the product concentration
C Non-competitive enzyme inhibitors bind to the active site of the enzyme
D Competitive enzyme inhibitors are always reversible
E The time of onset of action is always shorter for non-competitive than competitive enzyme inhibitors

2.5 The following statements about receptor agonists and antagonists are true:
A An agonist almost always results in an increase of cellular activity
B An antagonist almost always results in a reduction of cellular activity
C It is necessary for an antagonist to bind to an agonist to exert its pharmacological effects
D It is not possible for a substance to act as an agonist without binding to the receptor
E A partial agonist can produce a maximal response if present in a sufficiently high concentration

2.6 Factors associated with increased permeability of a drug to the plasma membrane include:
A A high lipid solubility
B A high water solubility
C A high molecular weight
D A high proportion of the non-ionised form of the drug
E The presence of specific carrier systems

2.7 Antagonism between two drugs:
A Is defined as the effect of two drugs together being less than either of the two drugs alone
B May be due to one drug being antagonist to another at the same receptor site
C Does not occur if the drugs act on different receptors
D May involve the release of a mediator by one of the drugs
E Is synonymous with potentiation between two drugs

2.8 Modified-release capsules:
A Increase the rate of absorption of the drug through the stomach
B Increase the rate at which the drug dissolves
C Are indicated if the drug may be inactivated by acids

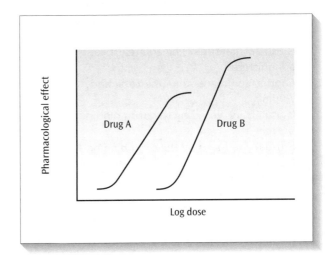

Fig. 2.1 Relationship between pharmacological effect and log dose for drugs A and B.

D Consist of numerous identical small granules
  E May result in a smooth sustained release of the drug

2.9 Drugs given via the following routes avoid first-pass metabolism by the liver:
  A Buccal mucosa
  B The skin
  C Respiratory mucosa
  D Subcutaneously
  E Intramuscularly

2.10 Systemic bioavailability of a drug administered orally may be:
  A Higher than that given intravenously
  B Reduced by poor gut absorption
  C Reduced by liver metabolism
  D Reduced by gut metabolism
  E Increased by binding with other substances in the gut lumen

2.11 The following statements about the effects of drug binding to plasma proteins are true:
  A Most drugs bind to plasma proteins irreversibly by covalent bonds
  B Most drugs do not bind to plasma proteins to any significant extent
  C The proportion of bound drug to total plasma concentration increases when the concentration of the drug is increased
  D Protein binding may smooth the free plasma concentration of a drug
  E The free concentration of a drug may be increased by the presence of another protein-binding drug

2.12 The apparent volume of distribution of a drug:
  A Is a measure of the extent of the drug distribution in the body
  B Is usually measured immediately after the drug is administered
  C Cannot be greater than the total body volume
  D Is usually increased by the drug binding to plasma protein
  E Is usually reduced by the drug binding to tissues

2.13 Renal clearance of a drug:
  A Is usually higher than hepatic clearance for lipid-soluble drugs
  B Decreases linearly with the concentration of the drug
  C Is defined as the rate of elimination of the drug by the kidney

  D Can be thought of as the volume of blood cleared of the drug by the kidney per unit time
  E Is the same as creatinine clearance if there is no net secretion or reabsorption of the drug into renal tubules

2.14 Renal clearance is higher:
  A For water-soluble than lipid-soluble drugs
  B For drugs with than those without active tubular secretion
  C In those with diseased kidneys than those with normal kidneys for a given drug
  D For acidic drugs the lower the urinary pH
  E For basic drugs the lower the urinary pH

2.15 The following statements about cytochrome P_{450} are true:
  A It is largely located at the nucleus of the cell
  B It is involved in the metabolism of endogenous substances
  C It is involved in the oxidation of many drugs
  D Activity may be increased or decreased by drugs
  E A reduction of activity may lead to a lack of drug effects

2.16 Significant factors determining the steady-state concentration of a drug when regularly repeated intravenous doses of a drug are given include:
  A The average rate of the drug given
  B The renal clearance of the drug
  C The hepatic clearance of the drug
  D The volume of distribution of the drug
  E Whether an initial large intravenous bolus of the drug (a loading dose) is given

2.17 The following statements about the elimination of a drug by zero-order kinetics are true:
  A The rate of elimination is faster the higher the plasma concentration of the drug
  B The elimination half-life of the drug is constant
  C The rate of elimination of the drug is constant over time
  D A steady-state concentration will be reached if an intravenous infusion is given at a rate above the current elimination rate
  E It occurs more frequently for therapeutic ranges than for toxic ranges of drugs

2.18 The following are relative indications for monitoring of the plasma concentrations of a drug:
  A The therapeutic effects are difficult to monitor clinically over a short time period
  B The toxic effects are difficult to monitor clinically
  C The therapeutic window is wide
  D The therapeutic index is low
  E The drug is eliminated by a first-order process

2.19 The following statements about the elderly compared with younger adults are true:
  A The metabolism of drugs is higher, which results in reduced bioavailability
  B The volume of distribution for water-soluble drugs is increased
  C The renal excretion of drugs is lower
  D The response to a given concentration of a drug is less
  E The doses required for a given drug are generally smaller

2.20 True drug allergy:
  A Is the commonest cause of adverse drug effects
  B Exhibits a graded dose–response relationship
  C Decreases in severity over time
  D Can be predicted from the mechanism of the therapeutic actions of the drug
  E Should be managed by a reduction in the dose of the drug given

2.21 The following statements about inverse agonists are true:
  A They are full agonists of different potencies
  B Their effects are inversely proportional to the concentration
  C The effects are inversely proportional to their potencies
  D They produce effects which are opposite to those of the agonists
  E They are synonymous with antagonists

2.22 The following statements about partial agonists are true:
  A They do not activate the receptors
  B They produce effects which are opposite to those of the full agonists
  C The maximal response is less than that of full agonists
  D The effect of a combination of a full and a partial agonist together is always greater than that of the full agonist alone
  E The effect of a full and partial agonist together is usually smaller than that of the partial agonist alone

2.23 The following reduce the systemic availability of an orally administered drug:
  A Low lipid solubility of the drug
  B Intestinal hurry
  C Binding of active drugs to food
  D Reduced liver metabolism of the drug
  E Instability of the drug under low pH

2.24 Drugs with a half-life of:
  A 10 min may be administered with a loading dose identical to the maintenance dose
  B 2 h may be administered orally three times a day
  C 12 h may be administered orally twice a day
  D 72 h may be administered intravenously
  E 120 h may be administered with a loading dose greater than the maintenance dose

2.25 Prolonged exposure to an agonist may result in:
  A Upregulation of receptors
  B An increase in the density of receptors on cells
  C A decrease in the capacity of the receptors to respond
  D An increase in the receptor occupancy
  E Patients tolerant and refractory to treatment by agonists of the receptors

2.26 The likelihood of the rebound phenomenon on withdrawal of drug is higher:
  A The longer the drug has been previously administered
  B The shorter the half-life of the drug
  C For a partial agonist than a pure antagonist
  D The more abrupt the withdrawal
  E For a drug with inhibitory than a drug with excitatory effects

2.27 Drug Y may increase the effect of drug X if drug Y:
  A Is a purgative and drug X is given orally
  B Binds to drug X in the gut lumen
  C Is an enzyme inducer and drug X is metabolised in the liver
  D Is an enzyme inhibitor and drug X is metabolised in the liver
  E Inhibits the active reabsorption of drug X across the renal tubular epithelium

2.28 A drug D with concentration x reacts reversibly with free receptors R to form complex DR. Assume that the concentrations of occupied receptors and total receptors are o and t, respectively.
  A Write out the reversible chemical reaction, indicating the concentration of each reactant and product. Assume that the rate constants for the forward and backward reactions are k_f and k_b, respectively.
  B Apply the law of mass action and write down the rate of forward and backward reactions.
  C Let the equilibrium constant for the reaction $K = k_b / k_f$. When the reaction is at equilibrium, use your results in (B) to write down an equation relating o, t, x, K.

2

Q

GENERAL BASIC MEDICAL SCIENCES

Pharmacology

D The fractional occupancy, p, is the proportion of receptors occupied (i.e. o/t). Use the equation obtained in (C) to express the fractional occupancy, p, in terms of x, the concentration of drug D.

E From your result in (D), sketch graphs to show the shape of the theoretical relationship between the fractional occupancy p and the following values:
  i   The concentration of drug D
  ii The logarithm of the concentration of drug D

F Does the shape of the graph in (E ii) resemble the dose–response curve?

G Can the model obtained in (D) be used to estimate accurately the affinity of a drug for a receptor from the dose–response curve? Give at least two reasons for your answer.

2.29 Table 2.1 shows the biological response (% maximum of that in the absence of Y) at various concentrations of the drug agonist X, with and without the presence of a drug Y.

A Plot the dose–response curve of drug X, in both the presence and the absence of drug Y.

B Is the slope of the dose–response curve of drug X significantly affected by the presence of drug Y?

C Is the maximal response of drug X significantly affected by the presence of drug Y?

D What type of drug is Y in relation to X? For example, state whether Y is an agonist or an antagonist; if an antagonist, whether it is competitive or non-competitive, reversible or irreversible.

E Give the approximate dose ratio of drug Y when X is between the following values.
  i 3.2×10^{-6} and $10^{-4}\,\mu mol/l$
  ii 10^{-4} and $3.2 \times 10^{-3}\,\mu mol/l$

F Estimate the biological response if the concentration of X and Y are $10^{-3}\,\mu mol/l$ and $10\,\mu mol/l$, respectively.

G Name three currently used drugs that act in a similar way to drug Y.

2.30 Table 2.2 shows the biological response (% maximum) at various concentrations of the drug agonist X, with and without the presence of antagonists A, B and C.

A Sketch the dose–response curve of drug X, together with the dose–response curves when antagonists A, B and C are present.

B Describe the effects of the antagonists A, B and C by writing 'yes' or 'no' in the blanks of the Table 2.3.

Table 2.1

	Agonist (X) concentration ($\mu mol/l$)							
	10^{-6}	3.2×10^{-6}	10^{-5}	3.2×10^{-5}	10^{-4}	3.2×10^{-4}	10^{-3}	3.2×10^{-3}
Biological response (% max.)	2	11	29	66	91	95	98	100
Biological response (% max.) in presence of Y at $1\,\mu mol/l$	0	2	12	30	65	92	96	99

Table 2.2

	Agonist (X) concentration ($\mu mol/l$)							
	10^{-6}	3.2×10^{-6}	10^{-5}	3.2×10^{-5}	10^{-4}	3.2×10^{-4}	10^{-3}	3.2×10^{-3}
Biological response (%. max)	2	11	29	66	91	95	98	100
Biological response (%. max) in presence of A	1	6	15	34	46	46	50	51
Biological response (%. max) in presence of B	0	1	2	12	30	65	90	96
Biological response (%. max) in presence of C	0	0	8	21	49	72	74	75

C Classify the antagonists A, B and C. (Choose from non-competitive, irreversible competitive and reversible competitive antagonists. Assume the phenomenon of spare receptors was not present.)

D Give examples of the types of antagonist, represented by A, B and C, used in clinical practice.

2.31 A non-steroidal anti-inflammatory drug X is used both as an analgesia and an antirheumatic agent. The drug is tested in two groups of adult patients: those with and those without a past history of suspected peptic ulcer. The results are as follows:

- Minimum dose for effective analgesic effect (both groups of patients): 20 g/kg body weight per day
- Minimum dose for effective antirheumatic effect (both groups of patients): 40 g/kg body weight per day
- Minimum dose for which toxic effects become manifest:
  no past history of suspected peptic ulcer: 80 g/kg body weight per day
  past history of suspected peptic ulcer: 60 g/kg body weight per day.

A Calculate the therapeutic index for both analgesic and antirheumatic effects for the following groups of patients.
  i Those with a past history of peptic ulcer.
  ii Those with no past history of peptic ulcer.

B Another drug Y has a therapeutic index of 8 for its analgesic effect for patients with no previous history of suspected peptic ulcer. What can you deduce, if anything, about the following characteristics relative to drug X?
  i Clinical usefulness
  ii Safety in accidental overdose
  iii Cost-effectiveness

C Give two limitations of the usefulness of therapeutic index in clinical practice.

D What precautions are often taken in the use of drugs with a low therapeutic index?

2.32 Drug [XH] is an acidic drug. Like most acidic drugs, the ionised form X⁻ has low lipid solubility, whereas the non-ionised form XH has high lipid solubility. There are no specific transport mechanisms. Answer the following questions using first principles:

A Compare the ionised, non-ionised and total concentration of the drug in the plasma and in the stomach.

B Compare the ionised, non-ionised, and total concentration of the drug in the plasma and in the alkaline renal tubule.

C What is the effect of an increase in urinary pH on the elimination of the drug from the body?

D What is the effect of an increase in plasma pH on the penetration of the drug into the central nervous system?

E State the effects of intravenous administration of the following substances on the plasma pH and the urinary pH. Explain the mechanisms involved.
  i Bicarbonate
  ii Acetazolamide

F Aspirin (salicylates) is an acidic drug. It has toxic effects on the central nervous system in high dosage. A patient is admitted with a serious aspirin overdose. Using information in (A) to (E) above, deduce the best way to treat the overdose.

2.33 100 g of drugs A, B, C and D were each injected intravenously into a 50 kg man. Five minutes later, blood and urinary samples were taken. The plasma and urinary concentrations of the drugs are shown in Table 2.4. Assume that the approximate volumes for the plasma, extracellular fluid and total body water are 0.05, 0.2 and 0.55 l/kg body weight, respectively.

Table 2.3

Antagonist	Significant effect of:		
	Right shift	Reduction in maximal response	Reduction in slope of dose–response curve
A			
B			
C			

Table 2.4

Drug	Plasma concentration (g/l)	Urinary concentration (g/l)
A	3.8	0
B	2.0	0
C	10.1	0
D	39.8	0

19

2

Q

GENERAL BASIC MEDICAL SCIENCES

Pharmacology

A Calculate the volume of distribution of the drugs A, B, C and D.

B With what anatomical compartments (if any) do these volumes of distribution correspond?

C Assuming your answers to (B) are correct, indicate the *probable* properties of the drugs by filling in the blanks in Table 2.5 table with 'yes', 'no' or '? (cannot be determined)'.

D A patient was admitted with a serious overdose of one of these drugs. For which one of the drugs is haemodialysis least effective in managing overdose?

2.34 10 mg of a drug D was administered intravenously to a 50 kg man; the concentrations of the drug were measured immediately after administration and every 3 h thereafter (Table 2.6). Answer the following questions by applying the single-compartment model.

A Calculate the apparent volume of distribution of drug D. What can you deduce about the property of the drug?

B By plotting an appropriate graph, or otherwise, describe the kinetics of the elimination of drug D. Justify your answer.

C Calculate the elimination rate constant k_{el}.

D How does the half-life vary with time? Calculate the half-life of the drug at around (1) 6 h and (2) 12 h.

E Assume that the bioavailability of the drug administered orally is 100%. Does the drug undergo first-pass metabolism? Explain.

F Compare the situation if the drug had been administered orally by stating whether each of the following measurements would have been greater, smaller or the same.
  i Initial concentration
  ii Duration of action
  iii Area under the concentration–time curve

G Give one advantage and one disadvantage of administering drugs intravenously compared with orally.

2.35 A young medical student weighing 50 kg quickly consumed 1.5 measures of beer (equivalent to 1 mol alcohol) one Saturday night at 11:00 p.m. Half an hour later, her blood alcohol concentration was 12 mmol/l. Another hour later, it was 8 mmol/l. The elimination of alcohol can be approximated by zero-order kinetics (saturation kinetics). Assume that alcohol is completely absorbed 30 min after ingestion.

A Explain the term zero-order kinetics, and why the elimination of alcohol can be approximated by zero-order kinetics.

B Estimate the time taken for the blood alcohol concentration to fall to 2 mmol/l.

C Is the half-time of the blood alcohol concentration constant?

D The student enjoyed her night and decided to increase her alcohol consumption on subsequent weekends. Assuming her alcohol elimination kinetics remain the same for all nights and weekends, calculate:
  • the initial alcohol concentration (i.e. concentration 30 min after ingestion)
  • the time she has to wait before she can legally drive.
  if she decided to consume 3, 4.5 or 6 measures of beer, and complete Table 2.7. Ignore the time taken to consume the alcohol. It is illegal to drive with a blood alcohol concentration of 17.4 mmol/l or above.

Table 2.5

Drug	Binding strongly to albumin	Very large molecules	High lipid solubility	Ability to enter CNS	Accumulate in body fat
A					
B					
C					
D					

Table 2.6

Time (h)	0	3	6	9	12	15	18
Concentration (mg/l)	4.0	3.0	2.3	1.7	1.3	0.9	0.7

Table 2.7

Beer consumption (measures)	3	4.5	6
Alcohol concentration (mmol/l) 30 min after consumption			
Time (h) the student has to wait before she could legally drive			

General principles of pharmacology

2.1 B
The relationship between pharmacological effects and the drug concentration is usually hyperbolic (Fig. 2.2). However, the relationship between pharmacological effects and log dose is usually sigmoid in shape, and the central proportion is almost linear. The maximal response is represented by the plateau of the curves, and is higher for drug B than drug A. The EC_{50} value is the concentration of drug which gives rise to 50% of the maximal response. The lower the value, the higher the potency. The value is lower for drug A. Hence, drug A is more potent. It is not possible to deduce the mechanisms of action from the log dose–response curve alone.

2.2 D
Sensitivity of target tissue reflects the concentration at which it responds to a drug. Loss of sensitivity results in a higher concentration of drug necessary to achieve the same effect. Hence, the EC_{50} value is increased. However, the maximal response is not affected. The log dose–response curve is shifted to the right.

2.3 B D E
A highly selective drug produces one pharmacological effect at a much lower dose than for other pharmacological effects. A formal definition of selectivity is the ratio of its potency for one effect to its potency for another effect. Hence, it has a lower EC_{50} value and a higher potency than for other effects. Selectivity does not compare the effect of one drug with another. The therapeutic index of a drug is its selectivity for its therapeutic effect. For a drug with a high therapeutic index, a wide range of concentrations can be tolerated without side effects. Conversely, for a drug with a low therapeutic index, there is a narrow range of concentrations for which the drug has therapeutic effect without side effects.

2.4 A B
The effects of enzyme inhibitors may be due to either increased concentration of the substrate (e.g. acetylcholinesterase) or to reduced concentration of the products (e.g. angiotensin-converting enzyme inhibitors). Competitive inhibitors bind to the active site, whilst non-competitive inhibitors bind to other sites. Although many competitive enzyme inhibitors are reversible, some are irreversible (e.g. organophosphorus compounds are irreversible competitive inhibitors of actylcholinesterases). This is because they form strong covalent bonds with the enzyme. Whilst the offset of action is longer for irreversible inhibitors, the onset of action depends mainly on the rate of the substrate to product reaction. Hence, the time of onset is independent of whether it is a reversible or irreversible enzyme inhibitor.

2.5 –
An active drug response may be produced by either increasing or decreasing cellular activities. An agonist produces an active response by activating receptors on the cell membrane. It may do so directly by binding to the receptor (e.g. adrenaline (epinephrine) binding to adrenergic receptors) or indirectly (e.g. tyramine promotes release of neuronal noradrenaline (norepinephrine)). An antagonist prevents agonists acting (e.g. by binding to the receptor), but does not produce an effect itself. A partial agonist produces an active response, although the response is less than that from a full agonist even when it occupies all the receptor sites.

2.6 A D E
Plasma membranes consist of a lipid bilayer with polar groups outside and non-polar groups inside. Lipid-soluble drugs (i.e. drugs with high lipid–water partition coefficient) are able to cross the plasma membrane by passive diffusion, and a low molecular weight is associated with more rapid diffusion. Very small water-soluble drugs (e.g. ethanol) can also pass through the membrane via small water-filled pores. Few drugs have specific carrier systems.

2.7 B D
Antagonism between two drugs is said to occur if the effect of the two drugs is smaller than the sum of their individual pharmacological effects. This may occur in many ways. The two drugs may be antagonists of each other at the same receptor (e.g. propranolol and adrenaline (epinephrine)), one drug may release a mediator which antagonises the effect of another drug (e.g. tyramine

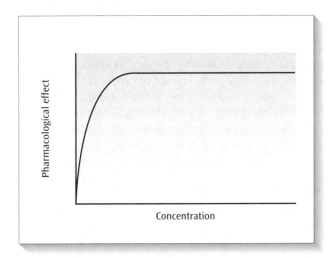

Fig. 2.2 Relationship between phamacological effects and concentration.

2

A

Pharmacology

GENERAL BASIC MEDICAL SCIENCES

releases noradrenaline (norepinephrine), which antagonises the effect of noradrenaline), or the two drugs may act at different receptors which gives rise to opposite effects (functional antagonist, e.g. propranolol, which reduces the heart rate by blocking the β_1 receptor, and atropine, which increases the heart rate by blocking muscarinic acetylcholine receptors in the heart). Potentiation is said to occur if one drug reduces the concentration of another drug necessary to produce a given pharmacological effect (e.g. anticholinesterases potentiate the effect of acetylcholine at the neuromuscular junction).

2.8   E
Modified-release capsules consist of numerous small granules which dissolve at different rates. This results in a smooth sustained release of the drug. If the drug can be activated by acids, enteric-coated tablets are indicated.

2.9   A B C D E
Drugs taken orally are absorbed via the gastrointestinal system. Since the venous drainage is via the hepatic portal system, they may be subjected to significant first-pass metabolism by the liver. Drugs given via other sites (e.g. sublingually via the buccal membrane, by inhalation via the respiratory mucosa, as a skin patch, intramuscularly or intravenously) will avoid first-pass metabolism since venous drainage is via the systemic circulation. Drugs given rectally are less predictable. In general, rectal mucosa of the lower rectum is drained directly to the systemic circulation, but the rest of the rectum is drained via the portal circulation.

2.10   B C D
Systemic bioavailability is the proportion of a drug administered that finally reaches the systemic circulation. For intravenous injection, the systemic bioavailability is 1. Systemic bioavailability for drugs given orally is often small for several reasons. The drug may not dissolve completely; it may be broken down in the gut lumen (e.g. benzylpenicillin); the absorption may be poor (e.g. aminoglycosides); it may bind to substances in the gut lumen (e.g. tetracyclines binding to calcium ions); and it may be metabolised either in the gut (e.g. levodopa) or in the liver (e.g. opiates). Hence, the dose of drugs given orally is often greater than that given via the other routes.

2.11   D E
Most drugs bind to plasma proteins (e.g. albumin) reversibly by non-covalent bonds. For lipid-soluble drugs, the proportion of bound drugs remains constant over the therapeutic range of concentrations. This is also true for polar drugs which bind to specific sites of a plasma protein, as there is often an excess of binding sites over drugs. Rarely, the drugs have a very high affinity for the receptors and they become saturated, and the proportion of bound drugs decreases with increasing concentration of drugs. Furthermore, the presence of another drug which competes for the same binding site may increase the free concentration of the first drug. Protein binding often smoothes out the plasma concentration and speeds up distribution of the drug.

2.12   A
The apparent volume of distribution of a drug is a measure of the extent of the drug distribution in the body at equilibrium. It is defined as the ratio of the amount of the drug in the body to the plasma drug concentration at equilibrium. Hence, if the drug distributes equally between all tissues and plasma, the volume of distribution is equivalent to the total body water. However, if the drug binds strongly to tissues, only a small proportion of the drug will be found in plasma, and the apparent volume of distribution can be much higher than the total body volume. Binding to plasma proteins will have no effect on the apparent volume of distribution.

2.13   D E
Lipid-soluble drugs are mostly metabolised by the liver into water-soluble substances. Water-soluble drugs and metabolites are mostly eliminated by the kidney. The clearance of a drug is defined as the rate of elimination of a drug divided by the plasma concentration of the drug. It can be thought of as the volume of blood cleared of the drug per unit time. The production of creatinine in the body is relatively constant, and it distributes throughout the extracellular fluid with minimal protein binding, and there is often no net secretion or reabsorption in the renal tubules. Hence, creatinine clearance is often used as a measure of GFR.

2.14   A B E
Three broad factors determine the rate at which a drug is excreted by the kidneys: its rate of filtration at the glomerulus, rate of reabsorption at the tubules, and the rate of secretion at the tubules. The rate of filtration depends on the proper function of the kidneys and the concentration of the drug in plasma. A high rate of tubular reabsorption reduces the renal clearance of a drug. Tubular reabsorption is usually passive, but may be active for a few drugs (e.g. thyroxine) which resemble physiological metabolites. Passive reabsorption is higher for non-polar, lipid-soluble drugs than highly polar water-soluble drugs. The proportion of non-polarised form of the drug is higher with low urinary pH for acidic drugs, and a high urinary pH for basic drugs. As only the polarised form of the drug is reabsorbed, the reabsorption rate is lower

(and the renal clearance is higher) for acidic drugs in the presence of a high urinary pH, and for basic drugs in the presence of a low urinary pH. Active secretion of drugs into the renal tubules (e.g. penicillin, salicylates) decreases the renal clearance.

2.15 B C D

The cytochrome P_{450} system is the most important mixed-function oxidase (MFO) system. This enzyme system is largely located in the smooth endoplasmic reticulum, but may also be present in the mitochondria (e.g. monoamine oxidase). The system is responsible both for the metabolism of endogenous substances (e.g. corticosteroids) and drugs. Most enzymes in the systems are involved in oxidation, although a few are involved in reduction. The system may be induced or inhibited by drugs. This is clinically important, as the therapeutic effects of drugs may be reduced if the enzymes are induced, and side effects may be enhanced if the enzymes are inhibited. Changes in drug doses are necessary to avoid this.

2.16 A B C

The steady-state concentration of a drug when regularly repeated intravenous doses of a drug are given depends mostly on the average rate of the drug given and the clearance rate from the plasma. The clearance rate from the plasma is largely contributed to by clearance from the kidneys and the liver. The volume of distribution of the drug determines the time taken to reach the steady-state concentration. The larger the volume of distribution, the longer is the time taken to reach steady-state concentration. However, the steady-state concentration is not affected. Similarly, an initial large intravenous dose of the drug will reduce the time taken to reach the steady-state concentration without affecting the actual steady-state concentration.

2.17 C

A first-order elimination process is said to occur if the rate of elimination is proportional to the plasma concentration. The elimination half-life (time taken for the plasma concentration to reduce to half) is constant. Since the rate of elimination increases with the concentration, a steady-state concentration will be reached even if the infusion rate is above the current elimination rate. By contrast, a zero-order elimination process is said to occur if the rate of elimination is constant and independent of the plasma concentration. The half-life is shorter for a smaller concentration of the drug. If the infusion rate exceeds the current elimination rate, the plasma concentration will continue to increase to a toxic level, and a steady-state concentration will never be reached. A zero-order elimination process usually occurs if the elimination is eliminated primarily by metabolism and the enzymes

responsible for the metabolism are saturated. This is more likely to occur if the concentration of the drug is high.

2.18 A B D

Monitoring of the plasma concentrations of a drug is useful in ensuring that the drug plasma level is between the therapeutic and the toxic level of the drug. It is particularly valuable if either therapeutic or toxic effects are difficult to monitor over a short period of time. For example, the effect of an anti-epileptic agent is difficult to monitor over a short period of time. Similarly, the toxic effect of aminoglycosides is difficult to monitor clinically. The therapeutic index is the ratio of the minimum therapeutic concentration and the minimum toxic concentration. The therapeutic window is the range of concentrations between the minimum therapeutic and toxic concentrations. Monitoring of plasma concentrations is more important for drugs with a low therapeutic index and a narrow therapeutic window.

2.19 C E

Compared with younger adults, the elderly are more likely to suffer from side effects of drugs. There are many reasons for this. The metabolism of drugs by the liver and the excretion of drugs by the kidneys are lower, which results in higher plasma concentrations. Furthermore, the response of the elderly to a given concentration of a drug is greater. Hence, the doses required for a given drug are generally smaller. As the proportion of body water decreases and that of fats increases in the elderly, the volume of distribution for water-soluble drugs is decreased, but that for lipid-soluble drugs is increased.

2.20 –

Most adverse drug effects can be predicted from the pharmacological properties of the drug. Amongst those adverse effects which are unpredictable, true drug allergy is the commonest. True drug allergy is due to one of the hypersensitivity reactions involving antigen–antibody reactions, and is unrelated to the mechanism of its therapeutic effects. A period of induction is required on primary exposure, but the side effects may be rapid and severe on re-exposure. True drug allergy is often over-diagnosed. However, with a history of true drug allergy, the drug should not be prescribed in future.

2.21 D

Agonists are substances which resemble the natural transmitter and activate the receptors. Antagonists are substances sufficiently similar to the natural transmitter to occupy the receptors without eliciting a response. Inverse agonists are substances which produce effects opposite to those of the agonists. An example is β-carbolines, which act on the benzodiazepine receptors. Benzodiazepines

Pharmacology

cause muscle relaxation whilst β-carbolines cause convulsions. However, they both act on the same receptors and through modulating the effects of the neurotransmitter GABA.

2.22 C

Partial agonists activate the receptors, but to a lesser extent than the natural transmitter. Hence, they produce maximal responses less than those of full agonists. The partial agonists also prevent the natural transmitters from reaching the receptors. Hence, they also act as antagonists. The effect of a combination of a full and a partial agonist may be less than that of the full agonist alone, as the partial agonists prevent the full agonists from reaching some of the receptors. However, the effect of a full and a partial agonist together is usually greater than that of the partial agonist alone. Partial agonists may be clinically useful. For example, oxyprenolol is a partial agonist whilst propranolol is an antagonist of the β-adrenergic receptors. On its own, oxyprenolol causes less bradycardia and patients on oxyprenolol have a higher resting heart rate than patients on equivalent doses of propranolol. However, oxyprenolol has the same protective effect as propranolol against the natural adrenaline (epinephrine) during exercise or under stressful situations. Substances which produce effects that are opposite to those of the full agonists are called inverse agonists.

2.23 B C E

In order for an orally administered drug to reach the systemic circulation, it must pass through the stomach intact, undergo absorption from the small intestine and pass through the liver without being metabolised. If the drug is unstable under low pH, it is liable to be inactivated by gastric acid. Slow gastric emptying, intestinal hurry or binding of the active drugs to food tends to reduce absorption of the drug from the intestinal wall. Lipid-soluble drugs are easier to absorb from the gut. Metabolism through the liver is the single most important reason for the low systemic availability for orally administered drugs.

2.24 A C E

Drugs are usually given by an initial loading dose followed by maintenance doses at regular intervals. The half-life of a drug is the time it takes for the plasma concentration to decline by half. As a rough general principle, intervals between maintenance doses may be approximately equal to the half-life of the drug. If a loading dose is not given (i.e. the loading dose being the same as the maintenance dose), it would take five half-life periods to achieve a steady-state concentration. Hence, for a drug with a half-life of 10 min, it may be acceptable not to give a loading dose as the steady-state concentration will be reached in

50 min. For a drug with a half-life of 2 h, it should be administered roughly every 2 h. Since this will not be acceptable to the patient, either sustained-release preparations should be given, or the drug should be given as a continuous infusion. A drug with a half-life of 12 h may be given twice daily. A drug with a half-life of 72 h should be given daily with the maintenance dose just sufficient to replace the amount eliminated in 24 h. A drug with a half-life of 120 h should be given a loading dose higher than the maintenance dose, as it would otherwise take 600 h to reach steady-state concentration.

2.25 C E

In general, the effect of the regulation of receptors is to restore the function of cells to its usual state. Hence, prolonged exposure to an agonist results in downregulation of receptors. This may be achieved by a decrease in the number of receptors, a decrease in the capacity of the receptors to respond, or a decrease in the receptor occupancy. Hence, patients can become tolerant or refractory to treatment by agonists. Conversely, prolonged exposure to an antagonist results in upregulation of receptors, which may be achieved by an increase in the number of receptors, an increase in the capacity of the receptors to respond, or an increase in receptor occupancy. Patients may become supersensitive to the effects of agonists.

2.26 A B D

The rebound phenomenon on withdrawal of a drug is due to the up or downregulation of receptors following prolonged use. For example, chronic use of β-blockers may result in upregulation of the adrenergic receptors. When administration of the drug is stopped, the effect of physiological β-adrenaline (β-epinephrine) and noradrenaline (norepinephrine) on the supersensitive receptors will be enhanced. The likelihood of the phenomenon is greater the longer the drug has been previously administered, the more abrupt the withdrawal, the shorter the half-life of the drug (as the withdrawal from the target organ is more abrupt), and if the drug is a partial agonist rather than if it is either a pure agonist or a pure antagonist. The rebound phenomenon is equally likely for drugs with inhibitory or excitatory effects.

2.27 D E

Drug interactions may occur at any stage from preparation to excretion. A drug which increases bowel motility is likely to reduce the absorption and hence the effects of orally administered drugs. Binding to another drug in the gut lumen will reduce the effect of both drugs. An enzyme inducer may decrease the effect of drugs by increasing the rate of metabolism in the liver, whilst an enzyme inhibitor may increase the effect of drugs by decreasing the rate of metabolism in the liver. Inhibition of the active transport of a drug across the renal tubular epithelium may increase its effect by reducing its rate of elimination.

2.28

A

$$D + R \underset{k_b}{\overset{k_f}{\rightleftharpoons}} DR$$

Concentration: x $(t-o)$ o

B

The law of mass action states that the rate of a chemical reaction is proportional to the concentrations of the reactants. Hence,

Rate of forward reaction $= k_f x (t - o)$

Rate of backward reaction $= k_b o$

C

At equilibrium, the rate of forward reaction is equal to the rate of backward reaction. Hence,

$$k_f x(t - o) = k_b o$$

Rearranging the equation gives

$$x(t - o) = (k_b/k_f)o = Ko$$

D

From the equation in (C),

$$xt - xo = Ko$$

$$xt = o(K + x)$$

Hence, $p = o/t = x/(K + x)$

E

i   See Fig. 2.3.

ii See Fig. 2.4.

F

Yes.

G

No. The affinity of the drug for the receptor cannot be accurately calculated from the dose–response curve using the theoretical relationship between fractional occupancy and log concentration. First, the relationship between the biological response and fractional occupancy of receptors is not usually linear. Second, the local concentration of drugs at the receptors is difficult to estimate, as drugs may be metabolised near the receptor sites. For example, acetylcholine is rapidly metabolised at the neuromuscular junction, and noradrenaline (norepinephrine) or adrenaline (epinephrine) are taken up at the sympathetic nerve terminals.

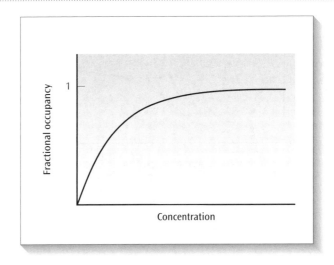

Fig. 2.3   Fractional occupancy versus concentration.

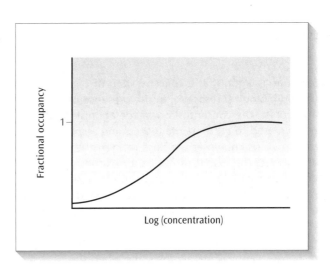

Fig. 2.4   Fractional occupancy versus log concentration.

2.29

A

See Fig. 2.5.

B

No. The slope of the dose–response curve is similar both with and without Y.

C

No. The maximal response is unaffected by the presence of Y.

D

Y is an antagonist as it shifts the dose–response curve to the right. It is a competitive antagonist as the slope of the

Pharmacology

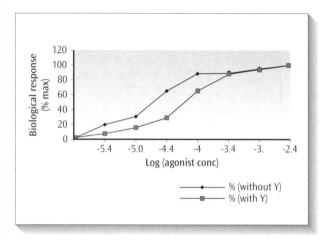

Fig. 2.5 Dose–response curve with and without Y.

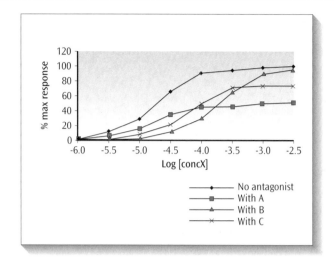

Fig. 2.6 Dose–response curve of drug X, with and without antagonists A, B and C.

dose–response curve is unaffected by Y. It is reversible because the maximal response is unaffected.

E

i Suppose an agonist at a concentration of c_1 achieved a certain biological response. In the presence of an antagonist, the concentration of the agonist needs to be increased to c_2 to maintain the same response. The ratio c_2 / c_1 is known as the dose ratio of the antagonist. The extent of right shift of the dose–response curve is a measure of the dose ratio (it is equal to the antilog of the degree of shift). When X is between 3.2×10^{-6} and 10^{-4} µmol/l, it can be seen either from the raw data or the dose–response curve that dose ratio is about 3.2. For example, the biological response is approximately the same when the concentration of X is 3.2×10^{-5} µmol/l without Y, and 10^{-4} with Y.

ii When X is between 10^{-4} and 3.2×10^{-3} µmol/l, the dose ratio is still about 3.2. It can be seen from the dose–response curve that the extent of the right shift is the same. Again, the dose ratio can be estimated from the raw data. For example, the biological response is approximately the same when the concentration of X is 10^{-4} without Y, and 3.2×10^{-4} with Y.

F

The dose ratio increases linearly with antagonist concentration. From (E), the dose ratio is 3.2 when Y is 1 µmol/l. The dose ratio will be 32 when Y is 10 µmol/l. Hence, when the concentrations of X and Y are 10^{-3} µmol/l and 10 µmol/l, respectively, the biological response is the same as with X at a concentration of ($10^{-3} / 32 = 3.2 \times 10^{-5}$ µmol/l) in the absence of Y. Thus, the biological response will be about 66% of maximum.

Table 2.8

Antagonist	Significant effect of:		
	Right shift	Reduction in maximal response	Reduction in slope of dose-response curve
A	No	Yes	Yes
B	Yes	No	No
C	Yes	Yes	No

G

There are numerous examples of competitive reversible antagonists; three of these are propranolol (at β-adrenergic receptors), tubocurarine (at nicotinic acetylcholine receptors) and naloxone (at opiate µ-receptors).

2.30

A

See Fig. 2.6.

B

See Table 2.8.

C

- A – irreversible competitive antagonist
- B – reversible competitive antagonist
- C – non-competitive antagonist.

It is clear that B is a reversible competitive antagonist as there is a right shift without a reduction in slope and maximum effect. It is also clear that A is an irreversible competitive antagonist as there is no right shift, and there is a reduction in the maximum effect. The effects of a non-competitive antagonist are a reduction in the maximum effect. There may also be a right shift or a reduction in the slope.

D

- Competitive reversible antagonist – e.g. propranolol at β-adrenergic receptors
- Competitive irreversible antagonist – e.g. monoamine oxidase inhibitors
- Non-competitive antagonist (i.e. antagonist which blocks the chain of events that leads to the production of a response by the agonist) – e.g. verapamil (which blocks the influx of calcium ions through cell membranes).

2.31
A
Therapeutic index is the ratio between the average minimum effective dose and the average maximum tolerated dose:

$$\text{therapeutic index} = \text{Maximun non - toxic dose/minimum effective dose}$$

i Therapeutic index for analgesic effects = 60/20 = 3. Therapeutic dose for antirheumatic effects = 60/40 = 1.5.
ii Therapeutic index for analgesic effects = 80/20 = 4. Therapeutic dose for antirheumatic effects = 80/40 = 2.

B
Drug Y has a higher therapeutic index than drug X.
 i No conclusions can be drawn about the clinical usefulness.
 ii Drug Y is safer in accidental overdose than drug X.
 iii No conclusions can be drawn about the cost-effectiveness.

C
1. It does not take into account idiosyncratic (non-dose dependent) toxic reactions.
2. The maximum non-toxic dose is usually based on animal study rather than clinical dose.

D
1. Monitor the function of organs which the drugs may damage (e.g. monitor renal function if gentamicin is used).
2. Monitor serum drug levels.

2.32
A
Only the non-ionised form of the drug can cross the cell membrane. Hence, the concentrations of the non-ionised form of the drug are equal in all compartments. For an acidic drug, the ionised form predominates over the non-ionised form in an alkaline (high pH) environment. Thus, both the ionised form and total concentration will be higher in an alkaline environment. The concentrations of both ionised and total concentration of an acidic drug are higher in the plasma than in the stomach.

B
The non-ionised form of the drug is the same in the plasma and in the renal tubule. The ionised form and the total concentration of an acidic drug are higher in the renal tubule than in the plasma.

C
An increase in the urinary pH causes an increase in the concentration of acidic drug in the renal plasma ('ion trapping') and hence increased elimination of acidic drugs from the body.

D
Increasing the plasma pH causes an increase in the proportion of the non-ionised form in the plasma and therefore extracts the drug from the central nervous system.

E
 i Intravenous administration of bicarbonate would increase the plasma pH by shifting the following reaction to the right:

$$H^+ + OH^- \rightleftharpoons H_2O$$

The urinary pH also increases as a result.
 ii Acetazolamide is a carbonic anhydrase inhibitor in the renal tubule. It inhibits the reaction:

$$H_2O + CO_2 \rightleftharpoons H^+ + HCO^-$$

An increased quantity of bicarbonate ions is excreted in the urine. Hence, the urinary pH increases and the plasma pH decreases.

F
Aspirin is an acidic drug. The aims are to extract the drug from the central nervous system to the plasma, and excrete the drugs in the urine. From (C) and (D), both plasma and urinary pH should be increased. From (E), intravenous administration of bicarbonate is the most effective treatment.

Pharmacology

2.33

A

The apparent volume of distribution of a drug (V_d) is the volume of fluid at the same concentration present in the plasma (C_p) which would contain the total amount of drug in the body (Q). In other words, $V = Q/C_p$. Thus:
- volume of distribution of drug A = 100/3.8 = 26.3 litres
- volume of distribution of drug B = 100/2 = 50 litres
- volume of distribution of drug C = 100/10.1 = 9.90 litres
- volume of distribution of drug D = 100/39.8 = 2.51 litres.

B

For the 50 kg man:
- the plasma volume = 0.05 × 50 = 2.5 litres
- the extracellular volume = 0.2 × 50 = 10 litres
- the total body water volume = 0.55 × 50 = 27.5 litres.

Hence, the corresponding anatomical volumes for the volume of distribution for:
- drug A is the total body water volume
- drug B does not exist (larger than the total body water volume)
- drug C is the extracellular fluid volume
- drug D is the plasma volume.

C

See Table 2.9.
- Drug A is a highly lipid-soluble drug, and can bind anywhere outside the plasma but without accumulating excessively in body fat.
- Drug B is similar to drug A, except that it accumulates in body fat.
- Drug C has a low lipid solubility and hence cannot enter cells easily. It does not consist of very large molecules and therefore can move from the plasma to the extracellular fluid compartment.
- Drug D consists of very large molecules, and/or it binds very strongly to plasma proteins. As a result, it is confined to the plasma volume.

D

Drug B. It is accumulated in body fat. Since haemodialysis results in lowering of the plasma concentration, it is inefficient in removing the drug from body fat.

2.34

A

Apparent volume of distribution of drug D = Q/C_p = 10/4 = 2.5 litres, where Q is the total amount of drug in the body and C_p is its plasma concentration. This is roughly equivalent to the plasma volume; thus, it may either consist of very large molecules, or it binds very strongly to plasma proteins.

B

See Fig. 2.7. This is almost a straight line graph; the elimination of the drug can be approximated by a single-compartment model with first-order elimination kinetics (i.e. the rate of elimination is directly proportional to drug concentration).

C

The elimination rate constant k_{el} can be calculated from the inverse of the slope of the plot of log concentration versus time in (B), i.e. k_{el} = −slope. Hence, the elimination rate constant k_{el} = 0.094.

D

In first-order kinetics, the half-life is constant. It can be calculated by:

$$\text{Half-life} = \ln 2/k_{el} = 0.693/0.094 = 7.4\,\text{h}$$

E

If the bioavailability of the drug is 100%, the drug cannot have been metabolised in the liver; hence, the drug does not undergo first-pass metabolism.

Table 2.9

Drug	Binding strongly to albumin	Very large molecules	High lipid solubility	Ability to enter CNS	Accumulate in body fat
A	No	No	Yes	Yes	No
B	No	No	Yes	Yes	Yes
C	No	No	No	No	No
D	?Yes	?Yes	?	No	No

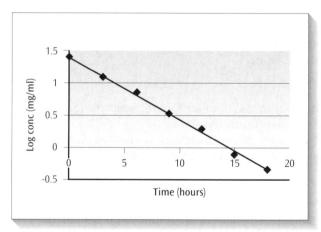

Fig. 2.7 Log concentration versus time.

F

  i Initial concentration would be lower.

  ii The duration of action would be longer.

  iii the area under the concentration–time curve is equivalent to the total amount of drug; hence, it is the same if bioavailability were 100%.

G

Advantages: rapid onset of action; higher initial concentration.

  Disadvantages: short duration of action; rapid fluctuation of concentration.

2.35

A

Zero-order kinetics (i.e. saturation kinetics) describes the elimination of drug eliminated at a constant rate independent of the plasma concentration. The elimination of alcohol can be approximated by zero-order kinetics because the limited availability of cofactor NAD^+ means that the oxidative actions of the enzyme alcohol dehydrogenase reach a maximum and cannot be increased by increased concentration of alcohol.

B

The rate of decrease of alcohol concentration is 12 – 8 = 4 mmol/l. The time taken for the alcohol concentration to fall from 8 to 2 mmol/l is (8 – 2)/4 = 1.5 h.

Table 2.10

Beer consumption (measures)	3	4.5	6
Alcohol concentration (in mmol/l) 30 minutes after consumption	24	36	48
Time (h) the student has to wait before she could legally drive	= (24 – 17.4)/4 =1.65	= (36 – 17.4)/4 = 4.65	= (48 – 17.4)/4 = 7.65

C

No, the half-time of the blood alcohol decreases with time.

D

See Table 2.10. If she doubles her consumption of alcohol from 3 to 6 measures, the time she needs to wait increases by more than double.

Nutrition and energy

3 **Q**

3.1 The following statements about the conversion of ATP into ADP and inorganic phosphate are true:
  A The reaction is endothermic
  B Free energy is required for the conversion
  C It may be coupled with an anabolic reaction
  D It has the highest free energy amongst all important biochemical reactions involving organophosphates
  E It occurs during muscle contraction

3.2 Sources of high-energy phosphates in the living cell include:
  A The urea cycle
  B Glycogenesis
  C Oxidative phosphorylation
  D Glycolysis
  E The citric acid cycle

3.3 The following statements about oxidative phosphorylation are true:
  A It occurs in the smooth endoplasmic reticulum
  B It may occur anaerobically
  C Water is formed as a by-product
  D Reducing equivalents (e.g. free electrons) are needed for the process
  E It is inhibited by cyanide

3.4 The following statements about the respiratory chain are true:
  A It consists of redox carriers which transport the reducing equivalents
  B It consists of no more than three components
  C The first component is the most electropositive
  D The inorganic phosphate to oxygen (P:O) ratio is higher for NAD-linked dehydrogenase than flavoprotein-linked dehydrogenase
  E The oxidation and phosphorylation processes occur simultaneously

3.5 Examples of monosaccharides include:
  A Glucose
  B Glycogen
  C Maltose
  D Fructose
  E Starch

3.6 The citric acid cycle may be involved in the oxidation of:
  A Glucose
  B Starch
  C Fatty acids
  D Lipids
  E Protein

3.7 The following statements about the citric acid cycle are true:
  A It occurs in the mitochondria
  B It provides reducing equivalents for oxidative phosphorylation
  C It may occur without oxygen
  D 12 ATPs are formed every full cycle
  E Two carbon dioxide molecules are formed every full cycle

3.8 The activity of the citric acid cycle is increased when energy is required (e.g. during muscular contraction). The following substances are likely to contribute significantly to this regulation of the citric acid cycle:
  A NADH
  B ADP
  C Calcium ions
  D Glycogen
  E Glucose

3.9 The citric acid cycle plays a role in the following processes:
  A Gluconeogenesis
  B Nucleic acid synthesis
  C Fatty acid synthesis from glucose
  D Lactic acid synthesis
  E Non-essential amino acid synthesis

3.10 The following statements about the glycolysis pathway are true:
  A It is the main mechanism for the metabolism of glucose
  B It is the main mechanism for the metabolism of fructose
  C ATP is consumed in the process
  D It is a more important pathway in the heart than in the brain
  E The quantity of lactic acid increases with the concentration of oxygen

3.11 The inability to metabolise pyruvate (into acetyl CoA by pyruvate dehydrogenase):
  A May occur with thiamine deficiency
  B May be inherited
  C Results in hypoxia
  D Results in accumulation of lactic acid
  E Results in adverse effects particularly on the brain

3.12 The following statements about glycogen are true:
  A It is a linear chain of monosaccharides
  B It is mainly found in the heart muscle
  C Liver glycogen provides an important source of energy for vigorous physical activities

D Disorders of glycogen storage result in muscle weakness

E Muscle glycogen store is usually significantly depleted after about 8 h of fasting

3.13 During starvation, the enzymes which catalyse the following carbohydrate metabolic reactions are inhibited:
A Conversion of glucose to glucose 6-phosphate
B Conversion of fructose 6-phosphate to fructose 1,6-bisphosphate
C Conversion of pyruvate to acetyl CoA
D Conversion of glycogen to glucose
E Conversion of phosphoenolpyruvate to pyruvate

3.14 The following statements about the source of fuel for the body during starvation are true:
A There is a net conversion of fatty acids to glucose
B Oxidation of glucose may be completely eliminated
C Glycogen is converted to glucose in preference to the breakdown of essential amino acids
D Free glucose is used in preference to fatty acids
E Free fatty acids are used in preference to ketone bodies

3.15 The energy expended by an individual is increased:
A By fever
B By high environmental temperature above 35%
C In males
D By increased physical activity
E By sleep

3.16 The following minerals must be present in the diet to maintain health:
A Phosphorus
B Magnesium
C Calcium
D Aluminium
E Iodine

3.17 The following statements about dietary proteins are true:
A All 20 types of amino acids must be present in the diet
B About 50% of the energy should be supplied by protein
C The quality of protein is measured by the amount of energy it contains per unit weight
D An adequate intake of carbohydrate and fat minimises the requirements for dietary high-quality protein
E Complementary proteins are defined as the combination of an animal and a plant protein

3.18 The following vitamins are water-soluble:
A Vitamin A
B Vitamin B_{12}
C Vitamin C
D Vitamin D
E Vitamin K

3.19 The following B vitamins are correctly matched to their functions:
A Thiamine (vitamin B_1) – provides one-carbon residues for nucleic acid synthesis
B Riboflavin (vitamin B_2) – prosthetic groups in flavoprotein enzymes in oxidoreduction reactions
C Pyridoxal phosphate (vitamin B_6) – coenzyme for amino acid metabolism
D Cobalamin (vitamin B_{12}) – coenzyme for oxidative carboxylation of α-keto acids and the pentose phosphate pathway
E Niacin (vitamin B_3) – coenzyme for oxidoreduction enzymes

3.20 The following vitamins are correctly matched to the clinical conditions associated with their deficiencies:
A Thiamine (vitamin B_1) – megaloblastic anaemia
B Niacin (vitamin B_3) – beriberi
C Cobalamin (vitamin B_{12}) – pellagra
D Vitamin A – night-blindness
E Vitamin C – scurvy

3.21 Ketone bodies:
A Include acetoacetate
B Are formed when fatty acid oxidation is inhibited
C Are mostly produced in skeletal muscles and kidneys
D Cannot be used as an energy source by any tissues
E Are produced in large quantities in untreated diabetes mellitus

3.22 Brown fat:
A Is mainly located around the buttocks
B Is not present below two years of age
C Is mainly innervated by parasympathetic nervous system
D Is metabolised by strict coupling with oxidative phosphorylation
E Produces more heat per ATP than white fat

3.23 The basal metabolic rate:
A Is determined whilst the subject is asleep
B Is determined whilst the subject is eating
C Is higher in women than in men
D Is higher in children than in adults
E Is increased during starvation

31

3

Q

GENERAL BASIC MEDICAL SCIENCES

Nutrition and energy

3.24 The respiratory quotient:
  A Is the ratio of the steady state of the volume of oxygen produced to the weight of food consumed per unit time
  B For carbohydrates is approximately 1
  C Is lower for fat than for carbohydrate
  D Is higher for protein than for carbohydrate
  E Is important in the calculation of heat energy released by combustion of foodstuffs using direct calorimetry

3.25 A young calorie-conscious medical student consumed one digestive biscuit, noting that the typical energy value of each biscuit was 60 kcal. She was thinking of getting rid of the energy by exercise (climbing stairs). She correctly calculated that 60 kcal was approximately equivalent to 250 kJ. Using the formula potential energy (J) = mass (kg) × gravitational constant (m/s^2) × height (metres) and taking $g = 10$ m/s^2, and mass = 50 kg, she reasoned that she would need to climb 500 m of stairs. She was very disappointed as this would mean climbing stairs from the ground floor to the 50th floor!
  A What is the definition of a kilocalorie (kcal)?
  B Describe how the energy value of the biscuit can be determined in the laboratory.
  C What gas will she consume and what gas will she produce on climbing the stairs?
  D What determines the proportion of the amount of the gas produced and the gas consumed?
  E Give a practical method to estimate her energy production while climbing stairs, bearing in mind your answer to (C).
  F Was her conclusion that she needed to climb 500 m of stairs to burn off the energy value of the biscuit correct? Explain your answers.

3.26 One hot summer's day, John, a young tall and athletic medical student pursuing his intercalated degree in physiology, spent the whole morning playing an important football match. After the match at noon, he suddenly remembered he had to attend a supervision with his supervisor at 1.00 p.m. As he had not given any thought to his research proposal on metabolism, he spent the next 45 min trying to collect some thoughts before running to his supervisor, Mary, a physiology professor with over 30 years experience, who was of short stature and led a sedentary lifestyle. Mary had been doing experiments that morning in her comfortable air-conditioned room, and had just finished lunch when John arrived. She had recently been diagnosed as suffering from hypothyroidism, but had not yet been treated with thyroxine. After about 10 min discussion

of John's research proposal, they decided to carry out a preliminary study, immediately before the end of the supervision that afternoon, by comparing their metabolic rates
  A How is metabolic rate usually measured in the laboratory?
  B List and comment on the factors that may cause John to have a higher metabolic rate than Mary.
  C List and comment on factors that may cause Mary to have a higher metabolic rate than John.
  D Describe hypotheses for the mechanisms by which thyroid hormones influence metabolic rates.

3.27 A healthy medical student fasted for 24 h. Blood glucose was 5.6 mmol/l before the fast and remained the same after the fast.
  A What is the main source of fuel for the brain during the fast?
  B Why did the plasma blood glucose level remain constant?
  The medical student continued a hunger strike for 15 days, during which time he did not consume any food, although he consumed water. At the end of the 15 days, ketones were detected in the urine.
  C What other mechanisms are available to increase the amount of glucose in the blood?
  D Why did ketones appear in the urine at the end of the fast?
  E What mechanisms are available to reduce the consumption of glucose?
  F What mechanisms are available to prevent the catabolism of protein in the brain and the heart?

3.28 An athletic medical student consumed several lumps of glucose 10 min before running a 100 m race.
  A What was the main biochemical pathway involved in metabolism of the glucose to derive energy during the race? Explain. What is the final product of this pathway?
  B What products from the biochemical pathway are rich in energy? Quantify each of these products per molecule of glucose metabolised.
  C Explain how this form of energy is used to help the student run.
  D What are the two most important enzymes regulating this metabolic pathway? Describe how the activity of these enzymes is controlled?
  E From your answer to (D), explain how this metabolic pathway was initiated during the race.

3.29 Another medical student consumed lumps of glucose during a 15 km race.

A What was the main energy-generating biochemical pathway for the metabolism of glucose for this student during this race? Explain. Give the overall substrates and products for this biochemical pathway, listing a few important intermediates.

B In which organelle did this main energy-generating biochemical pathway take place? Give the evidence that this organelle is of prokaryotic origin in evolution.

C What products from this biochemical pathway are rich in energy? Quantify each of these products per molecule of glucose metabolised.

D i How can high-energy phosphate substances (e.g. ATP) be derived from the products outlined in your answer to (C).

   ii Describe the mechanism involved.

   iii What are the overall substrates and products for this pathway?

   iv What factors control the rate of this process?

E What is the clinical consequence if the process in (D) is inhibited? Give an example of something that may inhibit this process.

F i What do 'uncoupling' of the process in (D) above mean?

   ii What are the consequences of uncoupling?

   iii Give one example of physiological uncoupling of this process.

3.30 John, a 30-year-old 1.8 m (6 foot) tall physically active medical student, has been a vegetarian for many years. John was referred by his general practitioner to a dietician as he was suspected to have a negative nitrogen balance. After performing a full history, the dietician calculated that John's average daily calorie intake was about 1500 kcal (50% from carbohydrates, 25% from fats, 25% from protein); the protein intake was about 70 g per day (recommended daily requirement for his sex and age 58 g per day) and was entirely made up of a very restricted range of grade II plant protein.

A What is meant by a negative nitrogen balance? How might it be manifested in severe cases?

B What are 'grade II proteins'? Explain whether they can be adequate in maintaining nitrogen balance?

C Why might John have a negative nitrogen balance? Give at least two reasons.

GENERAL BASIC MEDICAL SCIENCES

---

example, it may play a role in gluconeogenesis by the conversion of oxaloacetate into phosphoenolpyruvate, and into the main gluconeogensis pathway. Acetyl CoA, an important component of fatty acid synthesis, is formed by the action of pyruvate dehydrogenase, which is a mitochondrial enzyme. Since the enzymes responsible for fatty acid synthesis are outside the mitochondria, the acetyl CoA is converted into citrate via the citric acid cycle, which is then transported out of the mitochondria to be reconverted into acetyl CoA. The citric acid cycle is also important in providing the carbon skeleton in the formation of some non-essential amino acids. Lactic acid may be converted into pyruvate and then enters the citric acid cycle.

3.10 A B
Glycolysis is the main mechanism for the metabolism of monosaccharides such as glucose, fructose and galactose. In the process, glucose is converted into pyruvate and ATP is produced. It may occur either aerobically or anaerobically. In the absence of oxygen, pyruvate is converted into lactic acid (lactate). In the presence of oxygen, pyruvate is converted into acetyl CoA in the mitochondria and enters the citric acid cycle. As it can produce energy rapidly in the absence of oxygen, it is especially important in the brain and in skeletal muscle during vigorous activity. However, only two ATP molecules are generated per glucose molecule. This is much less efficient than if it occurs under aerobic conditions when a total of 38 ATP molecules per glucose molecule are produced.

3.11 A B D E
Normally, pyruvate produced during glycolysis is converted into acetyl CoA by pyruvate dehydrogenase in the mitochondria. However, poisoning by mercuric ions, a deficiency of thiamine (e.g. dietary deficiency) or inherited pyruvate dehydrogenase deficiency may make this impossible. This results in the conversion of pyruvate into lactate (lactic acid). As the brain depends especially on glucose for its energy, neurological disturbances are particularly likely.

3.12 D
Glycogen is a branched polymer of α-D-glucose, and represents the principal store for carbohydrates in animals. It is mainly stored in the liver and muscle. The primary function of liver glycogen is to maintain a stable blood glucose, and fasting depletes liver glycogen. Muscle glycogen is an importance source of energy for vigorous physical activity, and is usually depleted after a period of strenuous exercise. In disorders of glycogen storage diseases, deficiency in enzymes responsible for glycogen metabolism results in either deficient glycogen

mobilisation or the deposition of abnormal forms of glycogen. They are usually inherited; muscle weakness is a characteristic symptom due to lack of mobilisation of muscle glycogen.

3.13 A B C E
Glucose is a very important source of energy for the body which the brain depends heavily on. If the glucose level falls below a certain level, brain dysfunction occurs and the patient may lapse into a coma. Hence there are elaborate mechanisms to maintain an adequate glucose concentration during starvation. Ketone bodies and fatty acids are oxidised in preference to glucose. All the principal enzymes responsible for regulating glycolysis (breakdown of glucose to pyruvate) and pyruvate oxidation are inhibited. The regulatory enzymes for glycolysis are glucokinase (which converts glucose to glucose 6-phosphate), phosphofructokinase (which converts fructose 6-phosphate to fructose 1,6-bisphosphate) and pyruvate kinase (which converts phosphoenolpyruvate). Pyruvate dehydrogenase converts pyruvate to acetyl CoA, which is used in the citric acid cycle. The conversion of glycogen to glucose is activated to maintain the level of blood glucose. If a patient lapses into coma due to low blood glucose, one of the treatments is glucagon, which converts glycogen to glucose.

3.14 C
Although carbohydrates can be readily converted into fatty acids via the citric acid cycle, the conversion of pyruvate to acetyl CoA by pyruvate dehydrogenase is essentially irreversible. Hence, there cannot be net conversion of fatty acids to glucose. Since the brain and red blood cells depend on glucose for their energy sources, there is an obligatory rate of oxidation of glucose for the body. During starvation, glycogen stores are mobilised. Ketone bodies are used in preference to fatty acids, which in turn are used in preference to glucose.

3.15 A B C D
The basal metabolic rate is the energy expended in maintaining basic physiological functions when a subject is at rest, awake and in a warm environment. The basal metabolic rate is higher in males, with increasing surface area of the body, in fever and in those with hyperthyroidism. Sleep reduces the basal metabolic rate. Physical exercise is the most important factor which increases the energy expended above the basal metabolic rate. Other factors which increase the energy expended above the basal metabolic rate include high environmental temperature and following a meal, due to energy expended on digestion (i.e. its specific dynamic action).

3

A

GENERAL BASIC MEDICAL SCIENCES

Nutrition and energy

3.16   A B C E
Several minerals are essential for both physiological and biochemical functions. For example, sodium is the principal cation in the extracellular fluid, and potassium is the principal cation in intracellular fluid. Calcium, magnesium and phosphorus are important constituents of bones and teeth. In addition, calcium plays an important part in regulating the function of nerves and muscles, and magnesium is essential for some enzyme cofactors. Iodine is an important constituent of thyroxine. Other important minerals include chloride, copper, iron, manganese, selenium, zinc and fluoride. Aluminium is not an essential mineral, but has been suspected to cause disease (e.g. renal damage and possible links with Alzheimer's dementia).

3.17   D
Dietary proteins are digested into individual amino acids to synthesise specific proteins required by the body. Although there are 20 different types of amino acids, only nine of these (essential amino acids) cannot be synthesised in the body and must be present in the diet. The others (non-essential amino acids) can be formed in the body. High-quality proteins are those with the appropriate proportions of essential amino acids, and include eggs, milk and meat. Proteins which are deficient in some essential amino acids (e.g. wheat) are not of high quality. However, the deficiency may be complemented by other proteins (e.g. beans) to yield a satisfactory protein diet. These proteins are said to be complementary. If the intake of carbohydrates and fat is inadequate, the proteins ingested may be used for gluconeogenesis.

3.18   B C
All the B vitamins and vitamin C are water-soluble. The remaining vitamins (A, D, E, K) are fat-soluble. The importance of classifying vitamins into these two categories is that water-soluble vitamins are excreted in urine and rarely accumulate in toxic concentrations. However, their storage is limited and they must be replenished regularly.

3.19   B C
The B vitamins are generally important coenzymes for important processes in the metabolism of carbohydrates, lipid and proteins. Thiamine (vitamin B_1) is a cofactor in oxidative decarboxylation of α-keto acids and for transketolase in the pentose phosphate pathway. Deficiency in thiamine results in accumulation in the substrates in these reactions (e.g. pyruvate, pentose sugars, leucine, valine) and a clinical picture known as beriberi. It affects the heart muscles, skeletal muscles and nerves, resulting in oedema and heart failure, muscle weakness, peripheral neuropathy and Wernicke's

encephalopathy. Riboflavin (vitamin B_2) forms the prosthetic groups in flavoprotein enzymes in oxidoreduction reactions. Surprisingly, in spite of the important role it has in many biochemical reactions, deficiency of riboflavin results in non-life-threatening symptoms such as angular stomatitis, glossitis and photophobia. Pyridoxal phosphate (vitamin B_6) is the coenzyme of several enzymes of amino acid metabolism, and of enzymes for breaking down glycogen. Deficiency states are rare and not well recognised. Cobalamin (vitamin B_{12}) and folate are essential constituents for nucleic acid synthesis. Hence deficiency results in impaired DNA synthesis and prevents cell division and formation of nuclei in new red blood cells. This results in megaloblastic anaemia. Active niacin (vitamin B_3) is NAD, and is a coenzyme to many enzymes for oxidoreduction. Deficiency results in a pellagra syndrome characterised by depression, dementia, diarrhoea and weight loss.

3.20   D E
See question 3.19 above for the B vitamins. Ascorbic acid (vitamin C) is a water-soluble vitamin and an antioxidant that maintains many metal cofactors in the reduced state, and which is required for collagen synthesis. Deficiency results in a clinical syndrome called scurvy. Scurvy is related to defective collagen synthesis, and is characterised by subcutaneous and other haemorrhages, swollen gums and loose teeth, and muscle weakness. Vitamin A is a fat-soluble vitamin and is a component of the visual pigment rhodopsin in the retinal rod cells. Hence, vitamin A deficiency results in night-blindness.

3.21   A E
Ketone bodies are produced in mitochondria in the liver when there is already a high rate of fatty acid oxidation through β-oxidation to acetyl CoA. Ketone bodies include acetoacetate, 3-hydroxybutyrate and acetone, and can be used by tissues outside the liver (e.g. skeletal and heart muscles). Since oxidation of fatty acids occurs during starvation, ketone bodies are mildly elevated. The level of ketone bodies is dramatically raised in untreated diabetes. This is because insulin has antilipolytic and lipogenic effects, and these are lost in untreated diabetes.

3.22   E
Brown fat consists of only a small proportion of total body fat, and is particularly important in regulating heat production. It is more abundant in infancy, and is mainly located in the nape of the neck, between the scapulae, and along the great vessels in the thorax and abdomen. It is extensively innervated by the sympathetic nervous system. Stimulation of the sympathetic nervous system releases noradrenaline (norepinephrine), which acts via the β_1-adrengeric receptors. Although the oxidative

phosphorylation pathway can be used in the metabolism of brown fat, another pathway which does not generate ATP can also be utilised. Hence, the amount of heat energy per ATP molecule produced is higher than in white fat. Brown fat is an important mechanism in animals and humans for adaptation to the cold.

3.23 D
The basal metabolic rate is the metabolic rate of a subject determined at rest at a temperature within the thermoneutral zone 12–14 h after the last meal. It is slightly higher than when the subject is asleep. The basal metabolic rate is determined 12–14 h after the last meal because energy is required in absorption and digestion of food (the specific dynamic action). The basal metabolic rate is higher in men than in women, and higher in infants than in adults. It is reduced during starvation, due partially to a reduction in the level of circulating catecholamines and thyroid hormones. This explains why the rate of weight reduction for weight-watchers is fast initially but rapidly slows down.

3.24 B C
The respiratory quotient is the ratio in the steady state of the volume of carbon dioxide produced to the volume of oxygen consumed per unit time. It differs according to the type of foodstuff consumed. The respiratory quotient for carbohydrates, fat and protein is approximately 1, 0.70 and 0.82 respectively, although it may rise above 1 for anaerobic respiration. Indirect calorimetry is used to calculate the energy released on combustion of foodstuff by calculating the amount of carbon dioxide produced from the amount of oxygen consumed. Hence, the respiratory quotient of the foodstuff is important. In direct calorimetry, the energy released is measured directly using a bomb calorimeter. Knowledge of the respiratory quotient is not required.

3.25
A
A kilocalorie (kcal) is a unit of heat energy equivalent to 1000 cal; 1 cal is the amount of heat energy required to raise the temperature of 1 g of water by 1°C.

B
The energy value of the biscuit can be determined by direct calorimetry. The food is placed in a metal vessel surrounded by water inside an insulated container. The food is ignited, and the energy value of the food can be calculated from the rise in water temperature:

$$\text{Energy} = \text{rise in temperature} \\ \times \text{heat capacity of water} \\ \times \text{mass of water in the container}$$

C
She will consume oxygen and produce carbon dioxide (and water vapour).

D
The ratio of the amount of the carbon dioxide produced to oxygen consumed is known as the respiratory quotient (RQ). The type of food metabolised determines the RQ; for example, the RQ for carbohydrates, fats and proteins is approximately 1, 0.7 and 0.8, respectively.

E
A practical method of estimating her energy production during exercise is to measure her oxygen consumption per unit time. By assuming that carbohydrates are metabolised, her energy production can be measured.

F
Her conclusion that she needed to climb 50 floors to burn off the energy contained in one biscuit is clearly an overestimate: most of the energy during exercise is produced as heat; only a small fraction results in external work (i.e. gain in gravitational potential energy). The ratio of useful external work to the total energy expended is also known as efficiency.

3.26
A
In the laboratory, metabolic rate is usually measured indirectly via the amount of oxygen consumption per unit of time. A spirometer is filled with oxygen and fitted with a system to absorb any exhaled carbon dioxide. Using such a device, the volume of oxygen consumed can be measured. This volume of oxygen is then corrected to standard temperature and pressure and converted to the equivalent energy produced.

B
- Recent physical exercise (running).
- Male sex.
- Young age.
- Larger surface area (as John is taller).
- Higher level of anxiety causing increased discharge from the sympathetic nervous system.
- Environmental temperature has a U-shaped relationship with metabolic rate. When it is considerably lower than the body temperature, shivering occurs and metabolic rate increases. However, when the environmental temperature is above the body temperature, the body metabolic processes increase. Hence, it is possible that John may have a higher metabolic rate than Mary.
- Mary's untreated hypothyroidism.

3

A

GENERAL BASIC MEDICAL SCIENCES

Nutrition and energy

C

The only factor apparent in the question is that she was in a air-conditioned room. The environmental temperature might be considerably below body temperature. This might trigger shivering and other heat-conserving mechanisms and hence increase her metabolic rate.

D

Thyroid hormones increase metabolic rates and oxygen consumption of most tissues. Possible mechanisms of increased metabolic rates include:
- stimulation of the breakdown of fats and fatty acids
- increase in the activity of membrane-bound Na^+, K^+-ATPase in tissues.

3.27
A

The main source of fuel for the brain is plasma glucose.

B

The plasma glucose level remains constant because the student has a store of glycogen in his liver. During fasting, the liver glycogen is broken down and adds glucose to the bloodstream. This mechanism alone is sufficient in the first 24 h.

C

Other mechanisms include breakdown of muscle glycogen, gluconeogenesis from amino acids and glycerol.

D

Since there is a reduced supply of the products of glucose metabolism, less acetyl-CoA can be metabolised in the citric acid cycle. Hence, acetyl-CoA accumulates in the body. It condenses to form acetoacetyl-CoA and β-hydroxybutyrate and acetone in the plasma. These substances are known as ketone bodies and can appear in the urine.

E

Mechanisms available to reduce the consumption of glucose:
- conservation of glucose at the expense of fatty acids
- use of ketone bodies in tissues such as muscles
- in major starvation, the brain may derive up to 60% of its energy requirements from the oxidation of ketone bodies.

F

All the above mechanisms may prevent catabolism of brain proteins: breakdown of liver and muscle glycogen and use of fatty acids and ketone bodies as fuel. In addition, protein from liver, spleen and muscle is used in preference to protein from heart and brain.

3.28
A

The main biochemical pathway involved in metabolism of glucose to derive energy is glycolysis. In a short distance race, adequate oxygen required for the citric acid cycle is not available and hence glycolysis is the main metabolic pathway. The final product of glycolysis is pyruvic acid (pyruvate), which may be metabolised to lactate (lactic acid) in the absence of oxygen. The intermediates of this pathway include:

glucose (6 carbon) → glucose 6-P → fructose 6-P → fructose 1,6-biphosphate → glyceradehyde 3-phosphate (3 carbon) → ... → pyruvate.

B

The energy yield is in the form of ATP and NADH. For each molecule of glucose metabolised, there is a net yield of 2 ATPs and 1 NADH (which can be used to generate ATP from ADP).

C

The energy in the ATP is utilised in muscle contraction. ATP binds to the ATP-binding site of the myosin heads of the muscle. When hydrolysis occurs, the myosin heads are distorted and bind tightly to actin. The distortion of the head is then overcome, which creates movement of actin on myosin.

D

The two most important enzymes regulating glycolysis are hexokinase (which converts glucose to glucose 6-phosphate) and phosphofructokinase (which converts fructose 6-phosphate to fructose 1,6-biphosphate). Phosphofructokinase is the more important regulatory enzyme. It is activated by AMP but inhibited by ATP, citrate and hydrogen ions. Hexokinase is inhibited by its own product, glucose 6-phosphate.

E

Shortly after the race started, ATP is used up and AMP is produced. Phosphofructokinase is stimulated by an increase in AMP and a reduction of ATP. A reduction of citrate is also partly responsible. As a result, glucose 6-phosphate decreases and hexokinase activity is increased.

3.29
A

The main energy-generating biochemical pathway for the metabolism of glucose in a marathon race is the citric acid cycle, which requires the presence of oxygen. This pathway is much more efficient glycolysis pathway in generating energy from glucose metabolism. The overall substrates for this pathway are acetyl-CoA, NAD$^+$, GDP and FAD. The overall products are CO_2, NADH, GTP and FADH$_2$. The important intermediates are shown in Fig. 3.1.

B

This biochemical pathway takes place in the mitochondria. There is much evidence to support the endosymbiotic theory that mitochondria are of prokaryotic origin in evolution:

- The mitochondrion has its own small circular double-stranded DNA.
- Translation from DNA to mRNA is sensitive to chloramphenicol, as in prokaryotic cells.
- The mitochondrial inner membrane contains cardiolipin and lacks cholesterol. These features are similar to those of prokaryotic cells.

C

For each glucose molecule metabolised, 2 ATPs and 1 NADH molecule are generated in the glycolysis pathway before entering the citric acid cycle. Two molecules of acetyl-CoA enter into the citric acid cycle. For each molecule of acetyl-CoA entering the citric acid cycle, 3 NADH, 1 FADH$_2$ and 1 GTP molecules are produced.

Overall, for each molecule of glucose metabolised, 7 NADH, 2 FADH$_2$, 2 GTP and 2 ATP molecules are produced.

D

i   High-energy phosphate substances (e.g. ATP) can be derived from NADH and FADH$_2$ by the process of oxidative phosphorylation in the mitochondria.

ii Oxidative phosphorylation is driven by the oxidation of NADH and FADH$_2$ inside the mitochondria. This results in the transfer of protons (H$^+$) across the inner membrane (the cristae) of the mitochondria, creating an electrochemical potential difference across the inner membrane. This potential difference drives a reversible ATPase (ATP synthase) in the membrane to convert ADP and inorganic phosphate (Pi) to ATP.

iii The overall substrates are NADH or FADH, ADP, Pi and oxygen. The overall products are ATP, FAD and NAD. A by-product is water (H$_2$O).

iv The accumulation of ADP and the availability of oxygen to oxidise NADH and FADH$_2$ stimulate the oxidative phosphorylation process.

E

If oxidative phosphorylation is inhibited, oxygen cannot be utilised and the clinical picture is similar to hypoxia (e.g. confusion, drowsiness, coma and death) except that the patient may not be cyanosed. Examples include cyanide and carbon monoxide poisoning.

F

i   Oxidative phosphorylation is said to be 'uncoupled' if electron flow in the mitochondrial membrane is not coupled with ATP production. This occurs if the inner mitochondrial membrane becomes non-specifically permeable to protons from physical damage or chemical poisoning.

ii The consequence of uncoupling is that the energy in the electrochemical potential is dissipated as heat and cannot be utilised.

iii An example of physiological uncoupling of oxidative phosphorylation is the generation of heat from brown adipose tissue in infants.

3.30

A

Proteins are the main sources of nitrogen in our diet. A person is said to be in 'nitrogen equilibrium' if the amount of nitrogen excreted is balanced by the amount of nitrogen ingested. If the amount of nitrogen excreted exceeds that ingested, a state of 'negative nitrogen balance' is said to exist. In severe cases it may be manifested by visible muscle wasting, especially in the buttocks.

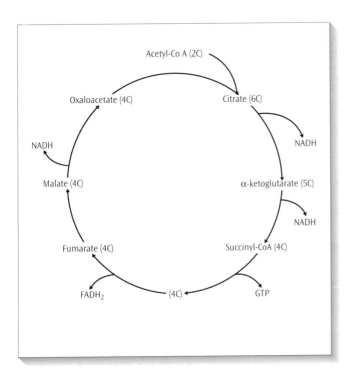

Fig. 3.1 The citric acid cycle.

3

A

GENERAL BASIC MEDICAL SCIENCES

Nutrition and energy

B

Grade 1 proteins include animal proteins in meat, fish, eggs and some plant proteins. They consist of amino acids in approximately the same proportions as those required for protein synthesis. Grade 2 proteins consist of different proportions of amino acids and may be lacking in one or more essential amino acids. They may be adequate to maintain nitrogen equilibrium only if they include a broad range and are taken in large amounts.

C

One reason why John might have a negative nitrogen balance is that his calorie intake was insufficient for his requirements. As a tall and physically active young male, at least 2500 kcal are necessary to meet his basal needs, and probably an extra 1500 kcal to meet his daily activities. As a result, proteins may be catabolised. A second reason is that his dietary protein intake may lack one or more essential amino acids. As a result, effective protein synthesis may be impossible.

General principles of pathological processes

4.1 Examples of external barriers against infection include:
A Lysozyme in tears
B Lactic acid in sebaceous secretions
C Cilia on respiratory epithelial cells
D Mucus secretion from epithelial cells
E Acid in gastric secretions

4.2 The following are phagocytic cells:
A Lymphocytes
B Eosinophils
C Polymorphonuclear neutrophils
D Macrophages
E Mast cells

4.3 The following statements about acquired immunological memory are true:
A The secondary response is usually slower than the primary response
B It extends to other unrelated antigens
C The memory cells are macrophages
D It forms the basis of vaccination
E The effectiveness of acquired memory remains constant throughout life

4.4 The following protect mainly against extracellular microorganisms:
A Antibodies
B T-helper cells
C Natural killer (NK) cells
D Complement-mediated system
E Soluble cytokines

4.5 The following statements about immunoglobulin are true:
A It consists of two identical heavy and two identical light chains joined by disulphide links
B All chains on an immunoglobulin molecule are coded for by the same chromosome
C There are about 100 different immunoglobulin molecules in normal human serum
D The variable region is responsible for complement fixation
E The constant region forms the antigen binding site

4.6 The following statements about classes of immunoglobulins are true:
A IgG crosses the placenta and confers passive immunity to the fetus
B IgM is usually produced early in the immune response
C IgD is the most effective class of immunoglobulin for agglutinating bacteria

D IgA exists as a dimer on seromucous surfaces
E IgE is important in cell-mediated immunity

4.7 The following are possible mechanisms for tolerance of T-cells to self-antigens:
A Separation of self-antigen from lymphocytes
B Deletion of self-reactive T-cells in the thymus
C Clonal anergy of T-cells
D Production of antibodies against self-antigens
E Production of autoantibodies

4.8 The following types of hypersensitivity and examples are correctly matched:
A Type 1 hypersensitivity – allergen-induced asthma
B Type 2 hypersensitivity – granulomatous reaction to tuberculosis
C Type 3 hypersensitivity – glomerulonephritis associated with systemic lupus erythematosus
D Type 4 hypersensitivity – rhesus incompatibility resulting in haemolytic disease of the newborn
E Type 5 hypersensitivity – hyperthyroidism caused by thyroid-stimulating autoantibody in Graves' disease

4.9 The following may reduce the risk of graft rejection after transplantation:
A Cross-matching donor and recipient for ABO antigens
B Cross-matching donor and recipient for major histocompatibility complex antigens
C Use of antimitotic drugs (such as azathioprine) after transplantation
D Use of ciclosporin A after transplantation
E Transfusion of blood from the donor before transplantation

4.10 Hyperplasia significantly contributes to the following tissue responses:
A Increase of breast tissue at puberty
B Increase of muscle bulk with exercise
C Enlargement of thyroid gland during pregnancy
D Enlargement of uterus during pregnancy
E Thickening of the left ventricular wall due to narrowing of the aortic valve

4.11 Dysplasia:
A Is associated with an increase in mitotic figures
B May be caused by chronic chemical injury
C Is always irreversible
D Is associated with a reduction in nuclear/cytoplasmic ratio
E Is a pre-malignant condition

41

4 **Pathological processes**

Q

GENERAL BASIC MEDICAL SCIENCES

4.12 Mechanisms of cellular injury may be mediated by:
A Osmotic pressure
B Glucose deprivation
C Damage to ion pumps
D Interruption of protein synthesis
E Free radicals

4.13 The following types of adult tissues heal by complete restitution:
A The skin epidermis
B Nerve cells
C Intestinal epithelium
D Striated muscles
E The heart

4.14 The following tissues are particularly susceptible to damage by ionising radiation:
A The liver
B The bone marrow
C The ovaries
D The uterus
E The intestinal epithelium

4.15 Necrosis:
A Is the inevitable consequence of any cellular injury
B May be caused by ischaemia
C May be caused by mechanical trauma
D Is often accompanied by inflammation
E Is usually associated with cell shrinkage

4.16 The following statements about apoptosis are true:
A It is usually triggered by cellular injury
B It is associated with leakage of lytic lysosome enzymes
C The dead cells are phagocytosed by macrophages
D Increased apoptosis may result in neoplasia
E Decreased apoptosis may result in tissue atrophy

4.17 The following types of necrosis and their causes are correctly paired:
A Coagulative necrosis – myocardial infarction
B Caseous necrosis – malignant hypertension
C Fibrinoid necrosis – tuberculosis
D Fat necrosis – acute pancreatitis
E Gangrene – *Clostridium perfringens* infection

4.18 Predisposing factors for thrombosis in an artery include:
A Laminar blood flow
B Fibrin deposition on the vessel wall
C Loss of endothelial cells
D Increased blood cholesterol level
E Decreased serum high-density lipoprotein level

4.19 The possible outcomes of thrombi include:
A Dissolution
B Embolism
C Organisation
D Apoptosis
E Recanalisation

4.20 Consequences of systemic emboli include:
A Pulmonary infarction
B A cerebrovascular accident
C Foot gangrene
D Ischaemic bowel
E Pulmonary hypertension

4.21 Possible sources of emboli include:
A Tumour
B Vegetations
C Amniotic fluid
D Gas
E Fat

4.22 Causes of acute inflammation include:
A Bacterial infection
B Acid burn
C Trauma
D Tissue necrosis
E Exotoxins

4.23 Characteristic physical features of acute inflammation include:
A Loss of function
B Pallor
C Coldness
D Swelling
E Pain

4.24 The following processes occur in the early stages of acute inflammation:
A A reduction in vascular permeability
B Persistent arteriolar constriction
C Formation of fluid transudate
D Accumulation of lymphocytes
E A reduction in blood viscosity

4.25 Chemical mediators of acute inflammation include:
A Histamine
B Prostaglandin
C C5a and C3a of the complement system
D Dopamine
E Bradykinin

4.26 In the presence of extensive necrosis, acute inflammation is particularly likely to result in:

A Suppuration
B Formation of granulation tissue
C Chronic inflammation
D Dystrophic calcification
E Fibrosis

4.27 Examples of chronic inflammation include:
A Anaphylactic reactions
B Crohn's disease
C Sarcoidosis
D Hashimoto's thyroiditis
E Pneumococcal pneumonia

4.28 In the presence of chronic inflammation, the following cells are often present in the cellular infiltrate:
A Neutrophils
B Multinucleate giant cells
C Lymphocytes
D Plasma cells
E Macrophages

4.29 The following tumour shapes are associated with malignancy:
A Ulcerated
B Papillary
C Fungating
D Sessile
E Pedunculated

4.30 The following histological features are more characteristic of benign than malignant tumours:
A Endophytic growth for tumours on mucosal surfaces
B Irregular outlines
C Presence of necrosis
D Multiple nucleoli
E Nuclear hyperchromaticism

4.31 Human tumours which may be caused by oncogenic viruses include:
A Cervical carcinoma
B Uterine carcinoma
C Hepatocellular carcinoma
D Nasopharyngeal carcinoma
E Breast cancer

4.32 The following statements about oncogenes and oncoproteins are true:
A Oncogenes may be absent in normal cells
B A larger quantity of oncoproteins may be produced in malignant compared to normal cells
C Oncoproteins produced from malignant cells may be different from those from normal cells

D All oncoproteins stimulate DNA synthesis
E Oncoproteins are important in regulating cellular growth and differentiation

4.33 Frequent sites for blood-borne metastases of common cancers include:
A The spleen
B The lungs
C Bone
D The liver
E The heart

4.34 By which of the following mechanisms can bacteria (including mycobacteria) cause disease in humans? For each mechanism you choose, give two examples of the bacteria and the diseases caused, and a brief description of how these diseases are caused:
• adhesion pili and adhesins
• inhibition of mitochondrial enzymes
• production of exotoxins
• production of endotoxins
• inhibition of transcription of mRNA
• inhibition of ATP production
• inhibition of protein synthesis
• production of aggressins
• induction of cell-mediated immunity response.

4.35 Chemical agents cause disease in different ways at the cellular level. Contrast how the following agents cause cellular injury by describing their mechanism of action:
A Alcohol
B Cigarette smoke (in causing lung cancer)
C Cigarette smoke (in causing heart disease)
D Acids (in causing burns)
E Drugs (e.g. rash caused by penicillin).

4.36 Briefly compare the body's attempts at repair when cells of the following organs are damaged by injury. Explain why the responses in these organs are different. In each case, name one other tissue that responds similarly to injuries.
A Gastrointestinal epithelium (damaged in gastroenteritis)
B Neurones in brain (damaged in head injury)
C Parathyroid gland (damaged by partial surgical removal during thyroidectomy).

4.37 A child is born with syndactyly (webbed finger) between the 4th and 5th fingers of the right hand.
A Name the process at the *cellular* level that has not taken place properly during the development of the fetus.
B Describe how the process occurs.

4 **Q**

Pathological processes

C Describe the factors controlling the regulation of the process.

D Give one other developmental abnormality contributed to by the failure of this process in fetal development.

E Give two groups of *acquired* diseases that may be associated with a reduction of this process.

4.38 A How do the growth mechanisms differ at the cellular level in the following physiological changes? Give appropriate terms to the growth mechanisms.

   i Breast enlargement in puberty.

   ii Enlarged muscle bulk in athletes.

B Give one example of growth in pathological processes for each of the two mechanisms.

C Give an example of growth involving a combination of the two mechanisms.

4.39 Compare and contrast the cellular processes of the following by filling in the blanks in Table 4.1.

A Disordered growth of cells in the uterine cervix associated with great variation in size and shape of cells and their nuclei.

B Change from ciliated respiratory to squamous epithelium in the trachea of smokers.

C Growth of breast tissue which invades surrounding tissues and spreads to other organs.

4.40 Contrast the main differences between the processes of cell death in the following by completing Table 4.2.

A Gangrene of the foot as a result of arterial obstruction.

B Death of unwanted lymphocytes in germinal centres of lymph nodes.

4.41 A patient suffering from malignant lymphoma was treated with a course of therapeutic irradiation.

A Describe the cellular and molecular mechanisms that might be helped by irradiation in the treatment of lymphoma.

B Why might it be possible for the malignant cells to be killed without similarly affecting the normal cells?

C Why might it be better to give therapeutic irradiation in several doses rather than in a single dose?

D What side effects are most likely to occur within the first few days of irradiation? Explain.

E How might irradiation induce another malignancy? When is it likely to occur?

4.42 The following are two examples of thrombosis:
- thrombus developing from an atheromatous plaque in the aorta
- thrombus developing in the femoral veins of the legs.

A What are the components of the Virchow's triad?

B Show how the Virchow's triad might contribute to the formation of the following.

   i Arterial thrombi in the aorta.

   ii Venous thrombi in femoral veins (less common than arterial thrombi).

C What are the consequences of embolism of the thrombi in each of the two examples?

4.43 A patient presents with cellulitis of the right arm – acute inflammation of the skin and underlying tissue secondary to infection. He was also noted to have a fever.

A Working from first principles, what symptoms and signs would you expect from this patient within the first 24 h of the illness?

Table 4.1

Process	A	B	C
Name			
Normal or abnormal			
Brief description			
Main histological features			
Reversible or irreversible			
How likely is it to give rise to malignancy?			
Give one other example of this process			

Table 4.2

Process	A	B
Name		
Extent (single cells/group of cells)		
Lysosomes intact		
Effects on cell membrane integrity		
Presence of inflammatory response		
How are the dead cells removed?		

B For each of the symptoms and signs listed, briefly outline the mechanisms involved at the cellular level. Name two chemical mediators that may be responsible for maintaining each of these effects.

C What would be the main cellular components if you examined the exudate under the microscope? Describe how these cells arrive at the site of inflammation.

D List the major systems of chemical mediators for acute inflammation.

E Describe the mechanism by which the patient developed a fever.

4.44 A lymph node biopsy was examined histologically. This showed features of granulomatous disease.

A What are the main features of granulomatous disease?

B What are the main cellular components in granulomatous disease? Why do the cells accumulate there?

C Name one possible product from these cells that may be measured in the serum. What disease is likely if the serum level of this product is raised?

D What particular features would you expect if it were due to tuberculosis?

E What are other possible causes?

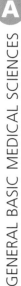

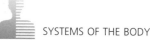

General principles of pathological processes

4.1 A B C D E
External barriers prevent microorganisms from gaining access to the body, and are first-line defences of infections. Two important external barriers are in the skin and in the respiratory epithelial cells. Fatty acids and lactic acid secreted by sebaceous and sweat glands in the skin inhibit bacterial growth. Cough and sneeze reflex, as well as mucus secretion and cilia of respiratory epithelium, form the external barriers against respiratory infection. Other external barriers include lysozyme in tears, acid in gastric secretions, and commensal bacteria which secrete substances (e.g. lactic acid by vaginal commensals and colicins by gut commensals) preventing opportunistic infections.

4.2 C D
The main phagocytic cells are polymorphonuclear neurtrophils and macrophages. These cells kill microorganisms by engulfing and digesting them. Polymorphonuclear neutrophils are found mainly in the bloodstream and are particularly important in the defence against bacterial infections. Macrophages are larger cells, and are present throughout the connective tissue and around the basement membrane of small blood vessels. They are particularly effective in killing microbacteria, viruses and protozoa.

4.3 D
Exposure to an antigen for the first time induces immunological memory, so that responses to future exposure to the specific antigen are faster and greater. The memory cells are lymphocytes. This forms the basis of vaccination, and explains why some vaccines (e.g. tetanus toxoid) need to be given more than once. The effectiveness of acquired memory declines slowly throughout life, and is only sustained by recurrent stimulation. Hence, booster vaccines are often needed.

4.4 A D
Immunological mechanisms to protect against extracellular organisms include antibodies, the complement-mediated system and neutrophil polymorphs. Intracellular organisms live inside host cells and antibodies cannot reach them. Cell-mediated immunity systems such as T-cells, macrophages and NK cells help to protect against them. Some organisms avoid the killing mechanisms of macrophages and survive inside them. T-helper cells, if primed to the antigen, can recognise and bind to the antigen with class 2 major histocompatibility complex (MHC) molecules on the macrophage surface and produce soluble cytokines, which may trigger intracellular killing of the organisms.

4.5 A
Immunoglobulins consist of four peptides – two identical heavy chains and two identical light chains – joined by disulphide links. Each chain is coded for by a different chromosome. The variable regions form the antigen binding sites, and are specific to a particular antigen. There are over 100 million different immunoglobulin molecules in human serum. The constant region carries out secondary biological functions such as complement fixation or binding to macrophages.

4.6 A B D
Of the five classes of immunoglobulins, IgG are the most abundant, and are especially important in neutralising toxins and fixing complement via the classical pathway in the extracellular fluids. Since IgG molecules are small, they can cross the placenta and provide passive immunity to the fetus. IgM are usually produced early in the immune response. Since they exist as pentamers, they are extremely effective in agglutinating bacteria and mediating complement-dependent cytolysis. IgA usually occur as dimers in seromucous secretions, and are important in the defence of external body surfaces against infections, especially in the gastrointestinal tract. IgD are present largely on lymphocytes. They are susceptible to proteolytic degradation, have a short half-life, and are likely to be cell surface antigen receptors for the control of lymphocyte activation and suppression. IgE bind to mast cells and binding to antigens leads to degranulation of mast cells and release of mediators such as histamine. They are important in allergic reactions.

4.7 A B C
T-cell tolerance to self-antigens is essential to avoid self-reactivity. This may be achieved either by compartmentalisation of self-antigens so that they are not exposed to T-lymphocytes (e.g. lens proteins or sperms), lack of major histocompatibility antigens, deletion of self-reactive T-cells in the thymus (i.e. negative selection process) and clonal anergy (paralysed T-cells) due to lack of stimulatory signals from antigen-presenting cells. Inability of T-cells to achieve tolerance results in the production of autoantibodies and possibly tissue destruction.

4.8 A C E
Type 1 hypersensitivity (anaphylactic hypersensitivity) is due to antigen interacting with specific IgE antibody binding to the mast cells, causing release of mediators such as histamines and leukotrienes. Clinical effects occur shortly after exposure to the antigen. Clinical examples are anaphylactic reactions and atopic allergy. Type 2 hypersensitivity (antibody-dependent cytotoxic hypersensitivity) is due to killing of cells bearing IgG by polymorphs, macrophages or K cells through an

extracellular antibody-dependent cell-mediated cytotoxicity mechanisms. Examples are haemolytic disease of the newborn through rhesus or ABO incompatibility. Type 3 hypersensitivity (complex-mediated hypersensitivity) is mainly due to activation of complement and attraction of polymorphonuclear cells due to antigen-antibody complexes. Examples are serum sickness following injection of large quantities of foreign proteins (e.g. antitetanus serum), and glomerulonephritis due to systemic lupus erythematosus. Type 4 hypersensitivity is due to interactions of antigens with primed lymphocytes, resulting in release of soluble cytokines which in turn activate macrophages inappropriately. Clinical effects may occur more than 24h after exposure to the antigen. Examples are Mantoux reaction to tuberculin and granulomatous reaction to tuberculosis. Type 5 hypersensitivity is due to an antibody which reacts with a surface receptor that activates the cell. An example is thyroid-stimulating antibody stimulating the thyroid gland, causing hyperthyroidism.

4.9 A B C D
Graft rejection after transplantation is mediated by lymphocytes. The major histocompatibility complex (the HLA in humans) antigens are responsible for the most severe graft rejections. Measures that may reduce the risk of graft rejection include matching donor and recipient for ABO and HLA antigens, producing general immunosuppression by drugs (e.g. corticosteroids, antimitotic drugs and ciclosporin A, which targets T-cells specifically). In animals, antigen-specific tolerance may be induced via suppression by regulatory T-cell by injection of donor's bone marrow or dendritic cell precursors, which display little or no MHC antigens.

4.10 A C D
Growth is brought about by either hyperplasia or hypertrophy. Both may occur due to either physiological or pathological conditions. Hyperplasia is growth by an increase in the number of cells. Examples include breast enlargement during puberty and pregnancy, and an increase in the number of bone marrow cells in haemolytic anaemia or at high altitudes. Hypertrophy is growth by an increase in cell size without an increase in the number of cells. Examples are increase in muscle bulk in athletes, and thickening of the left ventricular wall due to narrowing of the aortic valve. Enlargement of the uterus during pregnancy or puberty is caused by a combination of hypertrophy and hyperplasia.

4.11 A B E
Dysplasia is a pre-malignant condition, and may be caused by chronic inflammation or chronic exposure to physical or chemical injuries. It is characterised by increased mitosis,

abnormally large nuclei, and increased variations in the size and shape of cells and their nuclei. An important site for dysplasia is the squamous epithelium of the uterine cervix, and the long period of time between the development of dysplasia and neoplasia allows screening for cervical cancer by cervical smears.

4.12 A B C D E
Cellular injury may be mediated by a number of mechanisms. These include mechanical damage to cell membranes or interference with cell function, a deficiency of metabolities, damage to the energy generation process in the mitochondria, and interference to the DNA and protein synthesis process. Mechanical damage may be caused by sudden changes in the osmotic pressure of the intracellular and extracellular fluid. Damage to membrane integrity may be complement-mediated, perforin-mediated, or as a result of alteration to the membrane lipid or proteins, or blockage of the ion channels or ion pumps. Free radicals also damage cell membranes by damaging its fatty acids. Deprivation of essential metabolites such as vitamins, oxygen or glucose results in cellular damage.

4.13 A C
The cells in adult tissues can be classified into three types: labile cells, stable cells and permanent cells. Labile cells, such as the skin epidermis and intestinal epithelium, are constantly lost and replaced under physiological conditions. They heal by complete restitution. By contrast, permanent cells such as nerve cells, striated and cardiac muscle cells, and red blood cells, have no capacity to divide. They heal by forming fibrous tissues. Stable cells, such as the liver and the kidneys, divide at a slow rate physiologically. They have only a very limited capacity to regenerate.

4.14 B C E
All tissues are liable to damage by ionising radiation. However, tissues consisting of rapidly dividing cells are particularly susceptible. Hence the gonads, epidermis, intestinal epithelium and bone marrow are particularly susceptible to damage by ionising radiation.

4.15 B C D
Cellular injuries may result in healing, repair or cellular death. Necrosis is the death of tissues following cellular injury, and is always a pathological process. There are a large number of causes, which include ischaemia, trauma, infection and metabolic disturbances. Characteristically, there is a loss of cell membrane integrity, a leakage of lytic lyzosome enzymes, cell swelling and lysis. Inflammatory responses are usual, and the injured cells are often phagocytosed by neutrophils or macrophages. This

4 **Pathological processes**

contrasts with the process of apoptosis, another mechanism of cell death. Apoptosis is a physiological process to get rid of unwanted or abnormal cells, although it may also be triggered by pathological stimuli. It is initiated by energy-dependent fragmentation of DNA. It is associated with intact cell membrane, cell shrinkage and an absence of inflammatory response. The dead cells are phagocytosed by surrounding cells. Apoptosis is an important physiological process in controlling organ size and removing abnormal cells. Reduced apoptosis may result in inappropriate cell accumulation and neoplasia, whilst increased apoptosis may result in tissue atrophy.

4.16 –
See answer to question 4.15 above. Apoptosis can be a physiological process, is initiated by an energy-dependent fragmentation of DNA, and the dead cells are phagocytosed by surrounding cells. Increased apoptosis may result in tissue atrophy, and decreased apoptosis may result in neoplasia.

4.17 A D E
The type of necrosis is determined by the type of tissue involved and the cause of the cellular injury. Coagulative necrosis is the commonest. The outlines of the cells are preserved as the proteins coagulate. Necrosis following a myocardial infarction is a common example. Coagulative necrosis results from liquefaction of the tissues, and mainly occurs in the brain due to a lack of supporting structure. Fibrinoid necrosis is associated with a deposition of fibrin. It may occur in the smooth muscle walls of the arterioles in malignant hypertension. Fat necrosis results from the inflammatory response to a release of intracellular fat, and may occur after mechanical trauma to adipose tissues or following acute pancreatitis as a result of pancreatic lipase. Caseous necrosis describes a cheesy appearance with no recognisable structure. It commonly occurs in tuberculosis infection. Gangrene is necrosis of putrefaction of the tissues, and may be caused by clostridia. *Clostridium perfringens* is characteristically associated with gas gangrene.

4.18 B C D
Virchow first described the three general predisposing factors for thrombus formation: changes in the intimal surface of the vessel, changes in the pattern of blood flow and changes in blood constituents. In an artery, changes in the intimal surface of the vessel may include loss of endothelial cells, fibrin deposition and platelet clumping. Thrombus formation is more likely with turbulent than laminar blood flow. Changes in blood constituents may include increase in cholesterol and high-density lipoprotein levels and an increase in blood viscosity.

4.19 A B C E
Most thrombi are dissolved and cleared by the physiological fibrinolytic system. When this is unsuccessful, the thrombi are replaced by a scar and fibrous tissue in the process of organisation. Alternatively, the intimal cells within the thrombi may proliferate and new capillaries may grow into the thrombus to form a new channel. This is the process of recanalisation. Unfortunately, these protective mechanisms may fail. The thrombi may break off to form emboli, or the thrombi may cause ischaemia to vital organs, resulting in death.

4.20 B C D
Emboli in the pulmonary circulation (pulmonary emboli) usually arise from venous thrombi in the leg veins. Emboli in the systemic circulation (systemic thrombi) usually arise from the left side of the heart or major arteries. Pulmonary emboli may result in pulmonary hypertension or pulmonary infarction. Systemic emboli may be lodged in any systemic organs and cause ischaemic death (infarction). They may result in gangrene if lodged in the legs, a cerebrovascular accident (a stroke) if lodged in the brain, ischaemic bowel, or renal infarct it lodged in the kidneys.

4.21 A B C D E
Thrombi are by far the commonest source of emboli. Other sources of emboli include vegetations on heart valves, fat (e.g. release of fat into the bloodstream from the bone marrow following fracture of the long bones), gas (e.g. during surgical procedures such as laparoscopy), amniotic fluid (e.g. during delivery), tumour and foreign matter (e.g. contaminated intravenous fluid).

4.22 A B C D E
Acute inflammation describes the initial tissue reaction to injury, and may be caused by a variety of agents. Infection, especially bacterial and viral, is a common cause. Other causes include hypersensitivity reactions (other than type IV), physical injury (e.g. heat or cold injuries, direct trauma, ionising radiation), chemical injury (e.g. acids, alkalis, exo- or endodoxins) and tissue necrosis.

4.23 A D E
Celsus (first century AD) first described heat, redness, swelling and pain as the four characteristic features of acute inflammation. Loss of function is also characteristic.

4.24 –
In the early stages of acute inflammation, a brief and transient arteriolar constriction is followed by a longer period of arteriolar dilatation. This is accompanied by an increase in blood flow. This phase of hyperaemia is

followed by a slowing of blood flow due to increased vascular permeability, resulting in a higher proportion of blood cells to plasma in the vessel. The increased vascular permeability causes proteins to escape into the extravascular space, forming a protein-rich fluid exudate. Another component of acute inflammation is the formation of cellular exudate with the accumulation of neutrophil polymorphs.

4.25 A B C E
Chemical mediators play an important role in initiating vasodilatation, increased vascular permeability, and attracting neutrophils to the site of tissue injury. Chemical mediators may be released from the cells (e.g. histamine, prostaglandin, leukotrienes, serotonin and cytokines) or through the major cascade systems in the plasma (complement, kinin, coagulation and fibrinolytic systems). C3a and C5a mediate vascular dilatation and emigration of neutrophils, and are the most important mediators from the complement systems. Bradykinin is an important mediator of pain. Hageman factor (coagulation factor XII) can activate the kinins, coagulation and fibrinolytic systems.

4.26 B E
Acute inflammation usually results in complete resolution. However, in the presence of extensive necrosis, healing by organisation is likely. Hence the formation of granulation tissue and fibrous (scar) tissues is likely. Suppuration is likely if there is excessive exudate. Dystrophic calcification usually results from long-standing abscesses.

4.27 B C D
Chronic inflammation may occur with its characteristic features from the beginning of the course (primary chronic inflammation), or it may progress from acute inflammation. General causes of primary chronic inflammation include failure to eliminate infective agent or foreign body by phagocytosis or intracellular killing (e.g. tuberculosis, leprosy, asbestosis), autoimmune diseases (e.g. Hashimoto's thyroiditis, rheumatoid arthritis), and chronic inflammatory bowel diseases. Anaphylactic reactions are caused by type 1 hypersensitivity reaction, and is an example of acute inflammation. Pneumococcal pneumonia is a bacterial infection, and is a classical example of acute inflammation.

4.28 B C D E
The presence of lymphocytes, plasma cells and macrophages is characteristic of chronic inflammation. Macrophages may form multinucleate giant cells in chronic inflammation. Neutrophils are characteristic of bacterial infection.

4.29 A C
Tumour shapes are often associated with the malignant potential of the tumour. Ulcerated, fungating and annular tumours are more likely to be malignant. Papillary, sessile and pedunculated tumours are more likely to be benign.

4.30 –
Benign tumours are associated with slow growth, infrequent mitotic figures, smooth borders and a histological appearance similar to that of normal tissues. The presence of ulceration, necrosis or invasion into underlying structures indicates possible malignancy. Multiple nucleoli reflect increased DNA synthesis, and nuclear hyperchromaticism reflects an excess of DNA. Both features are characteristic of malignancy. For tumours on the skin or mucosal surfaces, tumours which grow into the underlying structure (endophytic growth) are more likely to be malignant than tumours which grow away from the underlying structure (exophytic growth).

4.31 A C D
DNA viruses may cause cancers by incorporating their viral genome into the host cell DNA. For RNA viruses, the RNA viral genomes have to be transcribed into DNA by reverse transcriptase before incorporation. Viruses which are known to cause cancers include hepatitis B virus (which may cause hepatocellular carcinoma), Epstein–Barr virus (which may cause Burkitt's lymphoma or nasopharyngeal carcinoma) and human papillomavirus (which may cause cervical cancer or warts). Kaposi's sarcoma is associated with HIV infection, although the mechanism is not entirely clear.

4.32 B C E
Oncogenes are DNA sequences controlling tumour growth. They are present in both normal and tumour cells. Oncogenes exert their effect through their gene products, called oncoproteins. Oncoproteins are important in regulating cellular growth and differentiation. Different oncoproteins have different functions. They may be stimulators of DNA synthesis, growth factors, receptors for growth factors, or they may bind to GTP, which has an important role in intracellular signalling. Tumour cells may either produce excessive amounts of normal oncoproteins, or they may produce a abnormal (mutant) form of oncoproteins.

4.33 B C D
Lung, breast and bowel cancers are the most common. Organs which are perfused by blood drained from the tumours are liable to be sites of metastasis. Frequent sites for blood-borne metastases include bone, the liver, the lungs and the brain. It is unclear why tumours rarely metastasise to the spleen.

4 GENERAL BASIC MEDICAL SCIENCES

Pathological processes

4.34 Bacteria may cause diseases by:
- adhesion pili and adhesins
- exotoxins
- endotoxins
- aggressins
- inducing immune responses with harmful consequences (including cell-mediated immune response).

(*Note* Inhibition of transcription and protein synthesis are the actions of many antibiotics.)

1. *Adhesion pili and adhesins.* Examples are β-haemolytic streptococci causing throat infection, meningococci causing meningitis, and enterobacteria causing gastroenteritis. Adhesion pili are processes on the surface of some bacteria that may be coated with recognition molecules (adhesins). They enable the bacteria to become fixed and infect target human cells.
2. *Exotoxins.* Examples are *Clostridium tetani* causing tetanus, *Staphylococcus aureus* causing scalded skin syndrome, *Vibrio cholerae* causing cholera, *Clostridium difficile* causing pseudomembranous colitis, and *Corynebacterium diphtheriae* causing diphtheria. Exotoxins are enzymes secreted by bacteria that may have specific local or general effects; for example, tetanospasmin produced by *Clostridium tetani* is neurotoxic. The synthesis of exotoxins is usually directed by the genes in the bacterial genome and occasionally in plasmids.
3. *Endotoxins.* Examples include *Escherichia coli* causing urinary or intra-abdominal infections, and meningococci causing endotoxic shock, disseminated intravascular coagulation and bilateral adrenal haemorrhage in Waterhouse–Friderichsen syndrome. Endotoxins are lipopolysaccharides (e.g. lipid A) from the cell walls of Gram-negative bacteria that are released after the death of the bacteria. They cause disease by activating the complement cascade, the coagulation cascades and interleukin-1 release from leukocytes.
4. *Aggressins.* Examples include *Staphylococcus aureus* producing hyaluronidase and coagulase in causing skin infection, and *Streptococcus pyogenes* producing streptokinase in causing cellulitis. Aggressins are bacterial enzymes that facilitate the growth and spread of the bacteria in the tissue; for example, coagulase induces the coagulation of fibrinogen, thus creating a barrier between the site of infection and the host's immune response. Hyaluronidase digests connective tissue, encouraging the invasion of the organisms in the tissue.
5. *Cell-mediated immune response.* Examples are *Mycobacterium tuberculosis* causing tuberculosis, and *M. leprae* causing leprosy. A component of the bacterium may induce a host cell-mediated immune response, involving macrophages and T-lymphocytes, that may result in severe tissue destruction.

4.35

A
Alcohol causes disease by interfering with metabolic pathways. There are several mechanisms: cellular energy may be diverted from essential metabolic pathways (e.g. fat metabolism) to the metabolism of alcohol. This explains the accumulation of fats in the liver. Products of alcohol metabolism (e.g. acetaldehyde) may bind to liver cell proteins, causing liver damage.

B
Cigarette smoke causes lung cancer via the carcinogens within the polycyclic aromatic hydrocarbon fraction of the smoke. The smoke causes cancer by binding to or altering DNA, resulting in its mutation.

C
Cigarette smoke causes heart disease via the carbon monoxide in the inhaled smoke. The carbon monoxide induces endothelial hypoxia in vessels, accelerating the development of atherosclerosis.

D
Acids cause cellular damage by direct corrosive effects on tissues. They cause digestion and denaturation of proteins.

E
Drug allergic reactions may cause cellular damage by inducing immune responses in the host. They may be antibody- or cell-mediated. Acute reactions due to penicillin are often due to immediate (type 1) hypersensitivity. In this type of hypersensitivity, antigens bind to IgE bound to mast cells. This triggers the mast cells to release their mediators (e.g. histamine) and causes an anaphylactic reaction.

4.36

A
Gastrointestinal epithelium responds to injury by rapid replacement of lost cells. This is because gastrointestinal epithelial cells are 'labile cells' which have a short life span and rapid turnover time. Epithelial cells of the skin and haemopoietic cells of bone marrow are further examples of labile cells.

B
Neurones in brain have very little capacity for regeneration. They repair by fibrous tissues. This is because neurones are 'permanent cells' which usually divide only during fetal life and cannot be replaced if lost. Other

examples of permanent cells include cardiac muscles and retinal photoreceptors of the eye.

C

Parathyroid gland cells normally divide very infrequently after fetal life but are stimulated to divide if injured. They are 'stable cells'; hence, if a parathyroid gland is partially removed, the remaining tissue is stimulated to divide to replace the lost tissue. The other parathyroid glands may also undergo hyperplasia to compensate for the loss. Other examples of stable cells include liver cells and the renal tubular cells in the kidneys.

4.37

A

The process that has not taken place properly is apoptosis.

B

Apoptosis is the process of individual cell death in morphogenesis. In apoptosis, activation of non-lysosomal endogenous endonuclease causes digestion of nuclear DNA into smaller DNA fragments and consequent cell death. The dead cells are phagocytosed and broken down by adjacent cells.

C

Cells in tissues may undergo both mitosis and apoptosis at the same time. Quiescent cells in G_0 phase of the cell cycle may be recruited into active G_1 state by growth factors. Whether they will undergo mitosis or apoptosis depend on three main groups of factors: apoptosis inhibitors, apoptosis inducers and genetic factors. Apoptosis inhibitors include growth factors, oestrogens and androgens. Apoptosis inducers include detachment from the matrix and cytotoxic drugs. Important genes include members of the *bcl-2* family.

D

Other developmental abnormalities caused by failure of apoptosis include spina bifida, bladder fistula and cleft palate.

E

Autoimmune diseases and malignancies may be associated with reduced apoptosis.

4.38

A

i   Breast enlarges by an increase in cell number induced by the action of hormones (e.g. prolactin, oestrogens, progesterone). The mechanism is known as hyperplasia.

ii Increased bulk in athletes is caused by an increase in muscle cell size. The mechanism is known as hypertrophy.

B

Examples of hyperplasia associated with pathological processes include psoriasis, Paget's disease of the bone, and enlargement of endocrine glands (e.g. parathyroid glands) due to low serum calcium level. Examples of hypertrophy associated with pathological processes include left ventricular hypertrophy secondary to myocardial infarct or right ventricular hypertrophy secondary to pulmonary hypertension.

C

An example of growth due to a combination of hyperplasia and hypertrophy is the growth of the uterus during pregnancy.

4.39

See Table 4.3.

4.40

See Table 4.4.

4.41

A

Tissues are made up mostly of water. When radiation passes through water, highly reactive radicals such as H· and OH· are formed. These radicals can then interact with DNA to cause breakage and cross-linking of DNA strands. DNA strand breaks may result in chromosome translocation or inversion. DNA strand cross-linking may prevent separation of the strand and the ability to make further copies. Hence, irradiation may result in death of the tumour cells and help in the treatment of the tumour.

B

The above mechanisms may occur both in tumour cells and normal cells. However, it may be possible to kill the tumour cells without similarly affecting normal cells if the tumour cells are more radiosensitive than normal cells. Tumour cells are frequently more radiosensitive as they have a much higher rate of mitosis.

C

It may be better to give irradiation in several doses than in a single dose because it allows time for normal tissues to repair any damage between doses. Normal tissues may be able to repair any damage caused by the irradiation better than tumour cells.

D

Early side effects are likely in organs with a high rate of cellular division, such as skin and intestinal epithelial cells: reddening of the skin and diarrhoea frequently occur in the first few days of treatment. Effects on bone marrow, kidneys and gonads occur later.

4

A

GENERAL BASIC MEDICAL SCIENCES

Pathological processes

Table 4.3

Process	A	B	C
Name	Dysplasia	Metaplasia	Neoplasia
Normal or abnormal	Abnormal	Normal	Abnormal
Brief description of process	Disordered growth and differentiation	Transformation of one type of fully differentiated cell into another type	Abnormal uncoordinated growth associated with genetic alterations
Main histological features	Increased growth; increased mitosis, pleomorphism (variation in size and shape); high nuclear/cytoplasmic ratio; increased nuclear DNA	Appearance of a cell type not characteristic of cells usually at the site (e.g. squamous cells in trachea)	Excessive uncoordinated growth which may invade surrounding tissue; high nuclear/cytoplasmic ratio; increased nuclear DNA
Reversible or irreversible	Only in the early stages	Reversible	Irreversible
How likely is it to give rise to malignancy?	Probable	Possible but unlikely	Definite
Give one other example of this process	Dysplasia of glandular epithelium of stomach	Metaplasia in transitional epithelium of bladder associated with stones	Carcinoma of lung, uterus, cervix, bone

Table 4.4

Process	A	B
Name	Necrosis (ischaemic in origin in this example)	Apoptosis
Extent (single cells/group of cells)	Group of cells	Single cells
Lysosomes intact	No. They leak lytic enzymes	Yes
Effects on cell membrane integrity	Lost	Intact
Presence of inflammatory response	Yes	No
How are the dead cells removed?	Phagocytosed by neutrophils and macrophages	Phagocytosed by neighbouring cells

E

Irradiation may induce malignancy by causing mutation of the normal cells by base alterations. Malignancies usually occur many years later (a mean of 6 years for leukaemia and over 20 years for solid tumours).

4.42

A

- Changes in the intimal surface of the vessel.
- Changes in the pattern of blood flow.
- Changes in the blood constituents.

B

It is important to note that the factors may aggravate one another.

i
- *Intimal surface*. An atheromatous plaque may cause a raised fatty streak on the surface of the vessel; turbulence of blood flow may cause loss of intimal cells.
- *Pattern of blood flow*. Enlarging atheromatous plaques may contribute to turbulent flow; platelet aggregates themselves added to the turbulent flow.
- *Blood constituents*. A person with high cholesterol or low-density lipoprotein levels would be at higher risk of thrombus formation.

ii
- *Intimal surface*. Valves protrude into the lumen. Vessel walls may be damaged by trauma or occlusion.
- *Pattern of blood flow*. Venous blood flow is dependent on the contraction and relaxation of calf muscles. Laminar blood flow may be lost if the blood pressure drops significantly or if the venous return is diminished through bed rest, occlusion or a prolonged fall in blood pressure.

- *Blood constituents*. Women on oral contraceptives are more likely to develop venous thrombosis.

C

Systemic embolism from arterial thrombus may result in ischaemia of the target organ involved; for example, a stroke may occur if the brain if affected. Venous thrombus enters the right side of the heart and hence embolises to the lungs to cause pulmonary embolism and infarct.

4.43

A

Celsus described four characteristic features of acute inflammation: redness, heat, swelling and pain. Virchow later added 'loss of function' to the list.

B

1. *Redness* may be due to vascular dilatation in acute inflammation. Vascular dilatation, resulting from opening of the precapillary sphincters, may be initiated and maintained by chemical mediators such as histamine, prostaglandins and nitric oxide.
2. *Heat*: local increase in temperature also results from vascular dilatation.
3. *Swelling* is due to vascular leakage of protein-rich fluid into the tissues. This results from increased vascular permeability of capillaries to large molecules such as proteins. The escape of proteins into the extravascular space increases the osmotic pressure and hence fluid accumulates in the tissue. The increase in vascular permeability is triggered by histamine and maintained by bradykinin, nitric oxide and C5a component.
4. *Pain* results partly from the mechanical stretching of the tissues due to swelling, and partly due to chemical mediators such as bradykinin, prostaglandins and serotonin.
5. *Loss of function* may occur if the movement of the arm is inhibited by pain.

C

The cellular component of the exudate would be mainly neutrophils. Neutrophils migrate by active amoeboid movement from the walls of venules and small veins. It appears that neutrophils are attracted to the site of inflammation by chemotactic factors (e.g. complement C3a and C5a, cytokines). Neutrophils may also migrate there randomly and be trapped by immobilisation factors.

D

- Kinin system.
- Fibrinolytic system.
- Complement system.
- Coagulation system.

E

The patient may develop a fever as a result of the neutrophil polymorphs producing endogenous pyrogens, which act on the hypothalamus to reset the themoregulatory mechanism.

4.44

A

Granulomatous disease is a form of chronic inflammation characterised by granuloma formation. A granuloma is an aggregate of epithelioid histiocytes. They are often elongated cells with large vesicular nuclei and frequently occur in clusters.

B

The main cellular component of granulomatous disease is the epithelioid histiocyte, which is a specialised form of macrophage. These cells accumulate there mainly via migration inhibition factors (MIFs), which trap macrophages in the tissue.

C

One possible product from the cells is angiotensin-converting enzyme (ACE). This enzyme is often raised in sarcoidosis and may be used as a marker for this disease.

D

If the granulomatous disease were due to tuberculosis, caseous (cheese-like) necrosis may be seen. The dead tissues appear to lack any structure.

E

Other causes of granulomatous disease include foreign bodies, leprosy, parasites and Crohn's disease.

5 General principles of infectious diseases

5.1 The following increase the likelihood of a particular type of bacteria infecting the lungs:
  A The ability of the bacteria to attach to a receptor molecule on the epithelial surface
  B Prior infection by measles virus
  C Suppression of the cough reflex
  D Impairment of the ciliary function
  E Increased activity of the alveolar macrophages

5.2 Viruses:
  A May consist of both RNA and DNA
  B May replicate without entering into host cells
  C May incorporate their genome information into the host DNA
  D Contain Golgi bodies
  E Contain mitochondria

5.3 Compared to Gram-positive bacteria, Gram-negative bacteria:
  A Have a thicker cell wall
  B Contain more lipopolysaccharide
  C Are more likely to cause fever and disseminated intravascular coagulation
  D Are more susceptible to destruction by penicillin
  E Possess an outer membrane

5.4 The following procedures are effective in sterilisation:
  A Ultraviolet radiation
  B Boiling in water
  C Hydrogen peroxide vapour
  D Washing in alcohol
  E Dry heat

5.5 Important host antibacterial defences include:
  A Neutrophils
  B Activation of alternative complement pathway
  C Non-killer cells
  D Antibodies
  E Interferon

5.6 Interferon:
  A Causes non-specific flu-like symptoms
  B Enhances T-cell recognition of the infected cells
  C Is a protein
  D May be released from B-cells, activated T-cells or macrophages
  E Increases the rate of protein synthesis

5.7 Important host antiviral defences include:
  A Antibodies
  B Neutrophils
  C Macrophages
  D T-cells

  E Activation of the classical and alternative complement pathways

5.8 Bacteria may alter their genetic information by:
  A Mutation
  B Taking up soluble DNA fragments from other species across their cell wall
  C Incorporation of human DNA from the host
  D Being infected by bacteriophages
  E Transfer of nucleic acid via plasmids

5.9 Gram-positive cocci include:
  A *Streptococcus pneumoniae* (pneumococcus)
  B *Neisseria meningitidis* (meningococcus)
  C *Clostridium tetani*
  D *Legionella pneumophila*
  E *Staphylococcus aureus*

5.10 Acid-fast bacilli:
  A Are easily seen after Gram staining
  B Include *Mycobacterium tuberculosis*
  C Include *Mycobacterium leprae*
  D Include *Bordetella pertussis*
  E Include *Mycoplasma pneumoniae*

5.11 Unlike *Staphylococcus epidermidis*, *Staphylococcus aureus*:
  A Forms white colonies
  B Is coagulase-positive
  C Does not possess DNase
  D Does not produce toxins
  E Commonly causes abscesses

5.12 Clostridia:
  A Are aerobic
  B Usually produce endotoxins
  C Seldom form spores
  D May be found in soil
  E Can be easily identified by Gram staining

5.13 The following types of clostridia and their associated clinical infection are correctly matched:
  A *C. tetani* – flaccid paralysis
  B *C. perfringens* – pseudomembranous colitis
  C *C. botulinum* – gas gangrene
  D *C. difficile* – food poisoning
  E *C. perfringens* – spastic paralysis

5.14 Diphtheria:
  A Is caused by a Gram-negative rod
  B May be transmitted via droplets
  C Can be prevented by a course of toxoid
  D Can be treated by metronidazole
  E May be associated with myocardial damage

5.15 *Listeria monocytogenes*:
A Is a Gram-negative bacillus
B May be transmitted via contaminated soft cheeses
C May cause abortion in pregnant mothers
D Particularly affects teenagers
E May cause meningitis in newborn babies

5.16 Meningococci:
A Belong to the genus *Neisseria*
B May be carried in the throat by healthy individuals
C Are often carried by farm animals
D May produce endotoxin
E May cause septicaemia without meningitis

5.17 *Haemophilus influenzae* type b:
A Is a Gram-positive bacillus
B Is capsulated
C Can be vaccinated against
D Infects teenagers more commonly than other age groups
E May cause epiglottitis

5.18 *Legionella pneumophila*:
A May cause atypical pneumonia
B Can be easily cultured
C Can only survive within human cells
D Is usually transmitted via droplets from person to person
E Can be effectively treated with erythromycin

5.19 *Bacteroides*:
A Are obligatory aerobic bacteria
B Should be vigorously treated if found in the stools
C May cause peritonitis
D Are Gram-positive bacilli
E Are most appropriately treated by penicillin

5.20 Bacteriophages:
A Are particular types of bacteria
B Allow accurate typing of some viruses
C May cause lysis of bacteria
D Have a very wide host range
E May be responsible for toxin production by some bacteria

5.21 Antibiotics which act by interfering with the cell walls of bacteria include:
A Penicillin
B Gentamicin
C Tetracycline
D Trimethoprim
E Cephalosporin

5.22 The following viruses and their associated diseases are correctly matched:
A Mumps virus – parotitis
B Respiratory syncytial virus – foot and mouth disease
C Coxsackie A virus – bronchiolitis
D Herpes simplex type 1 virus – shingles
E Herpes zoster virus – chickenpox

5.23 Diseases attributable to the Epstein–Barr virus include:
A Glandular fever
B Measles
C Burkitt's lymphoma
D Nasopharyngeal carcinoma
E Myeloma

5.24 The following viruses and their associated diseases are correctly matched:
A Parvoviruses – rubella
B Rotaviruses – pharyngitis
C Adenovirus – conjunctivitis
D Parainfluenza virus – gastroenteritis
E Small round virus – gastroenteritis

5.25 Human immunodeficiency virus (HIV):
A Contains DNA
B Contains reverse transcriptase
C May infect host T-helper cells (CD4 cells)
D Causes a reduction in host CD4 cells at late stages of the disease
E May be transmitted from mother to fetus during pregnancy

5.26 The following antiviral agents are effective against the corresponding viral infections:
A Amantadine – pneumonia due to cytomegalovirus
B Acyclovir – encephalitis due to herpes simplex
C Zidovudine – human immunodeficiency virus
D Interferon – influenza
E Ribavirin – bronchiolitis caused by respiratory syncytial virus

5.27 The following statements about plasmodia are true:
A They are fungi
B Sexual reproduction occurs in the human liver and red blood cells
C Asexual reproduction occurs in the intestines in mosquitoes
D They may cause anaemia in humans
E They characteristically cause continuous prolonged pyrexia

5

Q

GENERAL BASIC MEDICAL SCIENCES

Infectious diseases

5.28 The following diagnostic tests are useful for the corresponding purposes:
A Ziehl – Neelsen's (ZN) stain – detection of mycobacteria
B Electron microscopy – identification of fungus
C Immunofluorescence – detection of influenza virus
D Specific IgM antibodies – rubella immune status
E Specific IgG antibodies – detection of acute infections

5.29 The following are examples of passive immunisation:
A Protection against hepatitis A after exposure by administration of pooled human immunoglobulin
B An administration of three doses of hepatitis B vaccine
C Oral polio vaccine
D Mumps, measles and rubella (MMR) vaccine
E Immunity from measles in the first six months of life via maternal antibodies

5.30 Examples of toxoids include:
A Pertussis vaccine
B Cholera vaccine
C Diphtheria vaccine
D Tetanus vaccine
E BCG (bacille Calmette–Guérin) vaccine

5.31 Unlike killed vaccines, live attenuated vaccines:
A Can be given during pregnancy
B Can be given to leukaemic patients
C Usually require three doses
D Rapidly decline in efficacy
E Are usually more expensive

5.32 What is the difference between *disinfection* and *sterilisation*?
Describe methods in common use for each.

5.33 Suggest a suitable culture medium for the following:
A Growth of *Haemophilus influenzae*
B Growth of *Mycobacterium tuberculosis*
C Identification of lactose-fermenting enteropathogens
D Selection of *Salmonella* or *Shigella* species
E Growth of *Candida albicans*.

5.34 Suggest a staining method for microscopic identification of each of the following:
A *Staphylococcus aureus*
B *Pneumocystis carinii*
C *Cryptococcus neoformans*
D *Mycobacterium tuberculosis*
E *Legionella pneumophila*.

5.35 A How do viruses differ from bacteria in structure?
B How do they differ in metabolic activity?

5.36 How do Chlamydia and Rickettsiae differ from Mycoplasma?

5.37 Describe the process of viral cell entry and replication.

5.38 A Describe the main components of bacterial cell walls.
B How does this differ between Gram-positive and Gram-negative organisms?

5.39 For each of the following, state whether defence is provided against bacteria, viruses or both:
A Neutrophils
B Macrophages
C Complement
D Antibodies
E T cells
F NK cells
G Interferon
H Lysozyme.

5.40 What general first-line defences does the body have against invading bacteria?

5.41 Propose the mechanism(s) for increased susceptibility to bacterial infection in each of the following conditions:
A Severe burns
B Ventilation in an unconscious patient
C Achlorhydria
D Urinary catheterisation.

5.42 A Define the terms *virulence* and *virulence factor*.
B Give two examples of bacterial virulence factors.

5.43 What mechanisms exist for gene transfer between bacteria, allowing increased virulence and antibiotic resistance?

5.44 A What is interferon? Describe the role(s) of interferon in the context of viral infection.
B What side effects may be encountered with its therapeutic use as an antiviral agent?

5.45 Group the following antibiotic classes with their mechanisms of action.

A Cell wall (peptidoglycan) synthesis	Ciprofloxacin
B DNA gyrase	ß-Lactams, glycopeptides

C RNA polymerase   Aminoglycosides, macrolides
D Protein synthesis   Trimethoprim, sulphonamides
E Tetrahydrofolic   Rifampicin
    acid production

5.46 List the spectrum of action of the following antibacterial agents.
A Third generation cephalosporins
B Glycopeptides
C Metronidazole
D Erythromycin
E Aminoglycosides.

5.47 A How do the following display *natural* resistance to certain antimicrobial agents?
    i   *Mycoplasma pneumoniae*
    ii   Gram-negative organisms.
B Describe specific mechanisms of *acquired* antimicrobial resistance, giving an example of drug class in each case.

5.48 Describe the mechanism of action and spectrum of activity of the following antifungal agents.
A Amphotericin B
B Fluconazole
C Terbinafine
D Flucytosine.

5.49 A What characteristics comprise an 'ideal' vaccine?
B What difficulties are encountered with polysaccharide antigens when considering vaccine development and how may they be overcome?
C Describe the main types of vaccine currently in use and give examples for bacterial and viral pathogens.
D What is passive immunity?

5.50 A What are the advantages and disadvantages of live vaccines?
B In which circumstances are they contraindicated?

5.51 Describe the stages at which transmission of infectious agents may occur between mother and fetus or mother and neonate. In each case, give two examples of organisms that can be transmitted.

5.52 List the effects of congenital infection with each of the following pathogens.
A Rubella
B Cytomegalovirus (CMV)
C *Toxoplasma gondii*.

5.53 A List the population types vulnerable to infection with *Listeria monocytogenes*.
B How may infection occur?
C What disease processes does it cause?

5.54 Classify the following bacteria according to Gram stain and morphology and state the disease or disease process in each case.
A *Listeria monocytogenes*
B *Neisseria meningitidis*
C *Corynebacterium diphtheriae*
D *Clostridium difficile*
E *Leptospira interrogans*.

5.55 Match the following diseases with the appropriate class of virus and give the specific viral agent in each case.
A Molluscum contagiosum   Picornavirus
B Chickenpox   Retrovirus
C Poliomyelitis   Pox virus
D Hepatitis B (HBV)   Herpesvirus
E Hepatitis C (HCV)   Togavirus
F Acquired immune deficiency   Hepadnavirus
    syndrome (AIDS)

5.56 Interpret the Hepatitis B virus (HBV) serum antigen and antibody results given in Table 5.1.

5.57 What is the difference between exotoxin and endotoxin?

5.58 Give the infectious agent associated with each of the following rashes.
A Erythema marginatum
B Erythema infectiosum
C Pityriasis versicolor
D Erythema chronicum migrans
E Condyloma lata
F Erythema ab ignae.

Table 5.1

Result	HbsAg[a]	Anti-HBs[b]	Anti-HBc[c]
A	+	−	−
B	+	−	+
C	−	−	+
D	−	+	+

[a] Hepatitis B antigen.
[b] Antibody to HBsAg.
[c] Antibody to Hepatitis core antigen.

5

Q

GENERAL BASIC MEDICAL SCIENCES

Infectious diseases

5.59 A What is the incubation period for **infectious mononucleosis**? What is the causative agent and how is it spread?
   B Give two laboratory methods used in its diagnosis.
   C What complications of infection may occur?

5.60 A How does 'meningism' differ from 'meningitis' and what are its clinical features?
   B Give the commonest:
      i   Bacterial causes
      ii Viral causes.
   C Give the characteristic CSF findings in the following diseases.
      i   Bacterial meningitis
      ii Viral meningitis
      iii Tuberculous meningitis.

5.61 A Give the incubation periods and clinical features for each of the following causes of food poisoning.
      i   *Campylobacter jejuni*
      ii   non-typhoidal *Salmonella* spp.
      iii *Staphylococcus aureus*
      iv   *Bacillus cereus*
      v   *Clostridium botulinum*
      vi   *Entamoeba histolytica*
      vii *Giardia lamblia*.
   B Which of these are notifiable?

5.62 A What methods are used to monitor progress in infection with Human immunodeficiency virus (HIV)?
   B What is HAART (highly active anti-retroviral therapy) and why is it employed?
   C i   What is an opportunistic infection?
      ii Give two examples that are AIDS-defining.

General principles of infectious diseases

5.1 A B C D
Defences of the respiratory tract against infection include the cough reflex, ciliated cells (which drive foreign particles upwards from the lungs to the back of the throat), mucus-secreting globlet cells, and the alveolar macrophages if microorganisms succeed in reaching the alveoli. Mechanisms which increase the likelihood of bacterial infection of the lungs include depressed cough reflex (e.g. due to stroke or after anaesthesia), the ability of the bacteria to attach to the epithelial cells (e.g. *Bordetella pertussis*), impaired ciliary function (e.g. due to cigarette smoke or atmospheric pollution) or reduced macrophage activity (e.g. concurrent infection by respiratory viruses).

5.2 C
Viruses consist of a genome of either DNA or RNA (but not both) enclosed in a shell of protein and sometimes a lipid membrane. They do not contain protein or energy production machinery (e.g. Golgi bodies and mitochondria) and must depend on the biochemical mechanisms of the host cell for replication by incorporating their genome into the host DNA. (They are obligatory intracellular parasites.) Viruses are reproduced by assembling individual components produced by the host cell biochemical machinery rather than by binary fission.

5.3 B C E
Bacteria may be classified into Gram-positive and Gram-negative depending on their ability to retain Gram stain. An outer membrane is present in a Gram-negative bacterium but not in a Gram-positive bacterium. The cell walls are thinner for Gram-negative bacteria, but are more complicated structurally than Gram-positive bacteria. Gram-negative, but not Gram-positive bacteria, contain lipopolysaccharide (LPS), or endotoxin. Endotoxin activates the immune response and is liable to cause fever and disseminated intravascular coagulation.

5.4 A C E
Sterilisation is the total destruction of all microbes, including the more resistant bacteria spores and non-enveloped viruses. This may be achieved by physical means (e.g. dry heat or using steam under pressure, ultraviolet or ionisation radiation), gas vapour sterilisation (e.g. formaldehyde or hydrogen peroxide vapour) or by chemical means (e.g. hydrogen peroxide vapour). Only a maximum temperature of 100°C can be achieved by boiling in water, and is ineffective in destroying bacterial spores. Similarly, washing in alcohol is effective in destroying most, but not all, microbes. It is used as a disinfectant.

5.5 A B D
Important antibacterial defences against bacteria include neutrophils and macrophages which phagocytose bacteria by oxygen-dependent or oxygen-independent mechanisms, antibodies which bind to the surface structure of bacteria and facilitate opsonisation of bacteria, activation of the alternative complement pathway initially followed by the classical complement pathway by which chemotactic factors are produced, and enzymes such as lysozyme or lactoferrin. Non-killer cells and interferon are important for antiviral defences.

5.6 A B C D
Interferon is the body's first defence against viruses. Production is stimulated by double-stranded RNA. Interferon acts by activating the immune response by enhancing T-cell recognition of the infected cell, and inhibits viral replication by inhibiting protein synthesis in the cell. Interferon consists of a family of proteins produced by different cells (e.g. B-cells, macrophages, fibroblasts and activated T-cells) with different modes of action. It is partially responsible for non-specific flu-like symptoms in the patient.

5.7 A C D
Important host antiviral defences include interferon, antibodies (which may neutralise or opsonise viruses), T-cells (e.g. promote antibody and inflammatory responses and kill infected cell by CD8 cells), macrophages (which inactivate opsonised virus particles and present viral antigen to CD4 T-cells) and NK cells (which kill infected cells). Neutrophils and complements are important antibacterial but not antiviral defences.

5.8 A B D E
The ability of bacteria to change their genetic information is essential to their adaptation and survival in different environments, and determines their invasiveness and resistance to antibiotics. Bacteria may change their genetic information either through mutation or genetic transfer. Natural selection selects out mutants which have a selective advantage (e.g. increased invasiveness or resistance to certain antibiotics). Genetic transfer may be achieved either through taking up soluble DNA fragments from other species directly across their cell walls (i.e. transformation), through infection by viruses (i.e. bacteriophages) or by transfer of DNA via plasmids. Plasmids are extrachromosomal segments of DNA present in some bacteria which divide independent of the chromosome.

5.9 A E
- *Streptococcus pneumoniae* – Gram-positive coccus
- *Neisseria meningitidis* – Gram-negative coccus

59

5

A

GENERAL BASIC MEDICAL SCIENCES

Infectious diseases

- *Clostridium tetani* – Gram-positive bacillus
- *Legionella pneumophila* – Gram-negative bacillus
- *Staphylococcus aureus* – Gram-positive coccus

5.10 B C
Acid-fast bacilli include all bacteria of the genus *Mycobacterium*. They are characteristically difficult to Gram stain, and resist decolorisation by acid after staining with hot carbol fuchsin. They include *M. tuberculosis* (which causes tuberculosis), *M. leprae* (which causes leprosy) and atypical mycobacteria. Mycoplasmae are bacteria which do not form cell walls.

5.11 B E
S. aureus and *S. epidermidis* are the two main types of staphylococci, and they are different in several aspects. They can be distinguished in the laboratory in several ways. *S. aureus* forms golden-yellow colonies whilst *S. epidermidis* forms white colonies. *S. aureus* possesses the enzymes coagulase (which forms clots in plasma) and DNase, whilst *S. epidermidis* does not. Both exist as skin commensals. However, *S. aureus* may produce different types of toxins, and may cause boils, abscesses, osteomyelitis, septic arthritis and gastroenteritis. Infections by *S. epidermidis* are rarer, and this organisim may infect artificial heart valves and intravenous catheters.

5.12 D E
Clostridia are anaerobic spore-forming Gram-positive bacilli, and the spore can be seen at the one terminal of the bacillus. They can be easily identified by Gram staining as the bacteria take up the stain but the spores do not. They characteristically cause disease by the production of exotoxins.

5.13 –
- *C. tetani* – causes tetanus (spastic paralysis) by a powerful neurotoxin
- *C. perfringens* – may cause gas gangrene, food poisoning or cellulitis by production of α-toxins
- *C. botulinum* – causes botulism (flaccid paralysis) by a powerful neurotoxin
- *C. difficile* – causes pseudomembranous colitis especially in patients on broad-spectrum antibiotics, by the production of two toxins

5.14 B C E
Diphtheria is caused by the Gram-positive bacillus *Corynebacterium diphtheriae*. Symptoms are caused by an exotoxin which destroys epithelial cells. It causes infection in the upper respiratory tract, and affected patients may have pyrexia and acutely inflamed upper respiratory tract. In severe cases, the airway may be compromised, and the toxin may damage myocardial cells and neurones. A course

of toxoid may prevent the disease. Patients with suspected diphtheria should be admitted to the intensive care unit and treated with both antibiotics (penicillin or erythromycin) and diphtheria antitoxin.

5.15 B C E
Listeria monocytogenes is a Gram-positive bacillus which occurs naturally in the environment and in the gastrointestinal tract of some animals. It is usually transmitted via contamination of food products, especially soft cheeses. It may cause meningitis and septicaemia in the newborns and in immunocompromised individuals, but very rarely affects previously healthy subjects. However, it may cause abortion and premature labour in pregnant mothers. Hence pregnant mothers are often advised to avoid soft cheese.

5.16 A B D E
The *Neisseria* genus includes two important bacteria: gonococci (which cause gonorrhoea) and meningococci (which cause meningococcal septicaemia and/or meningitis). Humans are the only natural host for meningococci, which may be carried in the upper respiratory tract by up to 20% of the population. It is unclear why some individuals who carry the organisms develop the disease whilst others do not. Meningococcal septicaemia without meningitis often has a worse prognosis than with meningitis. Endotoxins are important in the pathogenesis of some meningococci.

5.17 B C E
Haemophilus influenzae type b is a capsulated Gram-negative bacillus, and the capsule confers its invasive properties. It particularly infects young children under the age of five years. It may cause meningitis, epiglottitis, otitis media and chest infection. However, the incidence has been declining in recent years due to the introduction of a vaccine against type b polysaccharide capsule which is offered to all children in the United Kingdom.

5.18 A E
Legionella pneumophila has been known only since 1976 when an outbreak occurred amongst the delegates at a conference in Philadelphia. This is because it has very particular requirements for its culture. The organism is found in the environment, and especially in water systems, such as fountains, water storage tanks and showers. It usually spreads by water droplets from these water sources, but is seldom transmitted from person to person. Erythromycin is the most appropriate treatment.

5.19 C
Bacteroides is a genus of Gram-negative anaerobic bacilli which form a large proportion of the normal gut flora.

Bacteroides may protect the gut against colonisation and infection by other more pathogenic bacteria. However, it may cause intra-abdominal sepsis, especially in bowel perforation and after bowel surgery. The most effective treatments are metronidazole and clindamycin.

5.20 C E
Bacteriophages are viruses which infect bacteria. Bacterial lysis may occur. Since the phages (viruses) have a very narrow host range, they allow accurate typing of some types of bacteria by observing which phages lyse the bacteria. The genome of the viruses may be incorporated into the bacteria. Some phages code for the production of toxin (e.g. diphtheria toxin) and cause the disease.

5.21 A E
The mechanisms of action of the antibiotics are as follows:
- Penicillin, cephalosporin – interfere with cell wall
- Aminoglycosides, tetracyclines, chloramphenicol – interfere with protein synthesis
- Sulphonamides and trimethoprim – interfere with DNA synthesis
- Rifampicin – interferes with RNA synthesis

5.22 A E
The correct answers are:
- Mumps virus – mumps (parotitis, meningitis, pancreatitis)
- Respiratory syncytial virus – bronchiolitis in infants
- Coxsackie A virus – hand, foot and mouth disease
- Herpes simplex type 1 virus – cold sores, keratoconjunctivitis
- Herpes zoster – chickenpox and shingles

5.23 A C D
The Epstein–Barr virus is a DNA virus. It commonly causes glandular fever with tonsillitis and lymphadenopathy. It may cause hepatitis and meningoencephalitis in severe cases. It is also implicated in Burkitt's lymphoma and nasopharyngeal carcinoma.

5.24 C E
The correct answers are:
- Parvoviruses – 'slapped cheek disease' in children, abortion in pregnant mothers
- Rotaviruses – gastroenteritis in children
- Adenovirus – pharyngitis and conjunctivitis
- Parainfluenza virus – tracheitis, bronchiolitis, pneumonia
- Small round virus – gastroenteritis

5.25 B C D E
Human immunodeficiency virus (HIV) is a retrovirus. It contains single-stranded RNA. cDNA is synthesised from the RNA by viral reverse transcriptase. The virus infects

mainly the T-helper cells (CD4 cells). The host CD4 cells decline at late stages of the disease, which is useful for monitoring the disease. CD4 cells may also fall during seroconversion in acute disease but this is a transient phenomenon. The virus is transmitted mainly via sexual intercourse (homosexual or heterosexual) and blood products. However, the virus is transmitted from mother to fetus during pregnancy, and rarely through breast milk.

5.26 B C E
The correct answers are:
- Amantadine and rimantadine – influenza
- Acyclovir – herpes simplex and zoster infections
- Zidovudine – human immunodeficiency virus
- Interferon-α – chronic hepatitis B and C
- Ribavirin – bronchiolitis due to respiratory syncytial virus

5.27 D
Plasmodia are protozoa (a type of parasite). Plasmodia cause malaria in humans. The life cycle of plasmodia can be divided into two stages: sexual reproduction occurs in the gut of mosquitoes, and asexual reproduction occurs in the human liver and red blood cells. Patients with malaria characteristically have bouts of pyrexia and sweating. These are due to the release of toxins when schizonts burst and release the merozoites. Anaemia occurs due to haemolysis of red blood cells.

5.28 A C E
The correct answers are:
- ZN stain – detection of mycobacteria
- Electron microscopy – identification of viruses
- Immunofluorescence – detection of viruses and chlamydia
- Specific IgM antibodies – detection of recent infection
- Specific IgG antibodies – detection of past infection or immune status

5.29 A E
Passive immunisation is the protection against infection by antibodies. This usually gives rapid protection, but lasts for only about half a year. Examples are protection against infection in the first six months of life by the transfer of antibodies via the placenta, and post-exposure prophylaxis by the administration of antibodies.

5.30 C D
Pertussis and cholera vaccines are killed vaccines. BCG is a live attenuated vaccine. Diphtheria and tetanus vaccines are inactivated bacterial toxins (toxoids).

5.31 –
Unlike killed vaccines, live attenuated vaccines are live organisms whose virulence has been reduced. Since they

Infectious diseases

replicate in the body in a similar manner to true infections, they are more effective, and usually only require one or two doses. Killed vaccines usually require several doses. Live attenuated vaccines are generally cheaper. However, mutation may occur in live attenuated vaccines and they may regain their virulence. Furthermore, they cannot be given to immunocompromised patients (as this may give rise to disease) or to pregnant mothers (as they may infect the fetus).

5.32

Disinfection inactivates vegetative (non-sporing) bacteria but is rarely capable of killing spores. Spores are survival mechanisms of genera *Bacillus* and *Clostridium* which are resistant to high temperatures and products that kill vegetative bacteria. Disinfection therefore renders materials safe but not sterile. Chemical agents are used, such as ethanol, chlorhexidine, povidone-iodine and gluteraldehyde.

Sterilisation is the complete destruction of all organisms, including spores.

Methods employed are physical and chemical:
- moist heat, e.g. autoclave (120°C)
- dry heat, e.g. oven (160°C)
- filtration, for heat-sensitive products (removes bacteria but not viruses)
- gamma irradiation
- vapour, e.g. ethylene oxide, formaldehyde.

5.33
A
Chocolate agar.

B
Löwenstein–Jensen medium.

C
MacConkey (pink colonies) or CLED agar (yellow colonies).

D
Desoxycholate citrate.

E
Sabouraud's agar.
Note It is useful to categorise different media according to use:
- **Enrichment** media, for fastidious organisms, e.g. *Haemophilus influenzae*, *Neisseria* and *Streptococcus* spp.
- **Selective** media, to separate pathogens from a mixture of organisms, e.g. from sputum or stool specimens

- **Indicator** media, to identify colonies of pathogens from organisms able to grow on selective medium. Indicator media are often also selective.

5.34
A
Gram stain.

B
Gomori–Grocott stain, immunofluorescence.

C
India ink.

D
Ziehl–Neelsen (staining with carbol fuschin, decolorisation with acid *and* alcohol, counterstaining with methylene blue or malachite green and observation for red bacilli against a blue background) *or* auramine (staining with auramine-phenol, decolorisation with acid and alcohol, application of potassium permanganate and observation for fluorescent yellow bacilli under ultraviolet light).

E
Direct immunofluorescence.
Note Staining and microscopy methods can be classified as follows:
- unstained preparations (for protozoa, helminths, pus cells)
- simple stains, e.g. Gram strain
- special stains e.g. Ziehl–Neelsen, auramine, Gomori–Grocott, India ink
- immunofluorescence (direct and indirect)
- electron microscopy.

5.35
A
- Viruses are smaller than bacteria (10–300 nm in diameter) and too small to be visible by light microscopy.
- Viruses contain only one kind of nucleic acid: *either* DNA *or* RNA. The nucleic acid is either double stranded (ds) or single stranded (ss). (ss RNA can be further divided into sense RNA (+), antisense RNA (–) and retro RNA.)

B
Viruses have neither mitochondria nor protein-synthesising apparatus and so are incapable of metabolic activity outside susceptible host cells. They reproduce by assembling components produced by host cell biochemical pathways.

5.36
Two main differences are size and growth requirements; all three groups tend to be handled in virus laboratories. Chlamydia and Rickettsiae are larger than viruses but smaller than Mycoplasma, which in turn are smaller than bacteria. Like viruses, Chlamydia and Rickettsiae are obligate intracellular organisms and so are unable to grow in inanimate media. Mycoplasma have evolved from bacteria but lack a peptidoglycan cell wall. They are the smallest prokaryotic organisms able to grow in cell-free culture medium.

5.37
There are seven stages:
1. *Adsorption*, to specific receptors on the host cell plasma membrane.
2. *Entry*, either by invagination of the host cell membrane around the virus particle followed by pinocytosis, or by fusion of the virus envelope with the cell membrane.
3. *Uncoating*, to render accessible the viral nucleic acid.
4. *Transcription* of the viral genome to produce mRNA. In *sense* ss RNA (+), the genome acts as mRNA without the transcription step.
5. *Synthesis* of virus components (nucleic acid and proteins).
6. *Assembly* of new virus genomes and proteins. This may take place in the cell nucleus, cytoplasm or at the plasma membrane.
7. *Release* of viral particles by budding or by sudden rupture.

Note Knowledge of these steps is useful when considering the mechanism of action of antiviral therapy.

5.38
A
The bacterial cell wall consists of two main layers, the **cytoplasmic membrane**, which encloses the bacterial cytoplasm, and an outer cell wall (**peptidoglycan**), which maintains bacterial structural integrity and prevents lysis by influx of water through the permeable cytoplasmic membrane.

B
Gram-positive organisms (Fig. 5.1a) have a **thick peptidoglycan** cell wall with surface proteins and polysaccharides called **teichoic acids**. Gram-negative organisms (Fig. 5.1b) have thinner peptidoglycan which is attached to an **outer membrane** containing **lipopolysaccharide** (LPS, also known as endotoxin). The outer membrane of Gram-negative bacteria is separated from the cytoplasmic membrane by the **periplasmic space**.

5.39
A
Bacteria (phagocytosis).

B
Both (inactivation of opsonised bacterial and viral particles and presentation of viral antigen to CD4 T-cells).

C
Bacteria, via the alternative and classical pathways.

D
Both. Defence against bacteria is by opsonisation, the classical complement pathway (if bound to bacterial

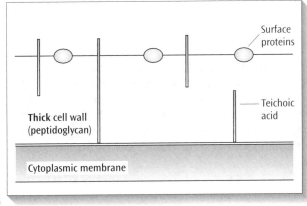 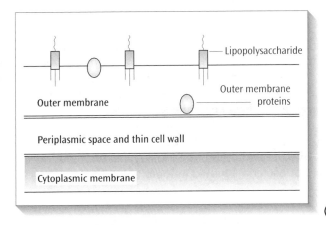

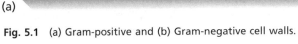

Fig. 5.1 (a) Gram-positive and (b) Gram-negative cell walls.

Infectious diseases

antigen) and binding to toxoid; antiviral defence is by neutralisation and cell-mediated cytotoxicity.

E

Viruses (by promotion of antibody and inflammatory response and killing of infected cells by CD8 cells).

F

Viral (killing of infected cells).

G

Viral (IFN is the first defence against viruses, appearing at sites of viral replication just after peak titres of virus and before the humoral antibody response).

H

Bacteria.

5.40

First lines of host defence can be divided into non-specific (intact skin, mucosal surfaces, washing action of fluid and antibacterial substances) and specific (e.g. secretory IgA, sIgA). Skin provides a physical barrier and has a number of surface properties, including low temperature (<37°C), dryness, continual sloughing of dead cells and colonisation by resident microflora (mostly Gram-positive). Antibacterial substances such as lysozyme and lipids protect pores and sweat glands, and bacteria that breach the skin surface are attacked by skin-associated lymphoid tissue (SALT). Mucosal surfaces are protected by a mucous layer and have additional defences, such as washing action of fluid, pH regulation and antibacterial enzymes, depending on the site within the body.

5.41

A

The protective barrier function of skin is broken, providing direct access of pathogens to subcutaneous tissues.

B

Insufficient oral hygiene allows growth of bacteria, which can then be inhaled. Lack of humidification of inspired air can cause drying and damage of the bronchial mucosa, impairing mucociliary blanket function and promoting adherence of inhaled pathogens.

C

Lack of gastric acid raises the intraluminal pH, reducing killing of bacteria ingested in foods.

D

The urinary catheter breaches the urethral sphincter, and constant drainage rather than intermittent purging allows microorganisms to adhere to areas of the bladder wall.

Infection may also occur in pools of stagnant urine, particularly in the supine patient.

5.42

A

Virulence, or pathogenicity, is the ability of a disease-causing organism to establish infection in a host. A *virulence factor* is a product or mechanism that contributes to virulence.

B

- **Pili** (for adherence to mucosal surfaces, e.g. *Pseudomonas aeruginosa*, *Neisseria gonorrhoea*).
- **Capsules** (for prevention of complement activation and phagocytic uptake, e.g. *Streptococcus pneumoniae*, *Haemophilus influenzae*, *N. meningitidis*).
- **Siderophores** (iron acquisition for growth, e.g. *Neisseria* spp.).
- **Surface antigen variation** and **surface coating** with host proteins (leading to evasion of antibody response e.g. *Staphylococcus aureus*).
- **Toxins** (causing epithelial cell damage, e.g. *P. aeruginosa*, *Streptococcus* spp.).
- **Survival inside host cells** (conferring protection from reactive forms of oxygen and low pH, e.g. *Salmonella* survival inside phagocytes).

5.43

- **Transformation**: uptake of exogenous bacterial DNA.
- **Transduction**: transfer of chromosomal DNA fragments by infection with bacteriophage (a virus that infects bacteria).
- **Conjugation**: transfer of plasmid DNA between bacteria by direct contact.
- **Transposition**: transposons or 'jumping genes' are sequences of DNA that can move between plasmids, or between plasmids and the bacterial chromosome, from one bacterial strain to another.

5.44

A

Interferons are a family of cytokines (small molecular weight proteins) synthesised by eukaryotic cells in response to various inducers. They cause biochemical changes leading to an antiviral state in exposed cells of the same species. They have antiviral, immunomodulatory and antiproliferative actions. Three types of IFN are described:

α- and β-IFN may be produced by nearly all cell types and have direct antiviral activity; γ-IFN, which is produced only by T-cells and natural killer (NK) cells, exerts a more immunomodulatory effect, involving macrophage activation, expression of MHC class II antigens and mediation of local inflammatory responses. The antiviral effects of IFNs take place at various stages of viral replication (viral penetration or uncoating, synthesis of mRNA, translation of viral proteins, viral assembly and release), depending on the virus and cell type. Most animal viruses are sensitive, although many DNA viruses are relatively insensitive.

B

α-IFN is the type most commonly used therapeutically. It reduces the metabolism of various drugs by the hepatic P$_{450}$ system so can significantly increase levels of drugs such as theophylline, and can increase the bone marrow toxicity of myelotoxic drugs such as zidovudine. Other side effects include neurotoxicity, characterised by somnolence, confusion, behavioural disturbance and rarely seizures, thyroid dysfunction, cardiotoxicity and general features of fatigue, malaise and weight loss.

5.45
A
Cell wall (peptidoglycan) synthesis: ß-lactams, glycopeptides.

B
DNA gyrase: ciprofloxacin.

C
RNA polymerase: rifampicin.

D
Protein synthesis: aminoglycosides, macrolides.

E
Tetrahydrofolic acid production: trimethoprim, sulphonamides.

5.46
A
Antibacterial spectrum is as for second generation (that is, wide range of Gram-positive and Gram-negative bacteria including *Haemophilus influenzae*) but with superior activity against *Staphylococcus aureus* and action in addition against *Pseudomonas aeruginosa*.

B
Gram-positive organisms only.

C
Anaerobes only (bacteria and protozoa).

D
Penicillin-like but with additional activity against *H. influenzae* and causative organisms of 'atypical'

pneumonia (*Legionella pneumophila*, *Mycoplasma pneumoniae*, *Chlamydia* spp.).

E
Gram-negative rods (coliforms and *P. aeruginosa*), staphylococci; no activity against streptococci or anaerobes. (Note that a similar spectrum is displayed in quinolones: activity against *Staphylococcus aureus* and Gram-negative bacteria, including *P. aeruginosa*, with less sensitivity in streptococci and resistance in anaerobes.)

5.47
A
i   Mycoplasma is resistant to the actions of ß-lactam antibiotics and other agents which interfere with cell wall metabolism because it lacks a cell wall.
ii Glycopeptides have no activity against Gram-negative organisms as they are unable to penetrate the Gram-negative outer membrane.

B
• Antibiotic inactivation, e.g. ß-lactams, aminoglycosides.
• Alteration of antimicrobial target molecules, e.g. penicillin.
• Entry restriction of the antibiotic to its target, e.g. imipenem.
• Bypassing of the metabolic pathway that is blocked, e.g. trimethoprim.

5.48
A
Amphotericin B is a polyene which binds to sterols in the fungal cell membrane. Active against most yeasts and systemic fungi.

B
Fluconazole is an azole which blocks biosynthesis of ergosterol in the fungal membrane, leading to disruption of function. Active against candida (some resistance in non-*albicans* spp.) and *Cryptococcus neoformans*; ineffective in aspergillosis.

C
Terbinafine is an allylamine which inhibits an enzyme important in fungal cell wall metabolism. Used to treat dermatophyte skin infections.

D
Flucytosine is a synthetic fluorinated pyrimidine which disrupts protein synthesis, by incorporation into fungal mRNA in place of uracil, and DNA synthesis by blocking

Infectious diseases

thymidylate synthase. Used in combination with amphotericin B in cryptococcosis and severe *Candida* spp. infection.

5.49

A

A vaccine should elicit a **strong immune response** to the **correct antigen** or antigens, promoting resistance which is **long lasting**. It should be prepared at **low cost** and be easily **stored** and transported. There should be no or minimal **side effects**, or at least side effects that are less harmful than the disease being vaccinated against.

B

Polysaccharides are less immunogenic than proteins and are processed in a way that bypasses T-cells. Because no memory cells are formed, immunity produced is short-lived. By covalently attaching a polysaccharide antigen to a protein this problem can be overcome, provided the structure of the native antigen is not altered in the process. Such a *conjugate* vaccine has been used successfully, for example against *Haemophilus influenzae* type b.

C

See Table 5.2.

D

Passive immunity is the injection of antibodies from another source to obtain an immediate bloodstream antibody response. It is used mainly for bacterial toxins.

5.50

A

Live vaccines are cheap, effective at stimulating the immune system and target appropriate tissue. There is a risk, however, that they may mutate to a virulent form following administration or that they may cause infection in people who are immunocompromised.

B

Although live vaccines have attenuated virulence, they may cause disease in individuals unable to mount an immune response. They are therefore contraindicated in anyone immunosuppressed, notably patients who are HIV-positive, those with chronic liver or renal impairment or with haematological or solid organ malignancy, transplant patients on immunosuppressive therapy, and those at extremes of age.

5.51

Transmission may be as follows:

1. **Transplacental**, e.g. rubella, CMV, HIV, VZV, Human parvovirus B19, *Toxoplasma gondii*, *Treponema pallidum*, *Listeria monocytogenes*
2. **Intrapartum**, e.g. HSV, HIV, HBV, Group B *streptococci*, *Chlamydia trachomatis*, *Neisseria gonorrhoea*, *Escherichia coli*
3. **Postpartum**, e.g. HIV, HBV, VZV, enteroviruses.

Note The term '*congenital* infection' is used for neonates who survive transplacental infection but may be left with permanent tissue damage (see question 5.52).

Table 5.2

Vaccine type	Bacterial	Viral
Live attenuated	Bacille Calmette–Guérin (BCG) *Salmonella typhi* Ty21a	Measles Mumps Rubella Polio (oral) Varicella zoster Yellow fever Influenza (live)
Heat inactivated	*Bordetella pertussis* *Salmonella typhi* *Vibrio cholerae*	Influenza (inactivated) Polio (inactivated) Rabies Hepatitis A Japanese encephalitis
Subunit	*Neisseria meningitidis*, A, C (polysaccharide) *Streptococcus pneumoniae* (polysaccharide) *Haemophilus influenzae*, type b Acellular *Bordetella pertussis*	Influenza Hepatitis B
Toxoid	*Clostridium tetani* *Corynebacterium diphtheriae*	

5.52
For each pathogen, the characteristic features of congenital infection are shown in bold print:

A
- **Cardiac**, including patent ductus arteriosus, pulmonary stenosis, ventricular septal defect and Fallot's tetralogy
- Ocular: **cataracts**, retinal or uveal tract dysplasias
- Neurological: **nerve deafness**, delayed motor and sensory development.

Note Congenital infection with rubella may occur during the first 16 weeks of pregnancy, after which time the fetus is not affected. As well as the defects above, there are also disorders due to generalised infection, including hepatosplenomegaly, thrombocytopenic purpura, low birth weight, jaundice, anaemia and lesions in the metaphysis of long bones. These features comprise the *rubella syndrome.*

B
- Ocular: choroidoretinitis (rare)
- Neurological: **nerve deafness**, upper motor neurone disorders, **psychomotor retardation**
- Other: **microcephaly**, **cerebral calcification**, myopathy (rare).

Note CMV during pregnancy is particularly problematic as: (1) the fetus may be affected during all three trimesters; and (2) maternal infection is almost always symptomless. Infants born with severe generalised infection or *cytomegalic inclusion disease* may have hepatosplenomegaly, jaundice and blood dyscrasias (thrombocytopenia and haemolytic anaemia) in addition to the above defects.

C
- Ocular: early or late **choroidoretinitis**, ocular palsy
- Neurological: cerebral palsy, epilepsy, deafness
- Other: **cerebral calcification**, **hydrocephalus** or **microcephaly**.

Note Toxoplasma may cause fetal infection throughout pregnancy. Although the chance of agent transmission increases with gestation, more serious defects occur as a result of *early* infection. Generalised infection may also occur in these infants, with features including fever, rash, hepatosplenomegaly and jaundice.

5.53
A
Extremes of age, immunocompromised individuals, pregnant women and neonates.
Note Infection in pregnancy is of greater danger to fetus than to mother, with 25% of cases resulting in abortion and stillbirth.

B
Listeria is usually acquired by ingestion, although it may be transmitted by direct contact with animals and birds as well as transplacentally and perinatally. It is carried in the gut by around 5% of the adult population, although carriage is normally transient following ingestion. The infective dose is unknown but the likelihood of infection is clearly dose-related. It can multiply in many foods but particularly paté and dairy products and can multiply at low temperatures (4°C) to reach high numbers.

C
In the population types listed in (A):
1. Adults:
   a. meningitis, occasionally cerebritis or cerebral abscess
   b. more rarely, bacteraemia causes infective endocarditis, arthritis and hepatitis
   c. mortality is up to 50%.
2. Fetus and neonate:
   a. abortion and stillbirth
   b. sepsis with meningitis and pneumonia.

5.54
A
Gram-positive rod; food poisoning, meningitis, neonatal infection (see question 5.53).

B
Gram-negative coccus; meningitis.

C
Gram-positive bacillus; diphtheria.

D
Gram-positive, anaerobic, sporing bacillus; pseudomembranous colitis.

E
Spirochaete (Gram-negative, anaerobic); leptospirosis (Weil's disease).

Note The first four examples in this question are exceptions to the general rule that most *commonly* encountered human bacterial pathogens that are *cocci* are Gram-positive and most that are *rods* are Gram-negative.

5.55
A
Pox virus (Molluscum contagiosum).

B
Herpesvirus (Varicella zoster virus, VZV).

Infectious diseases

C

Picornavirus (Polio virus).

D

Hepadnavirus (Hepatitis B virus).

E

Togavirus (Hepatitis C virus).

F

Retrovirus (Human immunodeficiency virus, HIV).

5.56
A

Early acute disease. The patient is infectious; HbeAg (blood-borne derivative of core antigen) is a marker of infectivity. Anti-Hbe usually appears in the first 1–3 weeks and HbeAg then becomes undetectable.

B

Acute disease or chronic carrier. Patient infectious. (Persistent carrier state is confirmed by the presence of HBsAg after >6 months following acute infection.)

C

Recent disease; HbsAg has disappeared but serum has been taken before the appearance of anti-HBs. Patient infectious.

D

Patient is immune, either by vaccination or previous disease (seen in convalescent phase of HBV infection; it is also possible for recovery to lead to loss of detectable anti-Hbc). In the case of immunity as a result of recognition anti-Hbs is present in the absence of anti-Hbc.

5.57

Exotoxins are toxic bacterial proteins produced by intact Gram-positive and some Gram-negative bacteria. Endotoxin is lipopolysaccharide (LPS), a component of the Gram-negative outer membrane, which is released only following cell lysis or death of the bacterium. The other main differences are listed in Table 5.3.

5.58
A

Streptococcus pyogenes; erythema marginatum is one of the major Duckett Jones diagnostic criteria of rheumatic fever. (Diagnosis requires 2 or more major or 1 major plus 2 or more minor criteria).

B

Human parvovirus B19; erythema infectiosum is also known as fifth disease.

Table 5.3

Property	Exotoxin	Endotoxin
Produced by	Gram-positive, some Gram-negative, bacteria	Gram-negative bacteria
Composition	Protein	Lipopolysaccharide (LPS)
Effect of heat	Labile	Strong
Antigenicity	Strong[1]	Weak
Range of effect	Wide[2]	Same physiological effect produced by all LPS

[1] Some toxins, e.g. diphtheria and tetanus toxins, can be converted to *toxoids* which remove the toxic effect while retaining antigenicity for use as antigens.
[2] Exotoxins can produce local and distant effects: the effect on different cells or organ types are specific for each exotoxin. The effects of LPS are all non-specific.

C

Malassezia furfur, a lipophilic yeast and normal skin commensal (previously called *Pityrosporum orbiculare*). Infection is confined to trunk and proximal aspects of limbs, leaving hair and nail plates unaffected.

D

Borrelia burgdorferi, the spirochaete responsible for Lyme disease.

E

Treponema pallidum; these warty plaque-like lesions found in moist body surfaces are a feature of secondary syphilis.

F

This is a reticulate, pigmented erythema due to damage from long-term exposure to local heat; it is not an infectious disease!

5.59
A

The incubation period for infectious mononucleosis (glandular fever) is *long*, 4–8 weeks. It is caused by Epstein–Barr virus (EBV), which is shed in pharyngeal secretions and is transmitted by close oral contact.

B

• Monospot test (for presence of heterophile antibodies).
• IgM anti-EBV capsid antigen (diagnostic of acute infection).
Note EBV culture, e.g. from throat swabs, is not useful as it is likely to be positive in asymptomatic individuals with latent infection.

C

• Threatened respiratory obstruction (caused by pharyngeal oedema).

Table 5.4

Organism	Incubation period	Blood	Vomiting	Fever
Campylobacter jejuni	3–10 days	✓	✓	✓
non-typhoidal *Salmonella* spp.	12–36 h	±	✓	✓
Staphylococcus aureus[a]	2–6 h	✗	✓	±
Bacillus cereus[a]	1–2 h	✗	✓	✗
Clostridium botulinum[a]	24–72 h[b]	✗	±	✗
Entamoeba histolytica	14–28 days	✓	✗	✗
Giardia lamblia	7–21 days	✗	✓	✗

✓ present; ✗ absent; ± may be present.
[a] Symptoms caused by toxin.
[b] Incubation period dependent on dose of ingested toxin. In food poisoning with *C. botulinum*, malaise and mild gastrointestinal features are followed by neurological disturbance characterised by *descending* paralysis. (*Note* The paralysis in Guillain–Barré syndrome, sometimes associated with *Campylobacter* infection, is *ascending*).

- Blood dyscrasias: thrombocytopenia, haemolytic anaemia (abnormal antibodies).
- Secondary infection of inflamed mucosae and sinus obstruction (for example, peritonsillar abscess or intracranial sinus infection).
- Splenic rupture. The enlarged spleen is friable and extends beyond the bony protection of the rib cage. Contact sports must be avoided until palpable lymphadenopathy has subsided (at least 1 month).
- Neurological sequelae: – self-limiting (lymphocytic meningitis, mononeuritis) – severe (encephalopathy).

5.60
A
Meningitis is inflammation of the meninges; the group of symptoms and signs which accompanies meningitis is *meningism*, which is characterised by:
- headache
- photophobia
- nausea and vomiting
- neck and back stiffness.

B
i Bacterial causes (in decreasing order of incidence in adults): *Neisseria meningitidis, Streptococcus pneumoniae, Staphylococcus aureus, Escherichia coli, group B streptococci, Haemophilus influenzae.*
ii Causes of viral meningitis include enteroviruses (echovirus, Coxsackie virus A, Poliovirus), herpes viruses (HSV-1 and -2, EBV), mumps, measles and HIV.

C
i Neutrophil pleiocytosis, ↑ protein, ↓ glucose.
ii Lymphocytic pleiocytosis, normal or ↑ protein, normal glucose.
iii Lymphocytic pleiocytosis, ↑ protein, ↓ glucose.

5.61
It is useful to consider gastrointestinal infection in terms of:
- presence or absence of dysentery (bloody diarrhoea) or fever
- whether the disease is a result of the organism itself or secondary to toxin production (Table 5.4).

B
All; 'food poisoning' is a notifiable disease.

5.62
A
- Viral load (number of HIV RNA copies per mililitre).
- CD4 lymphocyte count.
- Patient's clinical status.

B
HAART is the use of at least three antiretroviral drugs in HIV therapy. The rational for HAART is principally three-fold:
- reduce viral replication
- permit immune reconstitution (↑ CD4 count and function)
- minimise development of resistance to antiretroviral agents used.

C
i These are infections caused by microorganisms that are non-pathogenic in a normal host but may cause disease in patients with impaired immunity. Such infections may present with unusual symptoms and signs.
ii CMV retinitis, *Pneumocystis carinii* pneumonia, cerebral toxoplasmosis, mycobacteria (including pulmonary and extra-pulmonary TB, and *Mycobacterium avium-intracellulare*), systemic candidiasis (tracheal, bronchial, lung or oesophageal), extrapulmonary cryptococcosis, extrapulmonary or disseminated coccidiomycosis and extrapulmonary or disseminated histoplasmosis.

69

6 General principles of histology and embryology

6.1 The following statements about the epidermis of the skin are correct:
- A It is highly vascular
- B The outer layer (stratum corneum) is keratinised
- C The germinal layer (stratum germinativum) lies adjacent to the dermis
- D Melanocytes are found in the germinal layer (stratum germinativum) of the epidermis
- E Cells in the prickle cell layer (stratum spinosum) undergo continuous mitosis

6.2 The following statements about the dermis of the skin are true:
- A It meets the epidermis at the dermal papillae
- B It contains elastin
- C The cells of the dermis consist mainly of fibroblasts
- D It partly relies on the epidermis for metabolic support
- E It provides non-specific defence against infection

6.3 The following statements about arrector pili muscles are true:
- A Relaxation may cause hair erection
- B Contraction may cause 'goose-flesh appearance'
- C Contraction may result from an increase in environmental temperature
- D Contraction may result from fear
- E They are supplied by the parasympathetic nervous system

6.4 The following changes occur in the skin when the body temperature increases:
- A The hairs become more erect
- B The number of melanocytes decreases
- C The secretion from sweat glands increases
- D Blood flow to the skin decreases
- E The secretion from sebaceous glands decreases

6.5 Epithelial basement membranes:
- A Are made up of connective tissues
- B Provide structural support to the epithelium
- C May be breached by physiological epithelial growth
- D Are richly vascularised
- E May form a selective filter for the passage of substances from one body compartment to another

6.6 The epithelia at the following sites and the associated epithelial types are correctly matched:
- A Distal convoluted renal tubule – simple squamous epithelium
- B Capillary wall – simple cuboidal epithelium
- C Gallbladder lining – simple columnar epithelium (unciliated)
- D Bronchial lining – simple columnar ciliated epithelium
- E Oviduct lining – pseudostratifed columnar ciliated epithelium

6.7 The following statements about transitional epithelium are true:
- A It is a form of simple epithelium
- B It can withstand a greater degree of stretch than stratified squamous epithelium
- C The apparent number of cell layers decreases when stretched
- D The lining of the bladder is an example
- E The lining of the uterine cervix is an example

6.8 Intercellular adhering junctions:
- A Bind the cells of the epithelium together
- B Act as anchorage sites for the cytoskeleton of each cell
- C Include desmosomes
- D Include occluding junctions
- E Contribute to the resistance of the epithelium to mechanical stress

6.9 Communicating junctions:
- A Are also known as tight junctions
- B Allow electrical impulses to pass directly from one cell to another
- C Allow small positively charged ions to pass between epithelial cells
- D Are important for transfer of chemical signalling agents
- E Can be found in cardiac muscle

6.10 Unlike syncytiotrophoblasts, cytotrophoblasts in the second week of development:
- A Constitute the outer layer of the trophoblast
- B Are in direct contact with maternal sinusoids
- C Are multinucleated
- D Never contain mitotic figures
- E Produce human chorionic gonadotrophin (hCG)

6.11 Structures developed from the ectoderm include:
- A The aorta
- B The optic nerve
- C The peripheral nerves
- D Muscle fibres
- E The bladder

6.12 Structures developed from the endoderm include:
- A The heart

B The lungs
C Bones
D The stomach
E The liver

6.13 A baby was born with gross structural defects of the heart, gut and brain. The gestational period when these defects are induced may be:
A Two weeks
B Four weeks
C Six weeks
D 16 weeks
E 32 weeks

6.14 The following agents are teratogenic:
A Chickenpox virus
B X-rays
C Lithium
D Alcohol
E Rubella virus

6.15 The following statements about fetal development between the third and ninth month of gestation are true.

A The chambers of the heart are formed during the fifth month
B The rate of increase in fetal length is faster between the sixth and ninth month than between the third and sixth month of gestation
C The rate of increase in fetal weight is faster between the sixth and ninth month than between the third and sixth month of gestation
D Between the sixth and ninth month of gestation, the rate of growth is faster for the fetal head than the body
E The sex of the fetus can be determined by external ultrasound by about 12 weeks

6.16 A pair of twins can be confidently diagnosed to be dizygotic if:
A There are two placentas
B There are two chorionic cavities
C There are two amniotic cavities
D They are of different sex
E One twin is larger than the other

6 General principles of histology and embryology

A

GENERAL BASIC MEDICAL SCIENCES

6.1 B C D

The skin consists of the epidermis (superficial layer) and the dermis (the deeper layer). The epidermis has no blood supply. The cells in the outer layer (corneum) are keratinised, and are continuously shed. They are replaced by cells generated by mitosis in the innermost layer (stratum germinativum) of the epidermis, which lies adjacent to the dermis. Melanocytes, which produce the pigment melanin, are found in the stratum germinativum. The quantity of the pigment melanin determines the skin colour. Stratum germinativum is also known as stratum malpighii. The prickle cell layer (stratum spinosum) lies adjacent and superficial to the stratum germinativum, and is concerned with growth of the cells produced in the germinal layer.

6.2 A B C E

The dermis provides almost all the metabolic demands for the epidermis. It meets the epidermis at the dermal papillae, where the downward folds of epidermal ridges interdigitate with the upward projections of the dermis. This facilitates the adhesion between the epidermis and the dermis. There are two layers in the dermis: a superficial papillary dermis, and a deeper reticular layer. The papillary dermis consists mainly of collagen, and is highly vascular. The reticular layer consists of an interlacing arrangement of collagen fibre. Elastin is found in both layers, and accounts for the elastic property of the skin. The dermis provides non-specific defences against infection both as a physical barrier and via the tissue macrophages, white cells and mast cells.

6.3 B D

The arrector pili muscles originate from the sheath of hair follicles to the dermal papillae. The muscles are supplied by the sympathetic nervous system. Cold and fear cause contractions of the muscles, and results in 'goose-flesh' appearance of the skin as well as hair erection. Hair erection results in increased insulation due to more air being trapped by a thicker layer of hair. However, this effect is much less pronounced in humans than in other furry animals.

6.4 A C

When the temperature increases, heat loss from the skin increases via several mechanisms. Firstly, the sweat production increases, and heat loss via evaporation increases. Secondly, blood flow to the surface of the skin increases. Thirdly, the hairs become less erect, and a thinner layer of air is trapped. An increase in temperature per se does not alter the number of melanocytes, although increased exposure to sunlight may increase the melanocyte count. Sebaceous glands secrete sebum, an oily substance, onto the hair surface. The secretion of sebum varies little with temperature.

6.5 A B E

A basement membrane is a condensed layer of connective tissue at the boundary of epithelia or muscle fibres. The basement membrane is particularly important for the adhesion between cells and the support of epithelia as they are made up of closely packed cells. The basement membrane also acts as a control of epithelial growth, as physiological growth does not breach the basement membrane. Any growth of epithelial tissues which breaches the basement membrane is probably malignant. Basement membranes do not receive a blood supply, and they rely on nutrients diffused from the epithelium. In many tissues (e.g. the glomeruli), the basement membrane forms a highly selective filter for the passage of substances from one body compartment to another.

6.6 C

The correct matching is:
- Distal convoluted renal tubule – simple cuboidal epithelium
- Capillary wall – simple squamous epithelium
- Gallbladder lining – simple columnar epithelium (unciliated)
- Bronchial lining – pseudostratified columnar ciliated epithelium (i.e. one layer of cells, but nuclei are at different levels to give a false impression of more than one layer of cells)
- Oviduct lining – simple columnar ciliated epithelium

6.7 B C D

Transitional epithelium is a form of stratified epithelium, as not all the cells rest on the basement membrane. It is arranged so that the apparent number of cell layers decreases when stretched, although the total number of cells remains constant. Hence, it can withstand a greater degree of stretch. It is found almost exclusively in the urinary tract, where the epithelia also have to withstand the toxicity of urine. The lining of the uterine cervix consists of stratified squamous epithelium.

6.8 A B C E

There are three main types of intracellular junctions: occluding (or tight) junctions, adhering junctions, and communicating (or gap) junctions. The main function of occluding junctions is to prevent passage of substances from one side of the epithelium to the other. The main function of adhering junctions is to link the constituent cells of the epithelium together so that the whole epithelium functions together. This confers resistance to the epithelium against mechanical stress. This is achieved by the adhering junctions binding the constituent cells together, as well as acting as anchorage sites for the cytoskeleton of each cell. They may be of the continuous belt type or the spot type (desmosomes). Desmosomes are small circular patches circumferentially arranged around epithelial cells.

6.9 C D E
Communicating junctions are also known as gap (or nexus) junctions. They consist of numerous tiny pores allowing passage of substances from one cell to another. These substances include small ions or molecules important in the passage of chemical messengers and ions responsible for the depolarisation of cell membranes. Communicating junctions are also important for cell recognition. They also occur in cardiac and visceral muscle.

6.10 –
In the second week of development, the trophoblast differentiates into two layers: an outer layer (syncytiotrophoblast) and an inner layer (cytotrophoblast). The cells in the cytotrophoblast can undergo mitosis and divide, and migrate into the syncytiotrophoblast. The cells in the cytotrophoblast are mononucleated. The syncytiotrophoblast is in direct contact with maternal sinusoids. The cells in the syncytiotrophoblast have fused and lost their individual cell membranes. Hence, they are multinucleated. The two layers also have different functions. The syncytiotrophoblast produces (hCG) to maintain pregnancy. The cytotrophoblast later forms the primary villi.

6.11 B C
Major structures developed from the ectoderm include:
- The central nervous system
- The peripheral nervous system
- Pituitary glands
- Enamel of the teeth
- Sensory organs
- Epidermis

Major structures developed from the mesoderm include:
- The heart and blood vessels
- Muscle fibres
- Bone and cartilage
- Spleen
- Kidneys (not bladder)
- Gonads

6.12 B D E
See question 6.11 above. Structures developed from the endoderm include:

- Gastrointestinal tract and liver (being an outgrowth from the embryological gut)
- Respiratory tract
- Urinary bladder
- Parenchyma of thyroid and parathyroid glands, pancreas

6.13 B C
Gross structural defects of multiple major organs are most likely to be induced during the period of organogenesis, when the main organs in the body are formed. The period of organogenesis is about three to eight weeks of gestation.

6.14 A B C D E
Teratogenic agents include radiation, drugs, hormones and infections. Many drugs are potentially teratogenic, and include alcohol (which results in fetal alcohol syndrome), lithium (which causes specific heart abnormality) and thalidomide (which causes limb defects). Infections causing congenital malformations include the TORCHS infection (toxoplasmosis, rubella, cytomegalovirus, hepatitis B, syphilis), chickenpox virus (which causes limb and brain abnormalities) and HIV.

6.15 C E
Nearly all major organs have been formed by three months gestation, and maturation of these organs and growth occur between the third and ninth months of gestation. The rate of increase in fetal length is faster, but the rate of increase in fetal weight is slower between the third and sixth months than between the sixth and ninth of months of gestation. The rate of fetal head growth declines rapidly after the fifth month. The external genitalia are visible on ultrasound by 12 weeks.

6.16 D
Whether a pair of monozygotic twins share the same placenta, chorionic cavity or amniotic cavity depends on when splitting of the zygote occurred. If it occurred at the two-cell stage, each twin will have its own placenta, amniotic cavity and chorionic cavity. If splitting occurred at a late stage of development, there will be only one placenta, amniotic cavity and chorionic cavity. Monozygotic twins share exactly the same genes, and hence must be of the same sex. In about 10% of monozygotic twins who share the same chorionic cavity, the blood flow to the placenta is such that one twin receives much more blood than the other. This results in one twin being larger than the other.

General principles of genetics

7 **Q**

GENERAL BASIC MEDICAL SCIENCES

7.1 The following statements about trinucleotide repeat amplification as a mechanism of length mutation are true:
- **A** It is inherited as a chromosome disorder
- **B** Longer trinucleotide repeats are generally more unstable
- **C** Longer trinucleotide repeats are associated with more severe disease
- **D** Members of the same affected family usually have the same number of repeats
- **E** Dystrophic myotonia results from trinucleotide repeat amplification

7.2 The following are appropriate uses of DNA analysis techniques:
- **A** To exclude or identify suspects in rape offences
- **B** To resolve paternity disputes
- **C** To determine the carrier status of an asymptomatic female with a family history of a sex-linked recessive inherited disorder
- **D** To identify meningococcal antigens in patients with suspected meningococcal disease
- **E** To diagnose an autosomal recessive disease in an asymptomatic individual before symptoms develop

7.3 The following statements about meiosis are true:
- **A** It occurs in all tissues
- **B** It results in the formation of two diploid daughter cells
- **C** It occurs throughout life in the adult male
- **D** It occurs throughout life in the adult female
- **E** Crossover allows wider variation of genetic make-up of the gametes

7.4 The following human karyotypes are examples of trisomy:
- **A** 69, XXY
- **B** 69, XXX
- **C** 47, XX, +21
- **D** 45, XO
- **E** 46, XY

7.5 The following human karyotypes are examples of polyploidy:
- **A** 47, XX, +18
- **B** 46, XX
- **C** 69, XYY
- **D** 92, XXYY
- **E** 47, XXY

7.6 The following statements about a mosaic are true:
- **A** It arises from more than one zygote
- **B** It almost always results in a non-viable fetus

- **C** A gonadal mosaic trisomy has a high risk of producing abnormal children
- **D** A gonadal mosaic trisomy can be easily diagnosed clinically
- **E** It is caused by double fertilisation of the egg

7.7 Jane suffers from a disease. Two of her three sons and one out of her three daughters also have the disease. Three of her seven grandsons and two of her three granddaughters have the disease. Likely modes of inheritance for the disease include:
- **A** Autosomal recessive
- **B** Autosomal dominant
- **C** Sex-linked recessive
- **D** Sex-linked dominant
- **E** Chromosomal disorder

7.8 Compared to autosomal recessive disorders, autosomal dominant disorders:
- **A** Are less severe
- **B** Tend to have a horizontal pedigree pattern
- **C** Have a higher risk of transmission to offspring
- **D** Are more likely to be associated with defective enzymes
- **E** Affect more males than females

7.9 Non-penetrance:
- **A** Usually occurs in autosomal recessive disorders
- **B** May give rise to individuals with a normal genotype but an abnormal phenotype
- **C** May give rise to individuals with an abnormal genotype but a normal phenotype
- **D** Implies that a phenotypically normal individual will not pass on an abnormal autosomal dominant gene to the offspring
- **E** Makes it easier to offer genetic counselling

7.10 The following statements about sex-linked recessive disorders are true:
- **A** They affect males and females with equal frequency
- **B** 50% of the sons of an affected father have the disease
- **C** 50% of the daughters of an affected father have the disease
- **D** 50% of the sons of a carrier mother have the disease
- **E** 50% of the daughters of a carrier mother have the disease

7.11 Amongst the offspring of a normal father and a mother who is a homozygote for a sex-linked recessive disorder:

A 50% of all children have the disease
B 25% of all children have a normal genotype
C 50% of all daughters are carriers
D 50% of all daughters have the disease
E 50% of all sons have the disease

7.12 The following statements about X-linked dominant conditions are true:
A They are commoner than X-linked recessive conditions
B They affect more males than females
C They have a knight's move pedigree pattern
D Females are affected more severely than males
E The severity of the condition is uniform amongst all females

7.13 A newly discovered disease can be shown to be multifactorial in inheritance by:
A Analysis of the pedigree of a single family
B Chromosomal analysis
C Twin concordance study
D Family correlation study
E Biochemical analysis of gene products

7.14 The following relations have a quarter of their genes in common:
A Mother and daughter
B Grandfather and grandson
C Brother and sister
D Uncle and nephew
E First cousins

7.15 The following statements about trisomy 21 are true:
A In over 50% of affected individuals, one of the parents is a carrier of balanced translocation
B The incidence is lower amongst spontaneous abortus than live births
C The incidence is lower amongst stillbirths than live births
D Overall, the risk of recurrence in future pregnancy is 25%
E Carriers of a balanced translocation can usually be diagnosed by physical examination

7.16 The offspring of the following have a significantly increased risk of Down's syndrome compared with the general population:
A A mother with Turner's syndrome
B A 40-year-old mother
C A carrier of balanced translocation involving chromosomes 21 and 22
D Parents with consanguineous relationships
E A father with spina bifida

7.17 The following statements about fragile X syndrome are correct:
A It is the commonest inherited cause of mental handicap in males
B It generally affects males more severely than females
C Prenatal diagnosis is possible
D It results from deletion of part of an X chromosome
E All females of the same family who inherit the condition are affected equally

7.18 Methods of prenatal diagnosis include:
A Fetal DNA analysis
B Amniotic fluid biochemistry
C Ultrasound scan
D Fetal enzyme assay
E Fetal karyotyping

7.19 The prevalence of an autosomal recessive disorder in a population is one in 2500. Assuming heterozygotes do not have selective advantages over normal individuals:
A The carrier frequency is one in 1250
B The risk of disease to the offspring of two carrier parents is one in two
C The risk of disease to the offspring of a carrier parent and a parent randomly chosen from the general population is one in 100
D The risk of disease to the offspring of an affected parent and a parent randomly chosen from the general population is one in four
E The risk of disease to the offspring of two affected parents is one in two

7.20 The ability to roll the tongue is inherited as an autosomal dominant. Assuming that the gene is in genetic equilibrium in a population, and that the current proportion of those who cannot roll their tongue is q^2:
A The current proportion of those who can roll their tongue is $1 - q^2$
B The current proportion of heterozygotes is $q(1 - q)$
C The current proportion of those who have two tongue-rolling genes is $(1 - q)^2$
D The proportion of heterozygotes in the next generation is $2q(1 - q)$
E The proportion of those who cannot roll their tongue in the next generation is $2q^2$

7.21 The following bases occur at the start of the coding region of an mRNA sequence for a specific protein.

7

Q

GENERAL BASIC MEDICAL SCIENCES

Genetics

AUGUGUUACAAGCCUAGUGGU . . .

Mutation occurs in the following individuals, and the resulting mRNA sequences are shown. For each, name the type of mutation and postulate the likely effects on the protein products (e.g. no effects; altered activity, function or stability; loss of activity, function or stability). Explain.

A AUGUUUACAAGCCUAGUGGU . . .

B AUGUGUUACAAAGCCUAGUGGU . . .

C AUGUGUUACAAACCUAGUGGU . . .

D AUGUGUAAGCCUAGUGGU . . .

E AUGUGUUACUGAAAGCCUAGUGGU . . .

F AUGUGUUAAUACAAGCCUAGUGGU . . .

G AUGUGUUACAUUAAGCCUAGUGGU . . .

H AUGCGUUACAAGCCUAGUGGU . . .

I AUGUGUUGUUGUUGUUGUUGUUGUUACAAGCCU AGUGGU . . .

You are given the genetic code in terms of RNA codons:

Amino acids	Codes
Lysine	AAA, AAG
Tyrosine	UAU, UAC
Isoleucine	AUU, AUC, AUA
Cysteine	UGU, UGC
Arginine	CGU, CGC, CGA, CGG
Chain termination	UAA, UAG, UGA, UGG

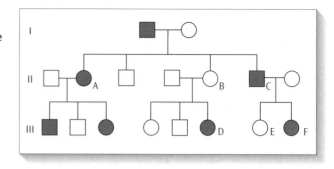

Fig. 7.1

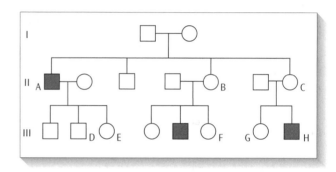

Fig. 7.2

7.22 The karotypes of seven individuals are shown below. For each, give the phenotypic sex, and whether the individual is normal. If abnormal, give the abnormality and the underlying mechanism for the abnormality.

A 46, XX

B 47, XY, +21

C 45, XO

D 47, XXY

E 69, XXY

F 46, XY, del(5p)

G 46, XX / 47, XX, +21

7.23 The family tree in Fig. 7.1 shows members suffering from a rare disease with single gene Mendelian inheritance. The family tree was constructed based on clinical diagnosis without knowledge of any genetic test results. Male and female members are shown by squares and circles, respectively. Filled squares or circles indicate phenotypically affected individuals. Empty squares or circles indicate phenotypically normal individuals.

A What is the inheritance? Explain your answer.

B If A, C and F marry people in the general population, what is the risk that their sons and daughters will be affected by the disease?

C From the family tree, B is phenotypically normal but D is affected. Give two possible explanations for this phenomenon. Which of these explanation is more likely?

7.24 The family tree in Fig. 7.2 shows members suffering from a rare disease with single gene Mendelian inheritance. The family tree was constructed based on clinical diagnosis without knowledge of any genetic test results.

A What is the inheritance? Explain.

B If the following individuals marry people in the general population, what is the risk that their sons and daughters will be affected by the disease? Explain.

  i D

  ii E

  iii F

  iv G

  v H

C What genotypes would you expect the following individuals to show on genetic testing?

  i A

  ii B

  iii C

D Give a possible reason (using chromosome inactivation hypothesis) why B does not show any obvious signs of the disease. Is it possible that she may have mild abnormalities on careful examination or laboratory testing? What determines whether someone with the same genotype will show any clinical signs of the disease?

7.25 The family tree in Fig. 7.3 shows members suffering from a disease with single gene Mendelian inheritance. The prevalence of the disease amongst all births is 1 in 40 000. The family tree was constructed based on clinical diagnosis without knowledge of any genetic test results.
A What is the inheritance? Explain.
B A and B would like to have more children. What is the chance that they will be affected by the disease?
C C would like to have more children. What is the chance that they will be affected by the disease? State any assumptions you make.

7.26 The family tree in Fig. 7.4 shows members suffering from a disease with single gene Mendelian inheritance.

A Which two modes of inheritance are compatible with this family tree? Which is more likely, according to the following parameters. Explain:
  i The pattern of inheritance in the family
  ii How common the mode of inheritance is.
B Assume the mode of inheritance is that which would explain the greater proportion of affected females compared with affected males. What is the risk of the sons and daughters of the following individuals inheriting the disease?
  i A
  ii B
  iii C
  iv D

7.27 The blood groups of some members of the families shown in Fig. 7.5 are given in Table 7.1.
A Explain how the ABO blood group is inherited.
B What are the genotypes of individuals A, B, C, F and G.
C What are the possible blood groups for D? What are the possible genotypes?
D What are the genotypes of E and H? Explain.

7.28 There is a gene locus with two alleles *B* and *b*, where *B* is dominant over *b*. The genotypes of 1000

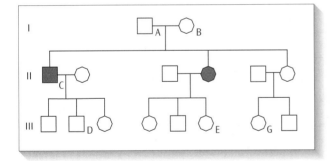

Fig. 7.3

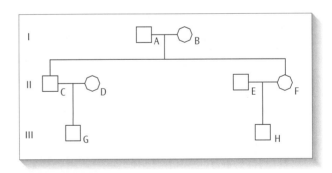

Fig. 7.5

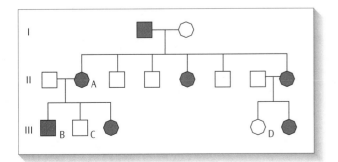

Fig. 7.4

Table 7.1

Individual	Blood group
A	A
B	B
C	O
E	A
G	A
H	B

individuals, randomly sampled from a population of 1 million on an isolated island, are tested. The results are:

Genotypes	Number
BB	487
Bb	422
Bb	91

A Estimate the gene frequencies of *B* and *b* (to one decimal place).

B Is the population in Hardy–Weinberg equilibrium? Explain.

C Estimate the gene frequencies in the next two generations. Explain.

D Assume that the population increases by 50% (to 1.5 million) in the next generation as a result of reproduction within the population. Estimate the number of people in the population with genotypes *BB*, *Bb* and *bb*.

7.29 The family tree in Fig. 7.6 shows members suffering from a disease with sex-linked recessive inheritance.

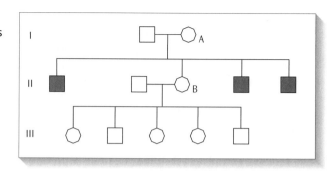

Fig. 7.6

Individuals with the disease can be diagnosed at birth, but the carrier state cannot be detected. Individual B sees you for genetic counselling. What is the chance that she is a carrier for the disease? What is the risk that her next child will be affected by the disease?

7

Q

General principles of genetics ⑦

7.1 B C E
Trinucleotide repeat amplification is a type of length mutation. Repeats of trinucleotides normally occur between and within genes. However, if the number of repeats is longer than normal, it may become unstable. Single-gene disorders result if it is associated within a gene. The longer the trinucleotide repeat, the more severe the disease. Different members of an affected family may have different lengths of repeats, and this explains the different degree of severity of the disease within the family. Examples of diseases associated with trinucleotide repeat amplification include dystrophic myotonia and Huntington's chorea.

7.2 A B C D E
DNA analysis techniques have been used for a wide range of purposes such as genetic counselling and research, detection of crime and to resolve paternity disputes. DNA analysis may be used to detect the carrier status of a female in a family with a sex-linked recessive disorder (e.g. haemophilia). It may also be used to diagnose a recessive condition before symptoms develop (e.g. cystic fibrosis).

   The two basic DNA analysis techniques are the Southern analysis and polymerase chain reaction (PCR) techniques. In Southern analysis, the DNA under analysis is cleaved into fragments using a specific restriction enzyme, the fragments are then separated according to size by electrophoresis. These are transferred to a DNA binding site filter, and the fragments may be identified by autoradiography. PCR analysis is more sensitive and faster. Two oligonucleotide primers complementary to the target segment of DNA are used. The primers initiate repeated DNA replication to produce numerous copies of the target sequence. The amplified DNA fragment can then be cleaved, separated by electrophoresis and directly visualised under ultraviolet light.

7.3 C E
Meiosis is a type of cell division which occurs in the gonads and results in the formation of gametes. It starts with a diploid cell and results in the formation of two daughter haploid gametes. It occurs after puberty in males and continues throughout life, although the rate declines in old age. In females, the maximum number of germ cells is less than 200 000 at puberty, and only about 400 will ovulate (about once a month) in her lifetime. Meiosis ceases after the menopause. Crossover during meiosis is the exchange of genetic material between the two chromosomes. This adds considerably to the variation of the genetic make-up of the resulting gametes.

7.4 C
Trisomy is the presence of an extra copy of a chromosome. Since the normal number of chromosomes in humans is 46,

trisomy results in a cell with 47 chromosomes. In 47, XX, +21, an extra number 21 chromosome is present, and is characteristic of Down's syndrome. 69, XXY and 69, XXX result from the presence of a complete extra set of chromosomes, and is known as triploidy. 46, XY is the karyotype of a normal male. 45, XO results from the loss of an X chromosome from the normal female, and is characteristic of Turner's syndrome.

7.5 C D
Polyploidy results from complete extra sets of chromosomes. 69, XYY is an example of triploidy with an extra set of chromosomes. The exact sex chromosome constitution depends on whether they are of maternal or paternal origin. 92, XXYY is an example of tetraploidy with two extra sets of chromosomes. 47, XX, +18 results from an extra number 18 chromosome, and is known as Edwards' syndrome. It is an example of trisomy. 47, XXY results from an extra X chromosome, and is known as Klinefelter's syndrome. 46, XX is the karyotype of a normal female.

7.6 C
A mosaic is an individual with two or more cell lines derived from a single zygote. It arises after fertilisation. A chimera is an individual with two cell lines derived from two separate zygotes, and could be caused by double fertilisation of the egg. A mosaic trisomy usually has a normal cell line and a trisomy cell line. The clinical features are usually less marked than a pure trisomy. A gonadal trisomy has trisomy cell lines confined to the gonads. Whilst they appear outwardly normal, they have a high risk of producing abnormal children.

7.7 B
In sex-linked recessive disorders, females who carry the affected gene in one of the chromosomes are carriers, and only males are affected. Sex-linked dominant disorders are rare. A father never transmits the disease to his sons. Autosomal recessive disorder is usually characterised by a horizontal pedigree pattern, and the risk of transmission to offspring is small. In autosomal dominant disorder, approximately half of the offspring are affected, and it occurs equally in each sex. Chromosomal disorder may occasionally transmit from parent to child (e.g. balanced translocation of trisomy). However, usually less than half of the children are affected.

7.8 A C
Autosomal dominant disorders are usually less severe than autosomal recessive disorders. Reproduction may not be possible in severe autosomal dominant disorders (e.g. Apert's syndrome), and new cases arise by mutation.

7 **Genetics**

A

GENERAL BASIC MEDICAL SCIENCES

Autosomal dominant disorders have a 50% risk of passing on to the offspring, and usually have a vertical pedigree pattern. It is usually associated with disorders of structural or receptor proteins, whereas autosomal recessive disorders are generally associated with defective enzymes. Both autosomal dominant and recessive disorders affect each sex equally.

7.9 C
Non-penetrance occurs in autosomal dominant disorders, when a person with the abnormal gene has the normal phenotype and appears clinically normal. Hence, a phenotypically normal but genetically affected individual has a 50% chance of transmitting the disease to his or her offspring. An example is the autosomal dominant inherited colonic cancer. Non-penetrance makes it difficult to offer genetic counselling, as affected individuals are difficult to distinguish from genetically normal individuals.

7.10 D
In sex-linked recessive disorders, a male with an abnormal gene in his X chromosome has the disease, where as a female with an abnormal gene in her X chromosome is a carrier. Hence, it occurs much more frequently in males than females. A father transmits his X chromosome to his daughters and his Y chromosome to his sons. Hence, none of his sons are affected, and all his daughters are carriers. A carrier mother has a 50% chance of transmitting her abnormal gene to both her sons and daughters. The sons with the abnormal gene will have the disease, whilst her daughters with the abnormal gene are carriers.

7.11 A
A mother who is a homozygote for a sex-linked recessive disorder has diseased genes on both her X chromosomes. Hence, one of the genes will be passed to all her children. All her daughters are carriers, and all her sons have the disease. Assuming half of her children are daughters, 50% of her children will have the disease.

7.12 –
X-linked dominant conditions are extremely rare. Examples are Xg blood groups and vitamin D-resistant rickets. A female has the disease if one or both of her X chromosomes contain the defective genes. Hence, the sex ratio is two females to one male. The pedigree pattern is vertical. It is similar to the autosomal dominant pattern except that there is no male-to-male transmission. Males are more severely affected than females. The severity of affected females is variable due to the process of inactivation of one of the X chromosomes in somatic cells in females (the process of lyonisation).

7.13 C D
Multifactorial disorders are determined by a number of genes at different loci as well as environmental factors. Each gene only has a small effect on the development of the disease. Hence, multifactorial disorders cannot be proved by analysis of the pedigree of a single family. Chromosomal analysis is also not helpful, as the genes involved are often unidentified. Twin concordance study compares the concordance rates between monozygotic and dizygotic twins in a large number of twins. Family correlation study compares the concordance amongst family members with the proportion of genes shared by them. Twin concordance and family correlation studies are the best tools to show multifactorial disorders.

7.14 B D
Monozygotic (identical) twins have 100% of their genes in common. First-degree relations (e.g. parents and child; siblings) have half of their genes in common. Second-degree relations (e.g. grandparent and grandchild; uncle/aunt and nephew/niece) have a quarter of their genes in common. Third-degree relations (e.g. first cousins) have an eighth of their genes in common.

7.15 –
About 95% of trisomy 21 cases result from non-disjunction at meiosis, most commonly at the first meiotic division. Both parents are normal in these cases. As chromosomal abnormalities often result in either spontaneous abortion or stillbirth, the incidence of all trisomies is higher amongst the spontaneous abortus than live births. For young parents who are not carriers of balanced translocations, the risk of recurrence is about 1%, although the risk is higher for older parents. Carriers of a balanced translocation are phenotypically normal, and cannot be diagnosed by physical examination. Chromosomal analysis is necessary.

7.16 B C
The incidence of Down's syndrome increases steeply with maternal age. The incidence is slightly higher in offspring of older fathers. A translocation refers to the transfer of chromosomal material between chromosomes. If the transfer results in no overall increase or reduction of chromosomal material, it is said to be a balanced translocation. The person appears normal. About 0.2% of the general population has balanced translocation. The offspring of carriers of a balanced translocation have a significantly increased risk of Down's syndrome. The risk depends on the type of balanced translocation. For example, the risk to the offspring of a parent with centric fusion of the chromosomes 13;14 is only 1%, whereas the corresponding risk for centric fusion 21;21 has a 100% risk.

7.17 A B C

Fragile X syndrome results from an unstable mutation of a trinucleotide CGG repeat in the X chromosome. In the pre-mutation condition, there are less than about 200 trinucleotide repeats. In the full mutation condition, there are over 200 repeats. Fragile X syndrome is the commonest inherited cause of mental handicap. The full mutation condition occurs in about one in every 1250 males, and the pre-mutation condition occurs in about one in 750 males. Males with the full mutation are mentally handicapped. Females with the full mutation may range from being normal to moderately mentally handicapped. This variability is partly due to lyonisation (inactivation of one X chromosome in the female), and partly due to different lengths mutation. Prenatal diagnosis is possible by DNA analysis of samples taken by chorionic villous biopsy.

7.18 A B C D E

Methods of prenatal diagnosis include fetal DNA analysis (e.g. for single-gene disorders such as cystic fibrosis), fetal karyotyping (e.g. for chromosomal disorders), fetal enzyme assay (e.g. for inborn errors of metabolism), amniotic fluid biochemistry (e.g. AFP level for increased risk of neural tube defect) and ultrasound scan (e.g. for structural abnormalities).

7.19 C

For autosomal disorders, the risk of the disease to the offspring from two carrier parents is one in four. If the carrier frequency is x, the expected prevalence of disease would be $1/4 \ x^2$. Putting $1/4x^2 = 1/2500$ gives the carrier frequency of one in 25. The same answer can be obtained using the Hardy–Weinberg law.

The risk of disease to the offspring of a carrier parent and a parent from the general population would be $1/4 \times 1/25 = 1/100$. The risk of disease to the offspring of an affected parent and a parent from the general population is $1/2 \times 1/25 = 1/50$.

The risk of disease to the offspring of two affected parents is 100%.

7.20 A C D

If the proportion of those with homozygous recessive gene is q^2, the proportion of those who can roll their tongue is $1 - q^2$. According to the Hardy–Weinberg law, the proportion of those with the two dominant genes is p^2 (where $p = 1 - q$), and the proportion of heterozygotes is $2pq$. (NB: the total is $p^2 + 2pq + q^2 = 1$.) If the population is in genetic equilibrium, these proportions do not change in subsequent generations.

7.21

A mutation is an alteration in genetic material. Mutations in the non-coding DNA generally do not have any phenotypic effects unless they occur in the promoter region which regulates gene expression. Mutations in the coding DNA may result in alteration or loss of function, activity and stability of the resulting protein.

In the coding region of the mRNA, each three-nucleotide bases (triplet or codon) codes for a particular amino acid. Chain termination is coded for by one of four termination codons. To determine the effect of a mutation in the coding region, it is important to determine:

1. Whether there is a shift in the reading frame (order of the triplet codons). Deletion or insertion of bases that are not in multiples of 3 will produce a shift in the reading frame. For example, if a deletion occurs in the sequence AUGAAAUACUAA to form AUGAAUACUAA, the original sequence will read as AUG-AAA-UAC-UAA, while the mutated sequence will read as AUG-AAU-ACU-AA, etc. A shift in the reading frame will inevitably lead to completely altered amino acid sequence.

2. Whether the mutation causes premature termination. If a mutation causes a codon coding for an amino acid to be changed to a termination codon, premature termination occurs. For example, the sequence AUGUGCGUU-codes for methionine-cysteine-valine-, whereas the sequence AUGUGAGUU-codes for methionine, and the chain is terminated by the codon UGA. Premature termination is likely to lead to loss of activity, function or stability of the resulting protein.

3. If there is no shift in the reading frame or premature termination, whether there is a change in the amino acid sequence. Substitution in the first or second bases in a codon almost always leads to a change in an amino acid. This may lead to an alteration of protein activity, function or stability of the resulting protein. Substitution in the third base in a codon may or may not change the amino acid coded. If it does not, the mutation is silent and no phenotypic or clinical effects are observed.

A

There is a deletion of G in the second base of the second triplet. This leads to a shift in the reading frame, and hence to a completely altered amino acid sequence.

B

There is an insertion of A in the third base of the fourth triplet. This leads to a shift in the reading frame, and hence to an altered amino acid sequence.

C

There is a substitution of AAA for AAG in the fourth triplet. From the genetic code given, both AAA and AAG code for lysine. Hence, the mutation is silent and there will be no phenotypic or clinical effects.

D

There is a deletion of the entire third triplet UAC. There is no shift in the reading frame, but there will be one amino acid less in the resulting polypeptide. This may lead to altered activity, function or stability of the resulting protein.

E

There is an insertion of UGA before the fourth triplet. Since UGA codes for chain termination, premature chain termination will occur, with resulting loss of function or activity of the resulting protein.

F

There is a substitution of UAA for UAC in the third triplet. From the genetic code given, UAC codes for tyrosine whereas UAA codes for chain termination. Hence, there will be premature chain termination with resulting loss of function or activity of the resulting protein.

G

There is an insertion of the triplet AUU before the fourth triplet. There is no shift in the reading frame, but there will be an extra amino acid (isoleucine) in the resulting polypeptide. This may lead to altered activity, function or stability of the resulting protein.

H

There is a substitution of CGU for UGU in the second triplet. This results in the substitution of the amino acid arginine for cysteine. This may lead to altered activity, function or stability of the resulting protein.

I

There are six extra repeats of the triplet UGU, which codes for cysteine. This is called a triplet amplification or expansion, and represents an unstable mutation. This leads to altered gene expression. Several diseases (e.g. Huntington's disease, myotonic dystrophy, fragile X mental retardation) have been identified to be due to triplet amplification, and almost all are associated with serious disorders of the central nervous system.

7.22

The karotype of an individual is usually represented by a chromosomal shorthand notation (e.g. 47, XY, +21). The figure 47 denotes that the individual has a total of 47 chromosomes. The symbol XY denotes the sex chromosomes. The symbol +21 denotes gain of an extra chromosome 21. Normal humans have a total of 46 chromosomes, and normal male and female karyotypes are 46, XY and 46, XX, respectively. The genetic sex is determined by the presence or absence of the Y

chromosome. Hence, XXY is genetically male, whereas XO is genetically female.

A

46, XX is a normal female karyotype.

B

47, XY, +21. The individual is a male as he has XY sex chromosome. He has a total of 47 chromosomes due to an extra chromosome 21. This is trisomy 21 or Down's syndrome. Individuals have short stature, characteristic facies, mental retardation, and there may be associated congenital abnormalities such as congenital heart disease. Most cases of Down's syndrome are due to failure of separation (non-disjunction) of one of the pairs of chromosome 21 during anaphase of maternal meiosis I. As a result, one gamete receives two copies of chromosome 21 and the gamete none. Occasionally, it may be due to non-disjunction of maternal meiosis II or of paternal meiosis. Rarely, Down's syndrome may result if one of the parents has a chromosome 21 transferred (translocated) to another chromosome (e.g. chromosome 14). The child may have trisomy 21 by receiving one chromosome 21 from each parent, in addition to the translocated chromosome.

C

45, XO. The individual is a female owing to the lack of a Y chromosome. She has 45 chromosomes as she only has one X chromosome. This is sex chromosome monosomy, or Turner's syndrome. As with trisomy, monosomy usually results from non-disjunction in meiosis. The gamete which receives two copies of a chromosome is responsible for trisomy and the gamete which does not receive a copy of the chromosome is responsible for monosomy.

D

47, XXY. The individual is a male owing to the presence of a Y chromosome. The disorder is Klinefelter's syndrome. Individuals may present with mild learning difficulties and clumsiness in childhood. Adults with the disorder usually have gynaecomastia (enlargement of breast tissue) and small infertile testes. The cause is non-disjunction at meiosis.

E

69, XXY. The individual has an extra set of all chromosomes. This is usually incompatible with life, and leads to abortion. It may be caused by failure to divide in meiosis, or rarely by fertilisation of an ovum by two sperm.

F

46, XY, del(5p). The individual is a male owing to the presence of a Y chromosome. The symbol del(5p) or 5p-denotes deletion of the short arm of chromosome 5. This individual is a male with cri-du-chat syndrome.

G

46, XX / 47, XX, +21. The symbol / stands for mosaicism – the presence in an individual of two or more cell lines derived from a single zygote but differing in their genetic composition. The individual is a female because the sex chromosomes in both cell lines are XX. The first cell line (46, XX) is that of a normal female karyotype. The second cell line (47, XX, +21) is that of a female with Down's syndrome. Hence, the individual is a mosaic Down's syndrome, and may have mild features of the disorder. Mosaicism usually results from non-disjunction after the zygote is formed, e.g. in an early embryonic mitotic division. It accounts for about 2% of all clinical cases of Down's syndrome.

7.23

A

According to the family tree, the disease can be traced through three generations and it is therefore likely that the disease is dominant (i.e. the disease is manifest in the heterozygous state). The disease can be passed from fathers to sons and daughters, and from mothers to sons and daughters. Hence, the gene is located in a autosomal chromosome: the inheritance is autosomal dominant.

B

Individuals A, C and F are all affected individuals (i.e. Aa where A is the disease allele). The probability of their sons or daughters inheriting the disease is 1/2.

C

From the family tree, individual D is affected, although neither of his parents were affected. The most likely reason is that individual B has the mutation genetically, but it was clinically undetectable. In other words, the disease is not 100% penetrant. This results in the disease skipping a generation. Another, much less likely, reason is that individual D has a new mutation. This is unlikely as we are told in the question that the disease in the population is rare; and a new mutation must therefore also be rare.

7.24

A

According to the family tree, the disease cannot be traced from one generation to another. Not all the affected individuals have an affected parent; therefore, the disease is inherited in a recessive manner. All the affected individuals are male, and the affected males inherit the disease from female members of the family. Hence, inheritance must be sex-linked recessive.

B

For diseases with sex-linked recessive inheritance, the risk of a carrier mother passing the disease to her sons is 1/2. Half of her daughters are carriers, but none are affected by the disease. An affected father never passes the disease to his sons, although all his daughters are carriers.

i   D is an unaffected male; hence, the risk of his children having the disease is zero.

ii E is a female, and the chance that she is a carrier is 1/2; the risk of E passing the disease to her sons is ($1/2 \times 1/2$) = 1/4. The risk of her daughters being affected by the disease is zero, although the risk that they are carriers is ($1/2 \times 1/2$) = 1/4.

iii F has an affected brother; hence, F's mother must be a carrier, and the chance that F is a carrier herself is 1/2. The chance that F's sons are affected is 1/4. The chance that her daughters are affected is zero, although the risk that they are carriers is 1/4.

iv G has an affected brother. The answer is the same as for F in (iii).

v   H is an affected male. The risk that his sons or daughters are affected is zero, but all his daughters will be carriers.

C

Let s be the affected allele and S be the normal allele.

i   Individual A is an affected male: his genotype is $X^s Y^s$.

ii Individual B is a carrier female: her genotype is $X^s X^S$.

iii Individual C is a also a carrier female: her genotype is also $X^s X^S$.

D

In 1961, Dr Mary Lyon proposed that, in females, one of the X chromosomes is inactivated in each cell in early embryogenesis. Either the maternally or paternally derived X chromosomes can be inactivated. This process is known as Lyonisation; it accounts for the presence of the Barr body in the nucleus of female cells, and the observation that the level of protein products derived from the X chromosomes (e.g. factor VIII) in females is similar to that in males.

Individual B is a carrier female. One would expect that in about 50% of her cells, the normal X chromosomes are active, while the diseased X chromosomes are active in the remaining 50%. The observation that she has no clinical signs for the disease could be explained in several ways. First, cells with active normal X chromosomes may have a selective advantage over cells with active diseased X chromosomes. Second, the relevant cells with the active normal X chromosomes may correct the defects in the adjacent abnormal cells. Third, the relevant protein products may usually be produced in excess, so that a reduction in the level of the protein products may not result in clinical symptoms or signs.

Genetics

It is possible that individual B may show mild features of the disease on careful examination or laboratory testing. Rarely, a female carrier shows mild or moderate features of the disease. This may occur if the production of relevant protein products are normally only just adequate. Alternatively, it may occur if by chance the normal X chromosomes are inactivated in significantly more than 50% of the cells.

7.25

A

According to the family tree, the disease cannot be traced from one generation to the next. Parents of the affected individuals appear to be normal: the disease is likely to be recessive. Both males and females may be affected: inheritance is autosomal recessive.

B

Both A and B must be carriers as they have two affected children: the risk of their children having the disease is 1/4.

C

C is affected: he is homozygous for the disease. The chance of his spouse being a carrier is that of the general population. We are told that the prevalence of the disease in the population is 1 in 40 000. Let p and q be the gene frequencies for the normal and disease genes respectively. Hence,

$$q^2 = 1/40\,000.\ q = 1/200,\ p = 1 - q = 199/200.$$

The chance of a person in the general population being a carrier is $2pq = 1/100$.
C's children will definitely inherit a disease gene from C. The chance that C's spouse will also pass on a diseased gene is $1/2 \times 1/100 = 1/200$; hence, the chance that a child of C will be affected by the disease is 1/200.

We have used the Hardy–Weinberg principle to calculate the carrier frequency and assumed that the population is in a state of Hardy–Weinberg equilibrium: no non-random mating, no selection, and no migration from populations with different gene frequencies.

7.26

A

From the family tree, the disease can be traced from one generation to the next. All affected members have one affected parent: the disease gene is dominant. Both males and females are affected: both autosomal dominant and sex-linked dominant inheritance are possible.

i Females are more likely to be affected than males. Furthermore, affected fathers pass on the disease to all their daughters, but not to their sons. Affected mothers pass on the disease to some of their sons and daughters. This pattern is characteristic of sex-linked dominant inheritance. One example of sex-linked dominant inherited disease is vitamin D-resistant rickets.

ii However, this does not exclude autosomal dominant inheritance altogether. The fact that only daughters are affected in the second generation might be due to chance. Autosomal dominant conditions are much more common than sex-linked dominant conditions.

B

Assume that the inheritance is sex-linked dominant. Fathers pass on the X chromosome to daughters and the Y chromosome to sons; hence, affected fathers pass on the disease to all daughters but to no sons. Affected mothers pass on the disease to half her sons and half her daughters.

i A is an affected female: half her sons and half her daughters will be affected.

ii B is an affected male: all of his daughters but none of his sons will be affected.

iii C is a normal male: none of his children will be affected.

iv D is a normal female: none of her children will be affected.

7.27

A

The ABO blood group is inherited, with the two alleles A and B being codominant, and the allele O being recessive to both A and B. Persons who possess the antigen A (but not antigen B) on the surface of their red cells have blood group A. Persons who possess antigen B (but not antigen A) have blood group B. Persons who possess both antigens have blood group AB. Persons who possess neither antigens have blood group O. The possible genotypes and their associated phenotypes are given in Table 7.2.

B

See Table 7.3. Note that:

• Individual C has blood group O: his genotype must be OO. His parents, A and B, must have the allele O in one of their chromosomes.

Table 7.2

Phenotype (blood groups)	Genotypes
O	OO
A	AA, AO
B	BB, BO
AB	AB

- H has blood group B. He must have inherited the allele B from his mother F, as his father E has blood group A. F must have inherited the allele B from her mother, and the allele O from his father. Hence, the genotype for F is BO.
- G has blood group A. His father C has genotype OO. Hence, G must have genotype AO.

C

G has genotype AO. He must have inherited the allele O from his father C, and the allele A from his mother D. D's genotype can be AO, AA or AB. Her blood group may be either A or AB.

D

The genotype of F is BO. Since E has blood group A, his genotype is either AA or AO. However, the first alternative is not possible, as his son H has blood group B; hence, E has genotype AO. H must have inherited the allele O from his father E and the allele B from his mother F; hence, H must have genotype BO.

7.28

A

The frequencies of the B allele in 1000 individuals (with 2000 alleles) are shown in Table 7.4.

The total number of copies of B out of 2000 alleles is $974 + 422 + 0 = 1396$. Hence, the gene frequency for B is $1396/2000 = 0.698 = 0.7$ (to 1 decimal place). The gene frequency for b is $1 - 0.7 = 0.3$.

B

Assume that the gene frequencies for B and b are 0.7 and 0.3 respectively (i.e. $p = 0.7$, $q = 0.3$). If the population is in Hardy-Weinberg equilibrium, the expected frequencies for the genotypes BB, Bb and bb and the expected numbers out of a 1000 population are shown in Table 7.5. The table shows that the actual number with each of the genotypes is very close to that expected from Hardy–Weinberg principles; hence, the population is in Hardy–Weinberg equilibrium.

C

By Hardy–Weinberg principles, the gene frequencies remain constant in all successive generations provided that there is no non-random mating, selection or migration; hence, the gene frequencies for B and b will remain 0.7 and 0.3, respectively.

D

If the population increases to 1.5 million by reproduction and not by migration, the gene frequencies for B and b will remain the same, and the proportion of the different genotypes will be the same as shown Table 7.5.

The expected number of people in the population with each of the genotypes are therefore:
- BB – $0.49 \times 1\,500\,000 = 735\,000$
- Bb – $0.42 \times 1\,500\,000 = 630\,000$
- bb – $0.09 \times 1\,500\,000 = 13\,500$.

7.29

A must be a carrier for the disorder as she has three affected sons. Hence, the chance of B being a carrier is 1/2. This is the prior probability. All of B's daughters are clinically normal. This would occur whether or not B is a carrier. However, more information can be derived from the fact that B has two unaffected sons. If B is a carrier, the chance that she has two normal sons is only 1/4.

Table 7.3

Individual	Genotype
A	AO
B	BO
C	OO
F	BO
G	AO

Table 7.4

Genotype	Number of copies of B	Number of individuals with the genotype	Total number of copies of B
BB	2	487	974
Bb	1	422	422
bb	0	91	0

Table 7.5

Genotype	Formula	Frequency	Expected number of people out of 1000	Actual number of people out of 1000
BB	p^2	0.49	490	487
Bb	$2pq$	0.42	420	422
bb	q^2	0.09	90	91

7

A

Genetics

However, if she is not a carrier, the chance of having two normal sons is 1. Intuitively, we would think that this fact implies that the chance of B being a carrier is less than 1/2. The probability of B having two unaffected sons, conditional on whether or not B is a carrier, is given in Table 7.6.

We know that B has two normal sons. Hence, her posterior probability that she is a carrier is 1/8 ÷ (1/8 + 1/2) = 0.2. (The knowledge that she had two normal sons reduces her chance of being a carrier from 0.5 to 0.2.) The chance that her next son will be affected by the disease is

Table 7.6

Probability	B is a carrier	B is not a carrier
Prior probability	1/2	1/2
Conditional probability of having two normal sons	1/4	1
Joint probability	1/8	1/2

$0.2 \times 1/2 = 0.1$; the chance that her next child will be affected by the disease is $0.1 \times 1/2 = 0.05$.

PART 2
SYSTEM-BASED MEDICAL SCIENCES

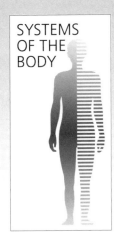

SYSTEMS
OF THE
BODY

Blood and bone marrow ⑧

8.1 Significant quantities of red blood cells are normally produced at the following sites in the fetus:
- A Bone marrow in tibia
- B Bone marrow in sternum
- C Bone marrow in vertebra
- D Liver
- E Spleen

8.2 Significant quantities of red blood cells are normally produced at the following sites in adulthood:
- A Bone marrow in tibia
- B Bone marrow in radius
- C Bone marrow in vertebra
- D Liver
- E Spleen

8.3 The following statements about normal blood cell formation are true:
- A Pluripotent stem cells which are capable of differentiating into red blood cells, white blood cells or platelets exist in the bone marrow
- B Once the bone marrow becomes depleted of functioning cells, it cannot produce blood cells even after the transfusion of functioning bone marrow cells
- C Megalokaryoblasts are the precursor cells for red blood cells
- D Lymphocytes and neutrophils share the same committed stem cells
- E Reticulocytes are the precursor cells for platelets

8.4 The following statements about blood cells are true:
- A There are more white blood cells than red blood cells in the circulation
- B There are more white cell precursors than red cell precursors in the bone marrow
- C The average lifetime for red blood cells in the circulation is about three years
- D The average lifetime for platelets in the circulation is about 200 days
- E The average lifetime for white blood cells in the circulation is about 120 days

8.5 The following cells contain a nucleus:
- A Erythrocyte
- B Megalokaryocyte
- C Platelet
- D T-lymphocyte
- E Neutrophil

8.6 The following features of red cells are characteristic of impaired splenic function:
- A Polycythaemia
- B Howell–Jolly bodies
- C Spherocytes
- D Target cells
- E Microcytes

8.7 The following red cell indices are generally higher in normal males than normal females:
- A Haemoglobin
- B Mean corpuscular volume
- C Mean corpuscular haemoglobin
- D Red cell count
- E Haematrocrit

8.8 The following statements about haemoglobin are true:
- A It is a globular molecule
- B There are two subunits in each molecule
- C The subunits share the same haem group
- D The globulin chains contain iron
- E The globulin portions consist of polypeptides

8.9 The haemoglobin in the fetus:
- A Is mainly haemoglobin A
- B Contains two β chains in each molecule
- C Contains two α chains in each molecule
- D Binds more tightly to 2,3-diphosphoglycerate (2,3-DPG) than adult haemoglobin
- E Contains more oxygen than adult haemoglobin given the same partial pressure of oxygen

8.10 Abnormally small red blood cells (microcytes) characteristically occur in:
- A Vitamin B_{12} deficiency
- B Drug-induced haemolysis
- C Iron deficiency
- D Bone marrow failure
- E Thalassaemia

8.11 The following statements about iron metabolism are true:
- A Over 95% of body iron is stored in the liver
- B Over 90% of the iron is normally stored as haemosiderin
- C The serum ferritin level is an accurate measure of total body iron stores
- D The terminal ileum is the main site for iron absorption
- E The total iron store is controlled mainly via the rate of urinary excretion

8.12 Recognised haematological findings in iron deficiency include:
- A Hypochromic red cells
- B Grossly increased reticulocyte count
- C Reduced mean cell volume (MCV) index

8 **Q**

SYSTEM-BASED MEDICAL SCIENCES

Blood and bone marrow

    D Increased mean corpuscular haemoglobin
       (MCH) index
    E Increased total iron-binding capacity

8.13 The following statements about vitamin B_{12}
    are true:
    A It is essential for DNA synthesis
    B It is available from most vegetables
    C Vitamin B_{12} absorption is not possible in the
       absence of intrinsic factor
    D Symptoms of vitamin B_{12} deficiency develop within
       a month of defective dietary intake
    E Milk can provide sufficient dietary vitamin B_{12} to
       prevent anaemia

8.14 Causes of vitamin B_{12} deficiency include:
    A Crohn's disease
    B Gastrectomy
    C Pernicious anaemia
    D Chronic gastrointestinal bleeding
    E Pregnancy

8.15 The following are recognised indications for iron
    therapy:
    A Iron deficiency due to heavy menstrual blood loss
    B Pregnant woman with a normal haemoglobin
       level
    C Anaemia due to increased haemolysis
    D Thalassaemia
    E Iron deficiency due to dietary deficiency

8.16 The following are valid indications for intramuscular
    rather than oral iron therapy:
    A Iron deficiency of nutritional deficiency origin
    B Past history of severe intolerable gastrointestinal
       side effects due to oral iron
    C Consistent lack of patient compliance
    D A quick response is desired
    E A haemoglobin level of below 9 g/dl

8.17 Recognised haematological findings in vitamin B_{12}
    deficiency include:
    A Reduced platelet count
    B Reduced white cell count
    C Multilobed nucleus in neutrophils
    D Low MCV index
    E Hypocellular bone marrow

8.18 The following conditions are associated with
    pancytopenia (anaemia, neutropenia and
    thrombocytopenia):
    A Antineoplastic chemotherapy
    B Ionising radiation to the bone marrow
    C Drug-induced haemolysis

    D Bone marrow infiltration by carcinoma
    E Folate deficiency

8.19 Causes of haemolytic anaemia include:
    A Spherocytosis
    B Thalassaemia
    C Iron deficiency
    D Sickle-cell disease
    E Mismatched blood transfusion

8.20 Features associated with abnormally excessive
    haemolysis include:
    A Increased conjugated serum bilirubin
    B Increased urine urobilinogen
    C Increased reticulocytes in peripheral blood film
    D Increased serum haptoglobin
    E Small spleen

8.21 Which of the following types of white blood cells
    and their associated features are correctly matched?
    A Monocytes – the commonest type of white cells
    B Mast cells – the largest type of white cells
    C Eosinophils – important for combating parasite
       infection
    D Basophils – histamine and heparin-containing
    E T-lymphocytes – precursor of plasma cells

8.22 In acute leukaemia:
    A Neoplastic proliferation of the precursors of white
       cells occurs
    B Anaemia is common
    C Reduced platelet levels rarely occur
    D Infiltration of the liver rarely occurs
    E Abnormal cells are almost always found in the
       peripheral blood

8.23 Known predisposing factors for leukaemic
    transformation include:
    A Irradiation
    B Exposure to certain viruses
    C Exposure to certain bacteria
    D Down's syndrome
    E Air pollution with sulphur dioxide

8.24 Multiple myelomas:
    A Are a malignant proliferation of T-cells in the
       bone marrow
    B Usually result in the accumulation of several
       different types of immunoglobulin chains
    C May result in increased urinary excretion of free
       light immunoglobulin chains
    D Are associated with greatly elevated erythrocyte
       sedimentation rate
    E Often result in anaemia

8.25 The following statements about lymph nodes are true:
- **A** Lymph enters the lymph nodes in the medullary area
- **B** The germinal centres contain mainly T-lymphocytes
- **C** The follicles are responsible for humoral response
- **D** The paracortex is responsible for cell-mediated immunity
- **E** Lymph leaves the lymph node via the efferent lymphatic at the hilum

8.26 The following statements about the circulation of lymph are true:
- **A** The total volume of lymph circulated is approximately 30 litres per day
- **B** Fluid enters the lymphatics from the interstitial space
- **C** Fluid drains into the aorta via the thoracic and right lymphatic ducts
- **D** All lymphatics have valves in their walls
- **E** The drainage of lymphatics in the collecting lymphatics is facilitated by contraction of the muscles associated with the organ

8.27 Causes of an enlarged lymph node include:
- **A** Epstein–Barr virus infection
- **B** Mycobacterial infection
- **C** Metastatic spread of leukaemia
- **D** Human immunodeficiency virus infection
- **E** Sarcoidosis

8.28 Hodgkin's disease:
- **A** Is a type of leukaemia
- **B** Spreads predominantly via the bloodstream
- **C** Occurs predominantly amongst those over 70 years of age
- **D** Is characterised by the presence of Reed–Sternberg cells
- **E** Is almost always associated with systemic symptoms such as weight loss or night sweats

8.29 The following statements about the thymus gland are true:
- **A** It develops from the sixth pharangygeal pouch
- **B** It is larger in the elderly than in adolescents
- **C** It contains mostly B-lymphocytes
- **D** Underdevelopment is associated with immunodeficiency disorders
- **E** Thymic hyperplasia or neoplasia is associated with autoimmune disorders

8.30 The rate of platelet production is controlled by:
- **A** A type of colony-stimulating factor
- **B** Erythropoietin
- **C** A type of interleukin
- **D** A type of prostaglandin
- **E** von Willebrand factor

8.31 The following statements about platelet aggregation following injury to a small blood vessel are true:
- **A** Thrombin is essential for platelet adhesion
- **B** Platelet activation is enhanced by von Willebrand factor
- **C** Platelets are activated by contact with collagen
- **D** Platelets produce ADP
- **E** Platelet-activating factor (PAF) is secreted by platelets

8.32 Drugs which inhibit platelet activity include:
- **A** Aspirin
- **B** Warfarin
- **C** Dipyridamole
- **D** Disopyramide
- **E** Ticlopidine

8.33 Recognised indications for anti-platelet agents include:
- **A** Myocardial infarction
- **B** von Willebrand disease
- **C** Transient ischaemic attacks
- **D** Unstable angina
- **E** Post-arterial graft surgery for peripheral vascular disease

8.34 The following statements about the clotting mechanisms are true:
- **A** A secure clot can be formed in the absence of platelets
- **B** The essential final step is the formation of fibrin
- **C** The intrinsic system is triggered by tissue damage
- **D** The extrinsic system is triggered by contact with collagen
- **E** Thrombin catalyses the conversion of fibrinogen into fibrin

8.35 The following statements about vitamin K are true:
- **A** The natural vitamin K is fat-soluble
- **B** It is converted into factor IX and X in the liver
- **C** Bile is necessary for its absorption
- **D** Gastrointestinal haemorrhage may occur in deficiency state
- **E** Prothrombin time is characteristically prolonged in deficiency state

8.36 Warfarin:
- **A** Acts within 24h of oral administration
- **B** Is a non-competitive inhibitor of vitamin K

8

Q

Blood and bone marrow

C Characteristically causes a high international normalised ratio (INR)

D Characteristically causes a prolonged activated partial thromboplastin time (APTT)

E May be used in the treatment of pulmonary embolism

8.37 The following are components of the fibrinolytic system:

A Binding of thrombomodulin to thrombin

B Inactivation of protein C

C Increase in the serum level of tissue plasminogen activator (t-PA)

D Conversion of plasmin into plasminogen

E Conversion of fibrinogen into fibrin

8.38 The following statements about heparin are true:

A Its effect may be reversed by protamine

B It is a competitive antagonist of antithrombin III

C It causes prolonged APTT

D It may be given orally

E It has a half-life of about 48 h

8.39 Which of the following drugs may remove thrombi?

A Streptokinase

B Tranexamic acid

C Aprotinin

D Tissue plasminogen activator (t-PA, such as alteplase)

E Urokinase

8.40 The following drugs may be useful in the management of haemophilia A (classical haemophilia):

A Factor IX concentrate

B Tranexamic acid

C Warfarin

D Desmopressin (DDAVP)

E Streptokinase

8.41 In an average adult male, 60% of body weight is water. Two-thirds of all total body water is intracellular. Plasma volume constitutes 25% of the extracellular body water. Using the dye Evans Blue, which binds to plasma proteins, the relevant body volume was estimated to be 3.5 litres. The haematocrit (% of blood volume made up of cells) is 40. From these figures, calculate the following volumes:

A Plasma volume

B Total blood volume

C Extracellular fluid volume

D Intracellular fluid volume

E Total body fluid volume

Draw a simple diagram to show the relationship between these volumes.

8.42 Which of the following sites would you expect to produce red blood cells?

A Liver in the fetus

B Spleen in the fetus

C Radius in a 4-year-old child

D Femur in a 4-year-old child

E Tibia in a 40-year-old adult

F Vertebrae in a 40-year-old adult

G Spleen in a healthy 40-year-old adult

H Spleen in a 40-year-old adult with bone marrow damaged by fibrosis

I Adult red marrow

J Adult yellow marrow

8.43 Three-quarters of the bone marrow cells belong to the myeloid series producing white blood cells, although there are about 500 times as many red cells as white cells in the blood. Explain this apparent contradiction.

8.44 Some of the red cell indices for two young adults, John and Ted, are shown in Table 8.1.

A Explain the term 'mean corpuscular haemoglobin'. Calculate the MCH for both John and Ted. Show your working

B Explain the term 'mean corpuscular volume'. Comment on the MCV for both John and Ted

C From (A) and (B), deduce the likely microscopic appearances of the red cells

D Give a likely cause for John's anaemia. How can the microscopic appearance explained by this cause?

8.45 A 33-year-old woman was noted to have a low haemoglobin concentration on a routine blood count.

A What is anaemia?

Table 8.1

Index	Normal values for males	John	Ted
Haemoglobin (g/dl)	13.0–17.0	10.0	10.0
Red cell concentration (×10^{12}/l)	4.3–5.7	4.2	3.5
Mean cell volume (fl)	78–98	65	103
Mean corpuscular haemoglobin (pg)	26–33		

B How does the body red cell mass in a healthy subject usually compare with that of an anaemic subject? Give an example where this relationship between anaemia and body red cell mass level does not hold.

C Why might anaemia cause fatty change in the liver?

D Why might anaemia be associated with heart failure?

The cause of the anaemia of the woman was found to be Addisonian pernicious anaemia.

E What is the basic defect in this disease? Explain carefully how this might cause anaemia.

F What is the likely microscopic appearance of the following. Explain.
i Erythrocytes in the peripheral blood.
ii Cells in the bone marrow?

G Would the production of white blood cells and platelets be affected? Explain.

H Who is at particular risk for Addisonian pernicious anaemia?

I What is the pharmacological treatment for this condition? What is the appropriate route of administration? Explain.

8.46 A 50-year-old man was diagnosed as having iron-deficiency anaemia owing to a dietary deficiency.

A What is the main source of iron in Western diet?

B Where is iron stored in the body? Explain how the body's iron store is regulated.

C Where is dietary iron usually absorbed? Can both ferric iron and ferrous iron be absorbed?

D What happens to the iron absorbed from the gastrointestinal tract?

E In what form is iron stored within the cell?

F How does the body get rid of excess iron?

G What is the treatment for iron-deficiency anaemia?

H What pharmacological interventions may be effective in a severe accidental overdose of iron tablets? Explain the mechanism of action.

8.47 A 10-year-old boy was diagnosed to be slightly anaemic due to hereditary spherocytosis.

A Briefly describe the three-dimensional shape of a normal erythrocyte. Explain the microscopic appearance of an erythrocyte.

B Can mature erythrocytes undergo cell division? Explain.

C What is the basic defect in hereditary spherocytosis? Explain why this may cause anaemia.

D What is the microscopic appearance of the erythrocytes in hereditary spherocytosis? Use your answers in (A)–(C) to explain this.

E What type of anaemia does this condition cause? What is the basic characteristic of this type of anaemia?

F Would you expect to find abnormalities of the following measures? Explain.
i Bilirubin level.
ii Reticulocyte count.

8.48 A 4-month-old Chinese boy was diagnosed to be severely anaemic due to β-thalassaemia major. The liver and spleen were both grossly enlarged and palpable.

A What is the basic defect in this disease?

B Why did the disease not present at birth?

C What would you expect to find for the following red cell indices?
i Haemoglobin concentration
ii Mean cell volume
iii Reticulocyte count
iv Mean corpuscular haemoglobin.

D What would you expect to find on haemoglobin electrophoresis?

E Explain why the liver and spleen were enlarged

8.49 A patient had an abnormally high haemoglobin level. Investigations did not reveal any myeloproliferative disorders.

A Give one physiological cause

B Give one pathological cause due to malignancy

C Give three pathological causes not due to malignancy

D For (A)–(C), briefly explain the mechanism for producing a raised haemoglobin level in these subjects

E Would you expect cigarette smokers to have a higher or lower haemoglobin level than non-smokers? Explain.

8.50 A 3-year-old boy initially presented acutely with anaemia, serious bacterial infections and bruising. After appropriate investigations, a diagnosis of acute lymphoblastic leukaemia was made. An enlarged spleen was palpable.

A What is leukaemia?

B Generally speaking, what are the known causes of leukaemia?

C Explain why the boy had anaemia, serious bacterial infections and bruising.

D What organs do leukaemic cells frequently infiltrate?

8

Q

SYSTEM-BASED MEDICAL SCIENCES

Blood and bone marrow

    E What abnormalities (if any) would you expect for the MCV and MCH for this boy?

    F What are the characteristic microscopic features of bone marrow cells in this boy?

8.51 A 70-year-old man was diagnosed as having multiple myeloma and rapidly developed anaemia and renal failure.

    A What is the basic defect in multiple myeloma?

    B What specific urine test is positive in this disease? Explain why this test is positive.

    C Why might the patient develop anaemia?

    D Why might the patient develop renal failure?

8.52 A 3-year-old child presented with bruises. He was noted to have a very low platelet count and was diagnosed as having idiopathic thrombocytopenic purpura. In this condition, there are autoantibodies to platelets.

    A Briefly describe the structure of platelets.

    B What substances do the granules in platelets contain?

    C Give a brief account of how platelets help to stop bleeding when a blood vessel wall is injured. Highlight the roles of von Willebrand factor and factor VIII.

    D How is platelet production usually controlled?

    E What is the approximate half-life of platelets? How soon would you expect his platelet level to rise once the disease activity ceased?

    F What are the precursor cells for platelets? Would you expect to see these precursor cells in the bone marrow of this child? Explain.

8.53 Figure 8.1 is a highly simplistic diagram of the coagulation and fibrinolytic pathways.

    A Name the substances (a)–(i).

    B Broadly speaking, which systems do the following clotting tests assess?

      i Activated partial thromboplastin time (APTT).

      ii Prothrombin time (PT).

    C What are the effects of the following drugs? Which systems do they act upon?

      i Warfarin.

      ii Heparin.

      iii Streptokinase.

      iv Tranexamic acid.

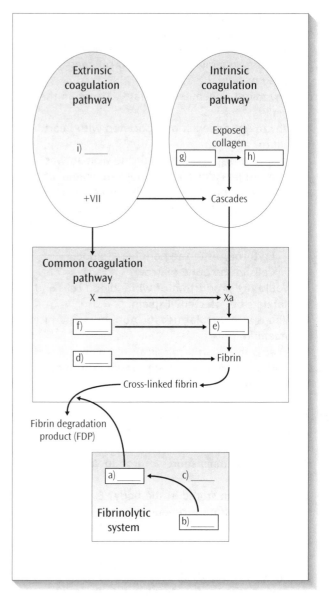

Fig. 8.1 Coagulation and fibrinolytic pathways.

Blood and bone marrow

8.1 A B C D E
In the fetus, blood cells are normally produced in all bone marrow cavities, the liver and the spleen. In childhood, blood cells are normally produced in all bone marrow cavities, but not in the liver and spleen. In adulthood, the marrow cavities of most long bones (except the femur and upper part of the humerus) become inactive, and become infiltrated with fat (yellow marrow). The marrow in the vertebrae, sternum, ribs, skull and pelvis are active, and is known as red marrow. This is important clinically. If the liver and spleen become active in producing blood cells in adulthood (extramedullary haematopoiesis), a disease affecting the function of the bone marrow (e.g. fibrosis of the bone marrow) is likely to be present.

8.2 C
See answer to question 10.1 above.

8.3 A
Red blood cells, white blood cells and platelets are derived from a common undifferentiated precursor cell (pluripotent stem cell). This explains why bone marrow transplantation is effective, where blood cell production resumes after infusion of normal bone marrow cells into a subject without functioning bone marrow. The pluripotent stem cell differentiates into differentiated lymphoid or myeloid stem cells. The lymphoid stem cells can differentiate further into B- or T-lymphocytes, whereas myeloid stem cells may differentiate into all other types of cells. Megalokaryocytes are differentiated precursors for platelets found in the bloodstream. In diseases with rapid destruction of platelets in the blood (e.g. idiopathic thrombocytopenic purpura), the number of megalokaryoblasts increases in the bone marrow. Reticulocytes are the precursors of red blood cells. In anaemia due to rapid destruction of red cells, reticulocyte count increases in an attempt to compensate for the anaemia.

8.4 B
Although there are about 500 times more red blood cells than white blood cells in the circulation, about three-quarters of the cellular components of bone marrow are white cell precursors. This is because the bone marrow acts as a reserve store for white blood cells, and respond rapidly to infection or tissue injury by the release of white cells. The white cells usually remain in the circulation for only a few hours. In contrast, there is almost no storage pool for red blood cells, and the average lifetime for red blood cells is about 120 days. This is important clinically, as diseases affecting the bone marrow may cause neutropenia very quickly, whereas it might take over a month before anaemia becomes apparent. The average lifetime for platelets is about 4–10 days.

8.5 B D E
All stem cells and precursor cells contain a nucleus. For red blood cells, the nucleus is lost in the final step in the maturation of reticulocyte into erythrocyte. Similarly, the nucleus is lost in the maturation of the megalokaryocyte into the platelet cell. Once the nucleus is lost in the erythrocyte and platelet cells, further division of the cell cannot take place, and their lifespan is limited. All white cells contain a nucleus.

8.6 B D
The erythrocytes are usually processed by the spleen before they are released into the circulation. Abnormal red cells may be destroyed by the spleen. For example, remnants of nuclear materials are removed, and red cells of abnormal shapes are removed. In the presence of impaired splenic function Howell–Jolly bodies which are remnants of nuclear materials may be present. Target cells with lack of central pallor may also be present. Impaired splenic function does not affect the size of the red cells. The haemoglobin concentration is also unaffected.

8.7 A D E
The proportion of cells in the blood is higher in men than women. Hence, the packed cell volume (haematocrit) and red cell count are higher in men than women. Since haemoglobin is found in red blood cells, the haemoglobin concentration is higher in men than in women. The normal haemoglobin level is between 13 and 16.5 g/dl for men, and between 11.5 and 15.5 g/dl for women. The mean corpuscular volume is a measure of the red cell size, and is obtained by dividing the haematocrit by the red cell concentration. The mean corpuscular haemoglobin is a measure of the amount of haemoglobin in a red blood cell, and is obtained by dividing the haemoglobin concentration by the red cell concentration. Both these values are the same in men and in women.

8.8 A E
Haemoglobin is the molecule responsible for carrying oxygen in the red blood cells. It is a globular molecule consisting of four subunits. Each subunit consists of a globulin chain (a polypeptide) and a haem group (which contains iron). There are two pairs of globulin chains in each haemoglobin molecule, each containing a different type of polypeptide. In normal adults, most of the haemoglobin is haemoglobin A, consisting of two α chains and two β chains.

8.9 C E
Haemoglobin in the fetus consists mainly of haemoglobin F. Each molecule of haemoglobin F contains two α chains and two γ chains. It binds less tightly to 2,3-DPG than adult haemoglobin. As a result, it holds on to oxygen

Blood and bone marrow

more tightly, and facilitates the transfer of oxygen from mother to fetus via the placenta. Haemoglobin F level normally declines rapidly after birth, and almost disappears by three months of age. It may persist in certain types of haemoglobinopathies.

8.10   C E
Microcytes result from extra cell division during red cell production. Cell division is usually inhibited by the haemoglobin concentration in the cytoplasm. Hence iron deficiency and thalassaemia result in extra cell division and microcytes. Vitamin B_{12} or folate and folate are essential for nucleic acid synthesis. Hence, in vitamin B_{12} or folate deficiency, mitosis is defective. This gives rise to large red cells (macrocytes). Bone marrow failure results in normal-sized red cells (normocytic anaemia). In haemolysis, the rate of red cell destruction is increased, but the red cell size is usually normal.

8.11   C
Iron absorption takes place mainly in the duodenum and upper jejunum, whereas vitamin B_{12} is mostly absorbed in the terminal ileum. It is excreted both in the urinary and the gastrointestinal tract as desquamated cells. Over half of the body iron exists in the form of haemoglobin in red cells, and less than a third is stored in liver, spleen and bone marrow. Iron is normally stored mainly as ferritin (a water-soluble protein–iron complex), and only a small proportion as haemosiderin (an insoluble aggregate). When there is iron overload, a higher proportion is stored as haemosiderin. The control of total body iron is important. On the one hand, iron is essential for the production of red blood cells; on the other hand, excess iron in tissues may cause damage to the heart, liver and pancreas (as in haemochromatosis). However, the body has little control over its excretion of iron, and its control on absorption is limited. Hence the body is vulnerable to iron deficiency whenever there is increased loss of iron.

8.12   A C E
In iron deficiency anaemia, the blood picture is typically microcytic and hypochromic. The microcytic picture reflects a low MCV whilst the hypochromic picture reflects a low MCH level. The reticulocyte count is usually low for the level of anaemia. This is because the bone marrow does not have sufficient iron to synthesise haemoglobin. The serum iron and ferritin level are usually low, but the total iron-binding capacity is high. Normally, the transferrin is about a third saturated. In iron deficiency anaemia, the total iron-binding capacity increases due to a compensatory increase in transferrin concentration.

8.13   A C E
Vitamin B_{12} is essential for DNA synthesis, and deficiency may cause anaemia and neurological dysfunction (e.g. subacute combined degeneration of the spinal cord, dementia). Vitamin B_{12} is found mainly in food of animal origin, and is absent in fruit and vegetables. However, eggs and milk provide sufficient vitamin B_{12} to prevent deficiency state. Hence only strict vegetarians are at risk of dietary vitamin B_{12} deficiency. The liver normally stores sufficient vitamin B_{12} for several years. Hence symptoms of deficiency do not occur for several years. Vitamin B_{12} is absorbed in the terminal ileum, but it must be bound to intrinsic factor before it can be absorbed. Intrinsic factor is produced by parietal cells in the stomach.

8.14   A B C
Causes of vitamin B_{12} deficiency include lack of intrinsic factor, malabsorption from the terminal ileum and dietary deficiency in strict vegetarians. The causes for lack of intrinsic factor include Addisonian pernicious anaemia, congenital lack of intrinsic factor, and after surgical removal of the stomach (gastrectomy). Causes of malabsorption from the terminal ileum include ileal resection and Crohn's disease. Chronic gastrointestinal bleeding and pregnancy do not give rise to vitamin B_{12} deficiency because the diet usually contains many times the body daily requirements, and the body stores for vitamin B_{12} are extremely large.

8.15   A B E
Recognised indications for iron therapy include iron deficiency and anticipated increased demand for iron (e.g. during pregnancy or in premature babies). Iron should be avoided in patients with haemolytic anaemia unless there is associated blood loss. This is because iron from the lysed red blood cells is still available and excess iron may result in haemosiderosis. This is especially true in thalassaemia, as patients often require blood transfusion and the risk of iron overload is high.

8.16   B C
Valid indications for intramuscular rather than oral iron therapy include consistent lack of patient compliance, past history of severe intolerable gastrointestinal side effects due to oral iron, and if iron cannot be absorbed from the gastrointestinal tract (e.g. after extensive small bowel resection). The response to intramuscular iron is not faster than that of oral iron. A haemoglobin level of 9 g/dl can usually be treated with oral iron. If the iron deficiency is severe or the patient develops serious symptoms due to anaemia, a blood transfusion should be given.

8.17   A B C
Vitamin B_{12} deficiency results in impaired DNA synthesis. This results in a reduction in mitosis, and affects all three

cell lines. Anaemia, reduced white cell count and low platelets may all occur to some extent (i.e. pancytopenia). The red cells are typically large (i.e. high MCV index) due to lack of mitosis, and the neutrophils characteristically show nuclear hypersegmentation (multilobed nucleus). In an attempt to compensate for the pancytopenia, the bone marrow is hypercellular. The developing red cells in the bone marrow are large (megaloblastic).

8.18   A B D E
In pancytopenia, all three cell lines are involved. This may be due either to bone marrow failure or to impaired DNA synthesis. Causes of bone marrow failure include anti-neoplastic chemotherapy, ionising radiation to the bone marrow or bone marrow infiltration by carcinoma or leukaemia. Causes of impaired DNA synthesis include vitamin B$_{12}$ or folate deficiency. Drug-induced haemolysis usually causes anaemia only.

8.19   A B D E
Red cell destruction is increased in haemolytic anaemia, and the red cell lifespan is reduced. Increased destruction may be due either to abnormalities of the red cells or to factors external to the red cells. Abnormalities of red cells which may lead to haemolysis include haemoglobinopathies (e.g. thalassaemia, sickle cell disease), enzyme defects (e.g. G6PD deficiency) and membrane defects (e.g. spherocytosis, elliptocytosis). Factors external to the red cells include antibodies (e.g. rhesus incompatibility, mismatched blood transfusion, drugs or toxins).

8.20   B C
In the presence of excessive red cell destruction, haemoglobin is broken down in the spleen to form haem and globin chains. The spleen therefore enlarges in haemolytic diseases. The haem is then broken down into unconjugated bilirubin. It circulates in the blood, and is then conjugated in the liver, and is excreted in the liver as urobilinogen. Serum haptoglobin binds to haemoglobin, and is therefore absent in the presence of excessive haemolysis. Red cell formation is increased in the bone marrow to compensate for the excessive destruction of red blood cells, and hence the number of reticulocytes increases.

8.21   C D
The commonest type of white cells are neutrophils, which normally constitute about 60% of white cells, and are essential for combating bacterial infections. Monocytes are the largest type of white cells, and are precursors of macrophages. Eosinophils combat parasite infections by producing leukotriene C$_4$ and platelet-activating factor. Both mast cells and basophils contain histamine and

heparin. Mast cells have IgE receptors on their cell membranes, and are important in producing an immediate allergic response. T-lymphocytes are important for cellular immunity, whilst B-lymphocytes are important for humoral immunity. Plasma cells produce antibodies, and are developed from B-lymphocytes.

8.22   A B
In most types of leukaemia, neoplastic proliferation of the white blood cells precursors occurs. However, the precursors of platelets and red cells are also affected in some types of leukaemia (e.g. chronic granulocytic leukaemia). The normal cells in the bone marrow are replaced by leukaemic cells, and hence bone marrow failure occurs. This may give rise to pancytopenia. Infiltration of the liver, spleen and lymph nodes is common, and invasion of meninges and the gonads may also occur. In the early stages of leukaemia, the abnormal cells may remain in the bone marrow and may not be found in the peripheral blood.

8.23   A B D
Known predisposing factors for leukaemia include both genetic and environmental factors. Patients with Down's syndrome have an increased risk of acute leukaemia. Reciprocal translocation between chromosomes 22 and 9 (Philadelphia chromosome) occurs in 95% of cases of chronic granulocytic leukaemia. Known environmental predisposing factors include irradiation, alkylating agents, some chemicals (e.g. benzene) and certain viruses (e.g. human T-leukaemia virus). There is as yet no proven association between leukaemia and bacteria or air pollution.

8.24   C D E
Multiple myelomas are a malignant proliferation of plasma cells in the bone marrow. Plasma cells are developed from B-cells. In most cases, only a single clone of cells is involved, which results in the accumulation of a single type of immunoglobulin. The whole immunoglobulin cannot be excreted in urine as the molecule is too large to be filtered at the glomerulus. However, the light chain can pass through the glomerulus. The high concentration of immunoglobulin increases the blood viscosity, and the red blood cells often have a tendency to adhere to each other. Anaemia is common as a result of interference with the bone marrow function.

8.25   C D E
The lymph node is a kidney-shaped structure. Lymph enters the node via afferent lymphatics to enter the marginal sinus. Beneath the marginal sinus lies the cortex. The cortex contains follicles which are packed with B-lymphocytes. The paracortex lies deep to the cortex, and

8

A

SYSTEM-BASED MEDICAL SCIENCES

Blood and bone marrow

contains large T-cells responsible for cell-mediated immunity. Towards the hilum of the node are medullary cords which are rich in plasma cells and lymphocytes. The associated sinuses are lined by histiocytes. The lymph leaves the node via the efferent lymphatic at the hilum of the node.

8.26 B E
The main function of the lymphatic circulation is to return excess fluid in the interstitial space back to the systemic circulation. The normal volume of lymph circulated is about 3 litres per day. There are two types of lymphatic vessels. There are no valves or smooth muscles in the walls of the initial lymphatics. The initial lymphatics drain into collecting lymphatics which have valves and smooth muscles in their walls. Hence contraction of the muscles associated with the organ may facilitate its drainage in the collecting lymphatics. The fluid is finally returned to the venous system via the thoracic and right lymphatic ducts.

8.27 A B C D E
The lymph node reacts to a large variety of stimuli (e.g. infecting agents, foreign bodies, neoplasia) by node enlargement. Lymph node enlargement may be a localised response (e.g. to local infection) or a generalised response (e.g. autoimmune disorders, sarcoidosis, HIV infection or Epstein–Barr virus infection). In order to diagnose the precise cause for the enlargement, a lymph node biopsy is needed, and the histological features in different parts of the lymph nodes may give valuable information about the aetiology.

8.28 D
Hodgkin's disease is a type of lymphoma – malignancies arising from cells in the lymph nodes. There are two main types of lymphoma: Hodgkin's disease and non-Hodgkin's disease. Unlike non-Hodgkin's disease, Hodgkin's disease occurs more commonly between 30 and 50 years old and is rare in childhood or in old age. Hodgkin's disease is characterised by a large, pale, multilobed nucleus known as Reed–Sternberg cells. In Hodgkin's disease, the lymph node capsule is very seldom breached. Hence only a third of patients suffer from systemic symptoms, and the disease spreads predominantly via the lymphatics.

8.29 D E
The thymus gland is developed from the third and fourth pharyngeal pouches. Its absolute weight increases after birth until puberty, and then gradually atrophies. The thymus is important for the maturation of T-cells and induction of the cell-mediated immune response. In the congenital DiGeorge syndrome, there is defective development of the third and fourth pharyngeal pouches. As a result, immunodeficiency and absent parathyroid

glands (which also develop from the third and fourth pharyngeal pouches) occur. Thymus abnormalities are also found in other forms of immunodeficiency.

Thymic hyperplasia is strongly associated with autoimmune thyroid disease, and thymoma (thymic neoplasia) is associated with a range of autoimmune diseases, including myasthenia gravis.

8.30 A C
The rate of platelet production is controlled by a type of colony-stimulating factor (granulocyte–macrophage colony-stimulating factor, or GM-CSF). Interleukin types 1, 3 and 6 (IL-1, IL-3, IL-6) increase the rate of conversion of uncommitted stem cells to committed platelet precursor. Thrombopoietin, which has recently been isolated, facilitates maturation of megakaryocytes. Erythropoietin increases the rate of red cell production. Platelets contain von Willebrand factor, which regulates the circulating levels of factor VIII.

8.31 B C D E
In response to small vessel injury, there are several intermediate steps of platelet aggregation. Firstly, platelets adhere to the exposed vessel wall. This initial step does not require any specific chemical activity. Platelets are then activated and produce ADP and thrombin. Activation may be brought about by binding to collagen or von Willebrand factor on the vessel wall. This causes release of platelet granules, which aggregate with other platelets. PAF is one of the many substances found in the platelets. It has inflammatory properties, and may increase platelet aggregation. This leads to a series of reactions resulting in the production of thromboxane A_2, which promotes vasoconstriction and further platelet aggregation.

8.32 A C E
Aspirin inhibits platelet function by inhibiting the synthesis of thromboxane and promoting the synthesis of prostacyclin. Dipyridamole inhibits the effect of platelets by reversibly inhibiting platelet phosphodiesterase, which in turn causes an increase in cAMP level. Ticlopidine acts by inhibiting the binding of fibrinogen to platelets. Warfarin interferes with the clotting mechanisms but has no effect on platelets. Disopyramide is an anti-arrhythmic agent.

8.33 A C D E
Anti-platelet agents are used to prevent further thrombi formation. Hence they are used in myocardial infarction, transient ischaemic attacks, unstable angina and peripheral vascular disease, especially following arterial graft surgery. There is a combination of clotting and platelet abnormalities in von Willebrand disease.

8.34 B E

The main function of the clotting mechanism is to convert the temporary clots formed by platelet aggregates into secure clots. There are two clotting systems (the intrinsic and extrinsic systems); both result in the conversion of soluble fibrinogen into insoluble fibrin with thrombin, and stabilised by cross-linkages to a tight aggregate. The conversion of fibrinogen into fibrin is catalysed by thrombin. The intrinsic system is activated when blood comes into contact with collagen fibres, or by the release of active factor XII. The extrinsic system is triggered by tissue thromboplastin, which is released in the presence of tissue damage.

8.35 A C D E

Natural vitamin K (K_1 and K_2) is fat-soluble, and bile is necessary for its absorption. Hence vitamin K deficiency may occur in long-standing obstructive jaundice or biliary fistula. Synthetic vitamin K (K_3) is water-soluble. Vitamin K is a cofactor for an enzyme responsible for metabolising glutamic acid residues in six of the clotting factors. Hence these clotting factors cannot be manufactured in the liver in the absence of vitamin K. Vitamin K deficiency may result in haemorrhage, especially in the gut. As the extrinsic system is mostly affected, the prothrombin time is characteristically prolonged in vitamin K deficiency.

8.36 C E

Warfarin is a competitive inhibitor of vitamin K. Since the synthesis of six of the clotting factors requires vitamin K, warfarin has anticoagulant properties which may be reversed by vitamin K. As warfarin affects mainly the extrinsic system, the prothrombin time is characteristically prolonged whilst the APTT is usually normal. The INR expresses the prothrombin time as a ratio of the control, and is usually used to monitor warfarin therapy. Warfarin is used to treat deep vein thrombosis, systemic or pulmonary embolism, and is occasionally used to prevent thrombosis in atrial fibrillation, transient ischaemic attack or valvular heart disease.

8.37 A C

To balance the clotting mechanism, there are in vivo body mechanisms to dissolve clots. The final pathway is to lyse fibrin. Several mechanisms are involved. Prostacyclin has an anti-aggregating effect which opposes the action of thromboxane A_2. Antithrombin III blocks the activity of clotting factors IX, X, XI and XII. Endothelial cells produce thrombomodulin. When thrombomodulin binds to thrombin, it activates protein C. This results in inactivation of factors VII and V, as well as increasing the effective concentration of t-PA. t-PA promotes the conversion of plasminogen into plasmin, which has the effect of lysing fibrin.

8.38 A C

Heparin acts mainly by making antithrombin III in the plasma more active. Antithrombin III acts as an inhibitor of thrombin and activated factor X. Heparin also acts by inhibiting platelet aggregation. As it affects the intrinsic system mostly, it is monitored by the APTT (or kaolin–cephalin clotting time). Heparin cannot be given orally as it is poorly absorbed from the gut. Its half-life is between 1 and 3h, depending on the dose given. Hence the effect of heparin wears off rapidly. This may be an advantage over warfarin when the dose required is uncertain, or if anticoagulation is required before an operation, but is undesirable during surgery. In the unlikely event that the effect of heparin needs to be reversed quickly, protamine may be used.

8.39 A D E

Plasmin destroys fibrin. Hence drugs which promote the formation of plasmin will remove thrombi (i.e. fibrinolytics). Plasmin is converted from plasminogen in the blood. Drugs such as streptokinase and urokinase are plaminogen activators, and hence tend to remove thrombi. Alteplase is a tissue type plasminogen activator and favours binding of plasminogen to fibrin. Hence it also tends to remove thrombi. By contrast, tranexamic acid blocks the binding of plasminogen to fibrin, and aprotinin is an inhibitor of plasmin. Hence they tend to favour formation of clots (antifibrinolytics), and are used in the treatment of severe haemorrhage.

8.40 B D

Haemophilia A (classical haemophilia) is a sex-linked inherited disorder caused by factor VIII deficiency, whilst haemophilia B (Christmas disease) is due to factor IX deficiency. Hence, moderate or major bleeding in haemophilia should be treated with injection of factor VIII concentrate. In the past, patients receiving factor VIII ran the risk of contracting hepatitis B or HIV infection. This should no longer be the case as factor VIII is now synthesised using recombinant DNA technique. Tranexamic acid stabilises any temporary clots formed by platelet reactions, and may be a useful adjunct. DDAVP is given intravenously, and it increases factor VIII activity by about five times. It is useful in patients with mild or moderate deficiency of factor VIII.

8.41

A

Since the dye Evans Blue binds to plasma proteins, the body volume measured was plasma volume; hence, the plasma volume is 3.5 litres.

Blood and bone marrow

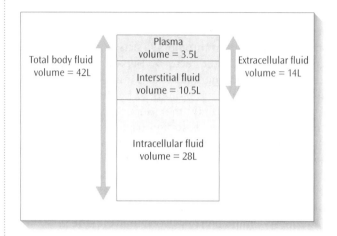

Fig. 8.2 Composition of total body water.

B

Haematocrit is the percentage of blood volume made up of cells. Since the haematocrit is 40, 40% and 60% of the total blood volume were made up of cells and plasma, respectively. Since the plasma volume is 3.5 litres, the total blood volume is 3.5/0.6 = 5.83 litres.

C

Since the plasma volume (3.5 litres) comprises 25% of the extracellular body fluid, the extracellular body fluid volume is 3.5 × 4 = 14 litres.

D

Since two-thirds of all total body fluid is intracellular, one-third of the total body fluid is extracellular. The extracellular body fluid volume is 14 litres, therefore the intracellular body water volume is 14 × 2 = 28 litres.

E

Total body water volume is 14 × 3 = 42 litres.

See Fig. 8.2 for a diagram describing the relationship between these volumes.

8.42

In the fetus, red blood cells are produced from all bone marrow as well as the liver and spleen. In healthy children, red blood cells are produced in all bone marrow, but not in the liver and spleen. In adulthood, the vertebrae and sternum are active in producing red blood cells; most long bones (apart from the femur and upper humerus) cease to be active in red cell production. Active cellular bone marrow is called red marrow; inactive marrow is called yellow marrow as the cells are infiltrated with fat. However, in children with severe haemolytic anaemia (e.g. thalassaemia), or in adults whose bone marrow is destroyed by fibrosis, the liver and spleen may become active in producing red blood cells. This is called extramedullary haematopoiesis.

The answers to the question are:

A Yes.

B Yes.

C Yes.

D Yes.

E No.

F Yes.

G No.

H Yes.

I Yes.

J No.

8.43

This apparent contraindication can be explained by the much longer average life span of red blood cells (about 120 days) compared with that of white cells (e.g. 6 h for neutrophils); hence, there is a higher requirement for the production of white blood cells.

8.44

A

Mean corpuscular haemoglobin is the average haemoglobin (in picograms) in a red blood cell. Hence:

$$\text{mean corpuscular haemoglobin}$$
$$= \text{haemoglobin concentration/red cell concentration}$$

For John,

$$\text{MCH} = 10\,\text{g/dl}/(4.2 \times 10^{12}/\text{l}) = 23.8 \times 10^{-12}\,\text{g} = 23.8\,\text{pg}$$

For Ted,

$$\text{MCH} = 10\,\text{g/dl}/(3.5 \times 10^{12}/\text{l}) = 28.6 \times 10^{-12}\,\text{g} = 28.6\,\text{pg}$$

B

Mean corpuscular volume is the average volume of a red blood cell. For John, the MCV is smaller than normal: John's anaemia is microcytic. For Ted, the MCV is larger than normal: Ted's anaemia is macrocytic.

C

From (A) and (B), John's red cell indices show a low MCV and MCH: his anaemia is microcytic and hypochromic. One would expect to find small and pale red cells microscopically. Ted's red cell indices show a high MCV and a normal MCH: his anaemia is macrocytic and one would expect to find large red cells microscopically.

D

John's anaemia is likely to be due to iron deficiency. (Thalassaemia may also cause microcytic hypochromic anaemia.) The small size of the red blood cells results from an extra cell division (in addition to the normal four) during red cell production. A high cytoplasmic haemoglobin concentration normally inhibits normoblast division; however, the failure of haemoglobin synthesis due to iron deficiency causes extra mitoses to occur, resulting in the production of small red cells.

8.45

A
Anaemia is usually defined as a haemoglobin concentration below the minimum expected for the age and sex of the individual (e.g. 13 g/dl for an adult male and 11.5 g/dl for an adult female).

B
Since the haemoglobin concentration is the body red cell mass divided by the plasma volume, the body red cell mass of an anaemic person is usually lower than that of a healthy person. However, in conditions where both the plasma volume and the red cell mass increase, but the former to a larger extent, anaemia may occur even though the red cell mass is high. Pregnancy is one such condition.

C
Anaemia may cause tissue hypoxia. This may result in fatty changes in the liver.

D
Anaemia may be associated with heart failure because the oxygen-carrying capacity of the blood is low; hence, the heart needs to pump more blood to maintain tissue oxygenation.

E
In Addisonian pernicious anaemia there is autoimmunity to the parietal cells in the stomach. This results in a lack of gastric intrinsic factor and a failure to absorb vitamin B_{12}. Since vitamin B_{12} is necessary for DNA synthesis, the body becomes unable to produce red blood cells if its store of vitamin B_{12} is exhausted.

F
Pernicious anaemia causes vitamin B_{12} deficiency.
i   In vitamin B_{12} deficiency, the erythrocytes are large (macrocytic). Due to impaired DNA synthesis, with normal RNA and protein synthesis, there is a reduction in the number of mitoses in red cell development.
ii The bone marrow shows extremely large red cell precursors (megaloblasts). There may be multilobed leukocytes.

G
Since vitamin B_{12} is required for all DNA synthesis, the production of white blood cell and platelet precursors may also be affected.

H
Since Addisonian pernicious anaemia is an autoimmune disorder, it occurs more commonly in young adult females. It often coexists with autoimmune thyroid disorders.

I
The treatment for Addisonian pernicious anaemia is vitamin B_{12}, which is normally given by intramuscular injection because there is usually a failure to absorb oral vitamin B_{12} in this disorder.

8.46

A
The main source of iron in the Western diet is meat. Although iron is also available in vegetables and cereals, they are mostly trivalent (ferric) and need to be reduced to the ferrous form for absorption.

B
About 60% of the body's iron is stored in the red blood cells. About 30% of the body's iron is stored in the bone marrow and the reticuloendothelial system as ferritin or haemosiderin. The body's iron store is mainly controlled by the rate of iron absorption via the gastrointestinal system. The exact control mechanism is still unclear, but the higher the rate of absorption, the lower the iron store and the higher the rate of red cell production.

C
Dietary iron is usually absorbed in the duodenum and the upper jejunum. Only ferrous iron can be absorbed. Ferric iron must be converted into the ferrous form before absorption.

D
Iron absorbed from the gastrointestinal tract may be either transported into the plasma or stored inside the cell as ferritin.

E
Iron is stored in the cell as ferritin (or rarely deposited as haemosiderin).

F
The body has no effective way of getting rid of excess iron other than by reducing the rate of absorption from the gastrointestinal tract or sloughing of ferritin-containing mucosal cells. Iron is not excreted in the urine.

G
The treatment for iron-deficiency anaemia is the treatment of the underlying disease and the administration of iron supplements. Iron is usually given orally as ferrous salts (e.g. ferrous sulphate). Only if the

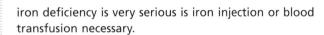

Blood and bone marrow

iron deficiency is very serious is iron injection or blood transfusion necessary.

H

In a severe accidental overdose of iron tablets, desferroxamine may be useful. Given via a gastric tube, it may bind iron in the gut lumen and prevent its absorption. Given intramuscularly, it acts as an iron chelator in the blood. It forms a complex with ferric iron and is excreted in the urine.

8.47
A

Red blood cells are non-nucleated, deformable, biconcave discs. Microscopically, they appear circular with a central pallor. The central pallor reflects the biconcave disc shape of the red cells. The surface area/volume ratio of a biconcave disc is much larger than a sphere. Hence, this facilitates oxygen transfer from the lungs to the blood, and from the blood to the tissue.

B

Reticulocytes (precursors of red cells) are nucleated but they lose their nuclei before entering the circulation. Mature red blood cells cannot therefore undergo cell division.

C

In hereditary spherocytosis, there is a defect in spectrin, a structural protein of the red cell membrane. As a result, biconcave red cells released from the marrow rapidly lose membrane and therefore assume a spherical shape. They are less deformable. This impedes their passage through the splenic microcirculation, where they remain for a longer than normal period of time and are liable to be phagocytosed prematurely. These abnormal red cells are more sensitive to osmotic stress, and their osmotic fragility can be tested in the laboratory.

D

In spherocytosis, the red blood cells ('spherocytes') appear smaller than the normal red cells, with loss of central pallor microscopically. This loss of central pallor reflects their three-dimensional spherical shape.

E

It causes haemolytic anaemia, in which there is reduced red cell survival. It usually results in raised unconjugated bilirubin in the blood and absent serum haptoglobin, which binds haemoglobin.

F
i   Serum unconjugated bilirubin would be raised due to haemolysis. Serum conjugated bilirubin would be normal.

ii   The reticulocyte count will be high. To compensate for the increased destruction of red blood cells, the bone marrow erythroid activity increases; hence, the reticulocyte count increases.

8.48
A

In thalassaemias, the synthesis of the globin chain of haemoglobin is abnormal. In β-thalassaemia, the synthesis of the β-globin chain is affected. It is caused by a single gene defect. In β-thalassaemia major, both genes are affected.

B

Normally, haemoglobin F predominates in the fetus. Haemoglobin F consists of 2 α chains and 2 γ chains; hence, it is not affected in β-thalassaemia. However, by 3–6 months after birth, adult haemoglobin (haemoglobin A, which consists of 2 α and 2 β chains) should have completely taken over. The disease therefore usually becomes manifest at this time.

C

Thalassaemia causes a picture of severe haemolytic anaemia with microcytic hypochromic anaemia. To compensate for the defective haemoglobin synthesis, the red bone marrow greatly expands. The red cell indices are expected to be as follows:
i   Severely reduced (to about 5 g/dl)
ii   Reduced
iii   Increased
iv   Reduced

D

Haemoglobin electrophoresis would show a lack of β-globin chain and an increase in the γ-globin chain in the blood.

E

In response to the low haemoglobin level, the liver and spleen enlarge in an attempt to synthesise haemoglobin. This is called extramedullary erythropoiesis.

8.49
A

An abnormally high haemoglobin level not due to polycythaemia rubra vera is usually known as secondary polycythaemia. It is usually seen in response to hypoxia. Living at high altitude is an example of a physiological cause.

B

Pathological causes due to malignancy include renal carcinoma, cerebellar haemangioblastoma and hepatocellular carcinoma. All these tumours may produce ectopic erythropoietin.

C

Pathological causes not due to malignancy include renal disease, cyanotic heart disease, chronic obstructive airways disease and severe hypoventilation due to scoliosis. In fact, any causes of chronic hypoxia may cause secondary polycythaemia.

D

The common mechanism causing secondary polycythaemia in the conditions given in (A)–(C) above is an increased production of erythropoietin, either due to inappropriate production by a tumour or in response to chronic hypoxia.

E

Cigarette smokers would be expected to have a higher haemoglobin level than non-smokers. The carbon monoxide in the tobacco smoke may reduce effective blood oxygenation and stimulates the production of erythropoietin.

8.50

A

Leukaemias are neoplastic proliferations of white blood cell precursors.

B

Generally speaking, the causes for most cases of leukaemia are unknown; however, factors that are known to cause leukaemia include irradiation, drugs (especially alkylating agents), exposure to chemicals (e.g. benzene), viruses (e.g. human T-cell leukaemia virus in T-cell leukaemia), and genetic factors (e.g. Philadelphia chromosome in chronic myeloid leukaemia, increased risk of leukaemia in Down's syndrome).

C

In leukaemia, the leukaemic cells may replace normal bone marrow. This results in bone marrow failure. The inability to produce red blood cells, white blood cells and platelets may result in anaemia, infections and bruising, respectively.

D

Leukaemic cells frequently infiltrate the liver, spleen, lymph nodes, gonads and meninges.

E

The anaemia in leukaemia is due to bone marrow failure. The red cell size and the haemoglobin concentration in each red cell are unaffected. Hence, MCV and MCH are normal.

F

The characteristic microscopic features of bone marrow cells include grossly increased cellularity with leukaemic blast cells.

8.51

A

In myeloma, there is malignant proliferation of plasma cells in the bone marrow.

B

The malignant plasma cells synthesise a monoclonal immunoglobulin or light chain. Although immunoglobulins are too large to pass through the glomerular filter, light chains may enter the urine. They are called Bence Jones proteins and may be detected in the laboratory.

C

Anaemia may be present in the late stage of the disease because the malignant myeloma cells may infiltrate the bone marrow and cause bone marrow failure.

D

Renal failure may occur for two reasons: (1) the Bence Jones proteins may cause atrophy of the renal tubular cells; (2) amyloidosis may develop in the kidneys.

8.52

A

Platelets are small (about $3\,\mu m$ in diameter) granulated bodies. They have a ring of microtubules around them. The cytoplasm contains actin, myosin, glycogen and two types of granules: dense granules and α granules.

B

The dense granules contain serotonin and ADP; the α granules contain secreted proteins such as clotting factors and platelet-derived growth factors.

C

When a blood vessel is injured, the three steps which help to stop bleeding are platelet adhesion, platelet aggregation and fibrin generation. In the first step, platelets adhere to the exposed collagen and von Willeband factor in the vessel wall via the receptor sites on the platelets. Von Willebrand factor is synthesised by endothelial cells and associates with factor VIII. This step does not require platelet metabolic activity. In the second step, platelets become activated. They change shape, put out pseudopodia and discharge their granules, such as ADP, serotonin, fibrinogen and von Willebrand factor. These factors, together with metabolism of arachidonic acid to thromboxane A_2, promote platelets to stick to one another via receptor sites which use fibrinogen as an

8

A

SYSTEM-BASED MEDICAL SCIENCES

intercellular bridge. In the third step, exposure of tissue factor activates the extrinsic coagulation system.

D

The production of platelets is controlled both by the colony-stimulating factors, which regulate the production of megakaryocytes, and thrombopoietin, which facilitates megakaryocytic maturation. Low platelet numbers appear to stimulate an increase in these factors.

E

The half-life of platelets is about 4 days. The platelet level could therefore be expected to rise a few days after the cessation of disease activity.

F

Megakaryocytes (giant cells) in the bone marrow are the precursors of platelets. In this child, platelets in the blood are destroyed by autoantibodies; hence, the number of megakaryocytes would be expected to increase in an attempt to replace the lost platelets.

8.53

A

The substances in the diagram are:
a) Plasmin
b) Plasminogen
c) Urokinase or tissue plasminogen activator
d) Fibrinogen
e) Thrombin
f) Prothrombin
g) Factor XII
h) Factor XIIa
i) Tissue factor.

B

i For the activated partial thromboplastin time (APTT), the intrinsic pathway is activated by contact (e.g. by addition of kaolin); hence, it generally tests the intrinsic coagulation pathway.

ii For the prothrombin time, tissue factor and phospholipid are added; hence, it generally assesses the extrinsic coagulation pathway. To be precise, it assesses factors II, V, VII and X.

C

i Warfarin is structurally similar to vitamin K. It interferes with the post-translation of glutamic acid residues in clotting factors II, VII, IX and X, and functions like a vitamin K inhibitor. As it interferes with the post-translation process, it takes several days for it to take effect and only acts in vivo. It inhibits coagulation by interfering with the extrinsic coagulation pathway.

ii Heparin inhibits coagulation by activating antithrombin III. Antithrombin inhibits thrombin and factor Xa; thus, it acts mainly via the intrinsic coagulation pathway.

iii Streptokinase is a fibrinolytic drug. It promotes the formation of plasmin from its precursor plasminogen. Since plasmin digests fibrin into fibrin degradation products, streptokinase may be used to dissolve clots (e.g. immediately after a myocardial infarct).

iv Tranexamic acid is an antifibrinolytic agent. It inhibits the formation of plasmin from plasminogen. It may therefore be used to treat conditions with a high risk of bleeding (e.g. to prevent haemorrhage after tonsillectomy).

The cardiovascular system

9.1 The following statements about cardiac muscle are correct:
  A There are no banding patterns in the sarcomere
  B The cardiac muscle fibres branch irregularly
  C T tubules are not present
  D Calcium ions are efficiently removed from the cytoplasm into the sarcoplasmic reticulum between contractions
  E The function of the intercalated discs includes rapid spread of contractile stimuli between cardiac muscle cells

9.2 The following statements about cardiac muscle are true:
  A Striations are absent
  B The muscle fibres branch and interdigitate
  C Gap junctions exist to allow impulses to travel from one cardiac fibre to another
  D It contains actin, myosin, troponin and tropomyosin
  E Over 25% of the energy is derived from anaerobic respiration

9.3 The sino-atrial (SA) node:
  A Is located at the junction of the superior vena cava and the right atrium
  B Contains the pacemaker cells
  C Is developed from the left side of the embryo
  D Is supplied by both the sympathetic and parasympathetic nervous system
  E Largely depends on influx of sodium ions for its action potential

9.4 The following statements about the SA node are true:
  A The cells in the SA node discharge spontaneously
  B Its impulse is slower than that of the atrioventricular (AV) node
  C Stimulation of the vagus nerve increases the rate of conduction through the SA node
  D Depolarisation spreads through the atria and converges directly on the Purkinje system
  E Disease affecting the SA node may lead to marked bradycardia

9.5 The following statements about the conduction of impulses from the SA node to the ventricles are true:
  A The time taken is represented by the PR interval on the ECG
  B It is slowed by adenosine
  C Stimulation of the vagus nerve increases the rate of conduction
  D Increased rate of conduction may result in supraventricular tachycardia

E Complete interruption of the conduction results in first-degree heart block

9.6 The following statements about atrial fibrillation are true:
  A It may be due to multiple re-entrant excitation waves in the atria
  B There are multiple P waves on the ECG
  C The ventricular rate exceeds the atrial rate
  D The ventricular rhythm is irregular
  E The cause may be myocardial ischaemia

9.7 Cardiac actions of calcium channel blockers may include:
  A Increased contractility
  B Positive chronotropic effect
  C Prolonging conduction in the AV node
  D Reducing the refractory period in the AV node
  E Terminating an attack of supraventricular tachycardia

9.8 Cardiac actions of cardiac glycosides (e.g. digoxin) may include:
  A Stimulation of membrane adenosine triphosphatase (ATPase)
  B Influx of calcium ions into cardiac cells
  C Negative inotropic effect
  D Enhancing vagal activity on the conducting system
  E Abolishing atrial fibrillation

9.9 The following increase the heart rate in sinus rhythm:
  A Atropine
  B Propranolol
  C Exercise
  D Expiration
  E Sleep

9.10 The following statements about ventricular systole are true:
  A The tricuspid valve is closed during a large part of this cardiac cycle
  B The pulmonary valve is closed during a large part of this cardic cycle
  C It is followed by atrial systole
  D It is indicated by the interval between the P and R waves on the ECG
  E The left ventricular pressure remains below 50 mmHg

9.11 The following statements about the mitral valve are true:
  A It is bicuspid

9

Q

SYSTEM-BASED MEDICAL SCIENCES

The cardiovascular system

    B It regulates the flow of blood from the right atrium to the right ventricle

    C It lies posterior to the sternum at the level of the fourth left costal cartilage

    D The associated papillary muscles are smaller than those of the tricuspid valves

    E Its closure is associated with the second heart sound

9.12 The following statements about the left atrium are true:

    A It forms the base of the heart

    B It receives blood from the superior vena cava

    C The pressure is significantly lower than that in the right atrium

    D The blood is desaturated with oxygen

    E A significant portion of the interior wall is smooth

9.13 Cardiac output:

    A Is the amount pumped out of the left ventricle per unit time

    B Is numerically the same as the stroke volume

    C Can be calculated from the amount of oxygen consumed per unit time and the arteriovenous difference in oxygen level

    D Can be estimated clinically using echocardiography and Doppler techniques

    E May be increased by more than three-fold on exercise

9.14 The following increases cardiac output in a normal heart:

    A Decrease in heart rate

    B Increase in stroke volume

    C Stimulation of the sympathetic nervous system

    D Increase in end-diastolic volume

    E Standing motionless

9.15 The following significant changes occur during exercise in a physically fit individual:

    A Cardiac output increases

    B Peripheral resistance increases

    C Diastolic pressure increases

    D The blood arterioles in the muscles dilate

    E The venous return increases

9.16 Cardiac failure:

    A Cannot occur if the cardiac output is over 5 litres per minute

    B May be compensated for in the early stages by increased ventricular end-diastolic volume

    C May be precipitated by severe anaemia

    D May be associated with a decrease in cardiac output on exercise

    E Often results in ventricular hypertrophy

9.17 Causes of predominantly left heart failure include:

    A Acute myocardial infarct

    B Severe aortic stenosis

    C Systemic hypertension

    D Chronic obstructive airway disease

    E Cardiomyopathy

9.18 The following classes of drugs used in the treatment of cardiac failure and their mechanisms are correctly matched:

    A Diuretics – reduction of afterload

    B Nitrates – reduction in afterload

    C Hydralazine – reduction of preload

    D Cardiac glycosides – increased contractility of myocardium

    E Angiotensin-converting enzyme (ACE) inhibitor – reduction of both preload and afterload

9.19 Consequences of cardiac failure include:

    A Pulmonary oedema

    B Enlarged liver

    C Increased loss of sodium and water from the kidneys

    D Increased pulmonary venous pressure

    E Dilatation of left ventricle

9.20 The following statements about the arch of the aorta are true:

    A It develops from the embryological sixth aortic arch on the left side

    B The left recurrent laryngeal nerve hooks around it

    C It is linked to the root of the left pulmonary artery by the ligamentum arteriosum

    D It gives off the left coronary artery

    E It gives off the left common carotid artery

9.21 The following statements about the pericardium are true:

    A It encloses the heart and the roots of the great vessels

    B The pericardial cavity is the space between the fibrous and serous pericardium

    C The pericardial cavity normally contains a small quantity of clear fluid

    D Inflammation of the pericardium may cause chest pain

    E Extensive fluid in the pericardial cavity may restrict the movement of the heart and cause circulation failure

9.22 The arterioles:

    A Contain a higher proportion of elastic tissue in their walls than the arteries

B Contain a higher proportion of smooth muscle in their walls than the arteries
C Contribute significantly to the total peripheral resistance
D Contribute significantly to the total blood capacitance
E Are constricted by noradrenaline (norepinephrine)

9.23 When other factors are kept constant, the arterial pressure increases with:
A An increase in cardiac output
B A decrease in peripheral resistance
C An increase in heart rate
D An increase in stroke volume
E Peripheral vasodilatation

9.24 The arterial blood pressure recorded is higher:
A In the arms than in the legs in the standing position on direct cannulation of the arteries
B The narrower the cuff used over the arm with the sphygmomanometer method
C In the arms than in the legs if the same cuff is used with the sphygmomanometer method in the lying position
D Using the auscultation rather than the palpation method with the sphygmomanometer
E If the mercury column is raised with the sphygmomanometer method

9.25 Clinical hypertension:
A Is universally defined as a blood pressure of 160/100 mmHg or above
B May be diagnosed with a single blood pressure reading of 160/100 mmHg
C Is more common with increasing age
D Is often caused by abnormally high peripheral resistance
E Is often caused by abnormally high cardiac output

9.26 Causes of secondary hypertension include:
A Chronic renal failure
B Addison's disease
C Aortic stenosis
D Corticosteroid therapy
E Acute glomerulonephritis

9.27 Patients with benign hypertension have increased risk for:
A Atherosclerosis
B Intracerebral haemorrhage
C Aortic dissection
D Subarachnoid haemorrhage
E Ischaemic heart disease

9.28 The following classes of antihypertensive drugs and their main mechanisms of action are appropriately matched:
A Calcium blockers – depletion of body sodium and reduction in plasma volume
B ACE inhibitors – reduction in peripheral resistance
C Nitrates – dilatation of capacitance vessels
D β-Adrenoceptor blockers – reduction in heart rate and myocardial contractility
E α-Adrenoceptor blockers – reduction in myocardial contractility

9.29 Atherosclerosis:
A Mainly affects arterioles
B Often begins as fatty streaks
C Is a major predisposing factor for ischaemic heart disease
D Predisposes to thrombi
E Predisposes to aneurysms

9.30 Factors associated with an increased risk of atherosclerosis include:
A Cigarette smoking
B Hypertension
C Female sex
D Raised HDL-cholesterol level
E Diabetes mellitus

9.31 The oxygen consumed by the heart per unit time decreases with increasing:
A Stroke volume
B Heart rate
C Arterial pressure (with constant cardiac output)
D Dilatation of the ventricles
E Sympathetic stimulation

9.32 Coronary blood flow normally increases with:
A Hypoxia
B Increased adenosine concentration
C Stimulation of α-adrenergic receptors
D Stimulation of β-adrenergic receptors
E Rising pH

9.33 Significant myocardial infarction is commonly caused by sudden obstruction of the following arteries:
A Right coronary artery
B Right marginal artery
C Diagonal artery
D Circumflex artery
E Left anterior descending artery

9.34 Causes of ischaemic symptoms of the heart include:
A Stenosis of the coronary artery
B Coronary artery thrombi

The cardiovascular system

C Severe aortic stenosis
D Coronary artery spasm
E Pericarditis

9.35 In the presence of a thrombus in a branch of the coronary artery, the following increases the size of a myocardial infarct:
A The involvement of a major branch of the coronary artery
B The presence of extensive anastomosis within the coronary arterial circulation
C Administration of intravenous streptokinase within an hour of obstruction
D Immediate administration of oral aspirin
E Continuous exercise in spite of ischaemic symptoms

9.36 The following anti-anginal drugs act at least partially via the corresponding mechanism:
A Nitrates – dilatation of the venules
B Nitrates – dilatation of the coronary arteries
C β-Adrenergic blockers – dilatation of capacitance veins
D Calcium channel blockers – dilatation of the venules
E Calcium channel blockers – dilatation of the coronary arteries

9.37 The following changes may occur within 24–48 h of acute complete obstruction of the right coronary artery:
A Pallor and oedema of the right ventricle
B Increased white cell count
C ST elevation in leads II, III, and aVF in the ECG
D Q waves in leads II, III, and aVF in the ECG
E Development of granulation tissue in the right ventricle

9.38 The following statements about the capillary circulation are true:
A About 20% of the circulating blood is in the capillaries
B There is a net movement of fluid from the capillary circulation to the interstitial fluid in the intestines
C The hydrostatic pressure gradient across the arteriole end is higher than the venule end
D Over 80% of the filtered fluid in the capillaries is returned to the circulation via the lymphatic system
E The net pressure gradient across the wall of a capillary is similar at the arteriole and the venule end

9.39 There is a net diffusion of the following substances from the capillaries into the interstitial fluid:
A Oxygen
B Carbon dioxide
C Glucose
D Lactic acid
E Albumin

9.40 The following statements about the circulation of blood in the adult heart are true:
A Deoxygenated blood enters the right atrium via the superior vena cava
B Deoxygenated blood enters the left atrium via the inferior vena cava
C Deoxygenated blood is ejected into the lungs by the right ventricle via the pulmonary veins
D Deoxygenated blood enters the left atrium via the pulmonary veins
E Oxygenated blood is ejected into the aorta by the left ventricle

9.41 The following sites contain well-oxygenated blood in the normal adult:
A Pulmonary arteries
B Pulmonary veins
C Inferior vena cava
D Left atrium
E Right atrium

9.42 The following statements about the fate of most of the blood entering the fetal circulation from the placenta are true:
A It enters the fetus via the umbilical arteries
B It passes through the right atrium
C It passes through the right ventricle
D It passes through the pulmonary arteries
E It supplies the heart and the brain via the ascending aorta

9.43 The following statements about the fate of most of the deoxygenated blood returning from the head and neck of the fetus in the fetal circulation are true:
A It enters the right atrium via the inferior vena cava
B It passes through the right ventricle
C It passes through the pulmonary circulation
D It passes through the left ventricle
E It is returned to the placenta via the umbilical veins

9.44 Blood at the following sites is mostly well oxygenated in the fetal circulation:
A Superior vena cava

    B Inferior vena cava
    C Ascending aorta
    D Descending aorta
    E Pulmonary veins

9.45 The following sites in the adult cardiovascular system and their approximate normal systolic pressures are correctly matched:
    A Right atrium – 50 mmHg
    B Left atrium – 10 mmHg
    C Right ventricle – 70 mmHg
    D Left ventricle – 120 mmHg
    E Pulmonary artery – 50 mmHg

9.46 The following events occur in congestive cardiac failure:
    A The sympathetic nervous system is stimulated
    B Aldosterone secretion is increased
    C Reabsorption of sodium in renal tubules is reduced
    D Glomerular filtration rate is increased
    E Total body sodium is increased

9.47 Pulse character can be accurately and reliably assessed at the following sites:
    A Radial pulse
    B Brachial pulse
    C Carotid pulse
    D Femoral pulse
    E Tibial pulse

9.48 A patient's hands are blue, but the lips and tongue are of normal colour. Possible causes include:
    A Chronic obstructive airway disease
    B Right-to-left shunting of blood
    C Cold hands
    D Raynaud's phenomenon
    E Cyanotic congenital heart disease

9.49 The internal jugular vein:
    A Is separated from the right atrium by one or more valves
    B Is less reliable than the external jugular vein in assessing a patient's venous pressure
    C Lies superficial to the clavicular head of the sternomastoid muscle
    D Lies deep to the sternal head of the sternomastoid muscle
    E Can be palpated with the patient lying at 45° to the horizontal

9.50 The following statements about the jugular venous pulse are true:
    A It can be seen when a healthy subject is sitting upright

    B It can be seen when a healthy subject lies horizontally
    C Examination is made easier if the subject turns the head as far left as possible
    D It may be undetected if the jugular venous pressure is extremely high
    E The jugular venous pressure is proportional to the distance between the jugular venous pulse and the sternal angle

9.51 The following phases of the jugular venous pulse and their causes are correctly matched:
    A 'a' wave – onset of ventricular systole
    B 'c' wave – onset of atrial systole
    C 'a–x' descent – atrial relaxation
    D 'v–y' descent – emptying of blood from right atrium into right ventricle
    E 'y–a' ascent – filling of the right atrium from the venae cavae

9.52 The following heart conditions and their associated jugular venous pulse abnormalities are correctly paired:
    A Atrial fibrillation – prominent 'a' waves
    B Complete heart block – cannon waves
    C Superior vena caval obstruction – raised venous pressure with exaggerated pulsation
    D Tricuspid stenosis – giant 'v' wave
    E Tricuspid incompetence – slow 'v–y' descent

9.53 The apex beat:
    A Is the point on the precordium where the cardiac impulse appears strongest
    B Normally lies near the fifth left intercostal space
    C Normally lies near the anterior axillary line
    D Is detected by auscultation with the stethoscope
    E May be displaced laterally in left ventricular enlargement

9.54 Cardiac thrills:
    A Do not occur during diastole
    B May occur in the absence of a cardiac murmur
    C Are vibrations synchronous with certain phases of the cardiac cycle
    D May occur in normal subject
    E Indicate the presence of turbulent blood flow

9.55 The first heart sound:
    A Is partly caused by the closure of the tricuspid valve
    B Is partly caused by the closure of the pulmonary valve
    C Is louder at the base than the apex of the heart

The cardiovascular system

   D Signals the end of ventricular systole

   E Has a higher pitch than the second heart sound

9.56 The second heart sound:

   A Is best heard with the bell than the diaphragm of the stethoscope

   B Is louder at the base than the apex of the heart

   C Is normally single on inspiration

   D Occurs at the beginning of ventricular diastole

   E Usually begins with the aortic component in physiological splitting

9.57 The following conditions and their associated abnormalities of the second heart sound are true:

   A Aortic stenosis – soft aortic component

   B Pulmonary hypertension – loud aortic component

   C Right bundle branch block – wide splitting

   D Left ventricular outflow obstruction – fixed splitting

   E Pulmonary stenosis – reverse splitting

9.58 The cardiac murmurs due to the following cardiac lesions and their sites of radiation are correctly paired:

   A Aortic stenosis – neck

   B Aortic regurgitation – neck

   C Mitral stenosis – apex of the heart

   D Pulmonary regurgitation – right sternal border

   E Ventricular septal defect – upper sternal edge

9.59 A 70-year-old woman was admitted to hospital complaining of sweating, breathlessness and ankle swelling. A doctor diagnosed congestive heart failure. The rhythm of the heart was normal. Among other drugs, the doctor prescribed digoxin.

   A What is cardiac output? How would you explain heart failure in terms of cardiac output?

   B Name three mechanisms by which the cardiac output can be increased under normal physiological conditions.

   C Give a brief reason that might explain the following.

     i   The patient was sweaty.

     ii The patient was breathless.

   D The patient had heart failure in spite of the mechanisms you listed in (B). Give two possible reasons for this. Give an example of a disease process for each.

   E Give the sequence of events starting at the cellular level that might lead to an increase in cardiac output when digoxin is given.

   F Name three other classes of drugs that may improve the patient's heart failure. How do they act?

9.60 In a closely supervised experiment, a medical student was attached to a cardiac monitor and was noted to be in sinus rhythm with a heart rate of 75 beats per minute. Vagal stimulation was performed by carefully massaging the student's right carotid sinus. The heart rate steadily decreased to just below 60 beats per minute.

   A Name the main structures and pathways for the normal conduction of electrical impulses in the heart.

   B Where are the two main 'nodes' of the conducting system anatomically?

   C Where is the cardiac pacemaker normally?

   D Sketch a graph showing the variation of the membrane potential of the pacemaker tissue with time. Label your sketch with the type of ionic conductance associated with each phase of the action potential. Which phase accounts for its 'pacemaker' role? Explain.

   E Which part of the conducting system is affected when the following are stimulated:

     • right vagus nerve

     • left vagus nerve.

   F In the experiment, explain why the heart slowed down, taking care to include the following details (if appropriate):

     • the neurotransmitter involved

     • the type of receptors involved

     • any second messengers involved

     • the types of ionic conductance affected.

   G In your sketch in (D) above, add one more action potential to demonstrate the effect of vagal stimulation. Would you still expect the student to be in sinus rhythm after vagal stimulation?

   H Name one drug that acts exactly opposite to vagal stimulation. When might this drug be indicated in clinical practice?

9.61 A 75-year-old man was admitted with a suspected myocardial infarct. The ECG showed ventricular tachycardia with a rate of 130 beats per minute. In order to minimise the risk of ventricular fibrillation, the patient was given intravenous lidocaine (lignocaine).

   A Which part of the ECG corresponds to ventricular depolarisation?

   B Describe the likely mechanisms for the ventricular tachycardia in this patient.

   C What is ventricular fibrillation? Why is it a serious condition? Why might electrical defibrillation be effective in treating this condition?

D In which class of antidysrhythmic drugs is lidocaine (lignocaine) in Vaughan Williams' classification? Explain why it might be beneficial in treating ventricular tachycardia or preventing ventricular fibrillation.

9.62 A 70-year-old woman was found at a routine clinic to have an irregularly irregular pulse at a rate of 100 beats per minute. The doctor diagnosed atrial fibrillation and prescribed digoxin.

A What part of the ECG corresponds to atrial depolarisation? What would you expect to find on the ECG in atrial fibrillation?

B Can the diagnosis of atrial fibrillation explain the patient's irregularly irregular pulse? Explain.

C What do you think were the approximate atrial and ventricular rates?

D Explain the mechanism for atrial fibrillation.

E Why might digoxin be useful for the treatment of atrial fibrillation?

F Name one other drug that might be useful for atrial fibrillation and briefly state its mechanism of action.

9.63 A patient suddenly became unwell. From the ECG recording, a doctor diagnosed supraventricular tachycardia. After initial treatment, a bolus of intravenous adenosine was given.

A How does supraventricular tachycardia differ from atrial fibrillation? How can one tell the difference from the ECG recording?

B How does supraventricular tachycardia differ from ventricular tachycardia? How can one tell the difference from the ECG recording?

C What simple treatment might be effective for the condition before resorting to drug treatment?

D Explain why adenosine might be effective in the treatment of this condition, taking care to include the following details (if appropriate):
  • the type of receptors involved
  • any second messengers involved.

E What is the main potential side effect of adenosine on the respiratory system? What is the mechanism for this side effect?

F Why would intravenous adenosine be preferable to other drugs, such as verapamil?

9.64 A 65-year-old woman was admitted after a fall. She was found to have a regular pulse of 25 beats per minute. Her ECG showed a complete (third-degree) heart block. The patient was given an isoprenaline infusion while cardiac pacing was arranged.

A Briefly distinguish between first-degree, second-degree and complete heart block.

B How can the three types of heart block be distinguished on the ECG?

C What is the effect of isoprenaline on the heart? What is its mechanism of action?

D Explain the falls experienced by this patient.

9.65 In a laboratory experiment to measure the cardiac output of a healthy subject, oxygen consumption and oxygen content of the arterial and venous blood were measured. Over a period of 4 min, 1 litre of oxygen was consumed. Oxygen content obtained from the femoral artery was 200 ml/l; that from the pulmonary artery was 150 ml/l. (All measurements were at standard pressure and temperature.)

A Explain the Fick principle.

B Calculate the cardiac output of this healthy subject.

9.66 An athlete had a cardiac output of 6 litres/min at rest; this rose to 24.4 litres/min during a 400 m race. This question explores how this increase in cardiac output could be achieved.

A What is stroke volume? Give the formula showing the relationship between cardiac output, stroke volume and heart rate. What are the units for these three variables?

B What is the effect of exercise on heart rate? What is the main mechanism for this effect?

C What factors determine the stroke volume?

D Briefly explain Starling's law of the heart. Sketch a graph to illustrate the law and label the axes.

E From your graph in (D), show how the stroke volume can be increased during exercise.

F i What do you understand by the terms 'preload' and 'afterload'?
   ii How does exercise increase the contractility of the heart? Include in your answer the types of receptors and the intracellular mechanisms involved

G Show the effect of increased contractility on your curve in (D).

H How does the 'afterload' change during exercise? Explain the physiological mechanisms for these changes. What effect does it have on cardiac output?

I Oxygen requirements for the heart increase dramatically during exercise. Explain the mechanisms for the increase in oxygen supply to the heart.

J Oxygen requirements for skeletal muscle increase dramatically during exercise. Explain the mechanisms for the increase in oxygen supply to muscle.

9

Q

SYSTEM-BASED MEDICAL SCIENCES

The cardiovascular system

9.67 A 55-year-old man suffered from symptoms of angina (myocardial ischaemia) caused by insufficient blood flow to the left ventricle to meet its oxygen requirements. Investigations showed that the coronary arteries were not obstructed. However, there was moderately severe aortic stenosis (narrowing of the aortic valve) and this was thought to be the cause of the patient's symptoms.

A Give estimates of the pressure (in mmHg) of the normal aorta in both systole and diastole.

B Give estimates of the pressure (in mmHg) of the normal left ventricle in both systole and diastole.

C Give estimates of the pressure (in mmHg) of the normal right ventricle in both systole and diastole.

D From your answers to parts (A)–(C), estimate the pressure differential (in mmHg) across the following
   i   The aorta and the left ventricle.
   ii The aorta and the right ventricle.

E In which cardiac phase(s) can blood flow from (1) the aorta via the appropriate coronary artery to supply the left ventricle; and (2) the aorta via the appropriate coronary artery to supply the right ventricle? From the point of view of blood supply, which of the two ventricles is more liable to myocardial ischaemia?

F From your answers above, what is the effect of aortic stenosis on the blood supply to the left ventricle? Explain.

G What is the relationship between the oxygen consumption per beat of the ventricle, the stroke volume and the intraventricular pressure? Explain.

H From your answer in (G), what is the effect of aortic stenosis on the oxygen requirement of the left ventricle? Give two reasons for your answer.

I From your answer to (H), what pathological change would you expect to find in the left ventricle?

9.68 A 45-year-old woman was found to have a raised blood pressure of 140/105 mmHg on three separate occasions. She was thought to have essential hypertension. It was explained to her that hypertension could have potential adverse effects on the cardiovascular system and she was treated with a thiazide diuretic drug.

A Blood pressure is almost universally measured by the auscultatory method, using an inflatable cuff attached to a manometer and wrapped around the arm.
   i   Describe how the systolic and diastolic pressures are determined.

   ii What are the 'sounds of Korotkoff'? What are they caused by? Explain using the term 'critical velocity'.
   iii Give two important precautions for measuring blood pressure by this method.

B State the formula relating blood pressure with two of the following three variables: cardiac output, peripheral resistance and heart rate. Which of these factors is likely to explain this patient's hypertension?

C Give a brief account of the following possible pathophysiological mechanisms underlying essential hypertension:
   i   Sodium homeostasis
   ii The sympathetic nervous system
   iii The renin–angiotensin–aldosterone system.

D What potential adverse effects does hypertension have on the left ventricle and its workload? Explain in terms of Starling's law and law of Laplace.

E What potential adverse effects does hypertension have on the small arteries? How might it further worsen hypertension?

F Explain the mechanism for the antihypertensive effect of thiazide diuretics.

9.69 A 55-year-old man suddenly developed severe chest pain. He was given oral aspirin immediately by his general practitioner and was admitted to the coronary care unit. The ECG strongly suggested a diagnosis of anterior myocardial infarction and he was given intravenous alteplase. He died 4 days later. At post-mortem examination, extensive atherosclerosis was found in the abdominal aorta.

A From where do the coronary arteries arise?

B Name the main coronary arteries and the branches obstruction of which account for myocardial infarction. Which of these coronary arteries (or branches) was likely to have been obstructed?

C List the important factors that determine the size of the infarct when a coronary artery or its branch is obstructed. Why might the rapid onset of the obstruction affect the size of the infarct?

D What was the most likely cause for the obstruction of the coronary artery?

E i   What types of vessel does atherosclerosis mostly affect?
   ii List the types of atherosclerotic lesions and briefly describe their histological appearance.
   iii List the risk factors associated with atherosclerosis.

F What macroscopic and microscopic changes would you expect to find in the left ventricle at post-mortem? What changes would you expect if the patient had died 2 weeks later?

9.70 An elderly patient suffered from frequent angina attacks and was prescribed a combination of isosorbide mononitrate, atenolol and diltiazem (a calcium antagonist). He suffered a headache as well as a fall in pressure due to postural hypotension (a fall in blood pressure when he stood up).

A Explain the mechanisms by which isosorbide mononitrate may be beneficial in angina. Describe the cellular mechanisms as well as the effects on the cardiovascular system.

B Why might isosorbide mononitrate have caused a fall in blood pressure when he stood up?

C Explain why atenolol may relieve symptoms of angina.

D Explain the mechanisms by which diltiazem may be beneficial in angina. Describe the cellular mechanisms as well as the effects on the cardiovascular system.

9.71 A 3-year-old boy was noted to have a heart murmur. The paediatrician made a diagnosis of ventricular septal defect (a defect in the membranous (fibrous) part of the interventricular septum).

A Describe the embryological development of the interventricular septum and explain how various defects may occur.

B Figure 9.1 outlines the flow of blood in the normal heart from the vena cavae to the aorta. Name the chambers or vessels, and state whether the blood is saturated or desaturated with oxygen in each case.

C The pressures in a 3-year-old child are approximately two-thirds those of an adult. Assume both the left and right ventricular pressures in this child are normal for his age. Estimate the pressures inside the left ventricle and the right ventricle during systole and diastole. In which direction would you expect blood to flow in systole and in diastole? Indicate, on Fig. 9.1, where this extra flow of blood occurs.

D What is the mechanism of a heart murmur? In which phase of the cardiac cycle would you expect the murmur to be present in this child?

E Generally speaking, a child may appear cyanosed (blue) if the blood in the aorta is desaturated with oxygen. Would you expect this child to be cyanosed? Explain.

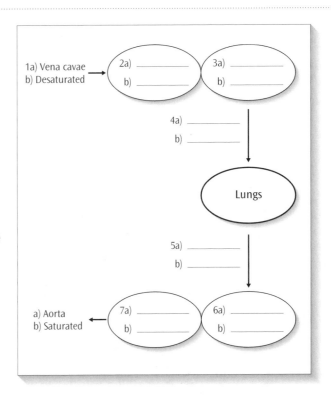

1a) Vena cavae
b) Desaturated

2a) _____
b) _____

3a) _____
b) _____

4a) _____
b) _____

Lungs

5a) _____
b) _____

7a) _____
b) _____

6a) _____
b) _____

a) Aorta
b) Saturated

Fig. 9.1 Adult circulation from the vena cavae to the aorta.

9.72 A newborn child was unwell and the paediatricians made a diagnosis of 'patent ductus arteriosus': the ductus arteriosus, which usually closes shortly after birth, remained open in this baby.

A Give a brief description of the anatomy of the ductus arteriosus immediately after birth. Which nerve hooks around it? What does the ductus arteriosus become after the newborn period?

B Give a brief account of the embryology of the ductus arteriosus and relate it to the anatomy as described in (A).

C In which direction would you expect blood to flow in this infant?

9.73 Figure 9.2 illustrates the fetal circulation for comparison with the adult circulation shown in question 9.71B.

A Name the structures (2) to (7).

B What are the structures in the fetus that allows blood to flow through (8) and (9) in Fig. 9.2?

C Trace the blood from the umbilical veins in the fetus. It passes through the ductus venosus. Using Fig. 9.2, indicate the various chambers and vessels the blood passes through before it reaches the aorta. Is this blood relatively well oxygenated or poorly oxygenated?

113

9

Q

SYSTEM-BASED MEDICAL SCIENCES

The cardiovascular system

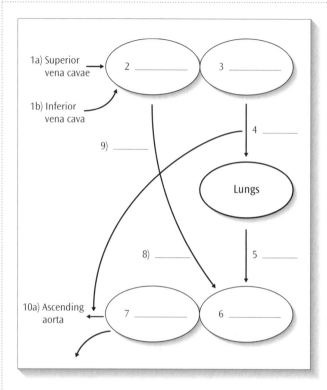

1a) Superior vena cavae

1b) Inferior vena cava

9) _____

2 _____

3 _____

4 _____

Lungs

8) _____

5 _____

10a) Ascending aorta

7 _____

6 _____

Fig. 9.2 Fetal circulation from the vena cavae to the aorta.

D Trace the blood returning to the superior vena cava via the fetus. Using Fig. 9.2, indicate the various chambers and vessels the blood passes through before it reaches the aorta. Is this blood relatively well-oxygenated or poorly-oxygenated?

E Explain why little blood passes through the channel (5).

9.74 A doctor detected a heart murmur in a patient and suspected that he might have narrowing of the mitral valve (mitral stenosis).

A Which two chambers of the heart does the mitral valve separate?

B Briefly describe the structure of the mitral valve.

C In which phase of the cardiac cycle is the mitral valve open and in which phase is it closed?

D What prevents blood from leaking back into the atrium?

E When a heart valve is narrowed (stenosed), blood flow through it is turbulent and causes a murmur. During which cardiac phase would you expect the murmur to be heard in this patient?

F What causes the first and second heart sounds? What abnormalities would you expect in this patient?

9.75 A 30-year-old man was admitted to hospital with serious bleeding into a fractured leg (femur) after a road traffic accident. He was cold and pale and had a heart rate of 130 beats per minute; however, his blood pressure was almost normal at 110/70 mmHg. It was estimated that blood loss amounted to 1 litre.

A What is hypovolaemic shock?

B Explain why he was cold and pale, and had a fast heart rate. How might these mechanisms compensate for the loss of blood volume?

C Explain the possible relevance of the following mechanisms in maintaining the blood volume in this patient in the short term.

  i Restlessness

  ii Rapid breathing

  iii Kidneys

  iv Renin and aldosterone.

The cardiovascular system

9.1 B E

Cardiac muscle fibres are similar to those of skeletal muscle in many ways. The arrangement of the contractile proteins is similar, and there are cross-striations in the cardiac muscle fibres. However, as the cardiac muscle fibres branch irregularly, the banding pattern is also irregular. T tubules and sarcoplasmic reticulum are present in cardiac muscle fibres. However, there is a slow leakage of calcium ions from the sarcoplasmic reticulum into the cytoplasm between contractions, and this accounts for the automaticity of cardiac contractions, and the inherent rhythm of the pacemaker tissues. Intercalated discs are specialised intercellular junctions between the ends of adjacent cardiac muscle cells. They allow rapid spread of contractile stimuli from one cardiac muscle cell to another, so that the cardiac muscle fibre functions as a syncytium.

9.2 B C D

Cardiac muscles are similar to skeletal muscles in many ways. Striations and Z lines are present. Although each fibre is enclosed in a cell membrane, the muscle fibres branch and interdigitate. The cell membranes at the ends of the muscle fibres form intercalated discs to maintain strong cell-to-cell cohesion, and gap junctions are formed in the cell membranes of adjacent fibres to allow electrical impulses to travel from one fibre to another. Like skeletal muscles, cardiac muscles contain actin, myosin, troponin and tropomyosin. The heart relies almost exclusively on oxidative phosphorylation for its energy supply, and the cardiac cells contain numerous mitochondria.

9.3 A B D

The SA node is located at the junction of the superior vena cava and the right atrium, and is developed from the right side of the embryo. Consequently, it is innervated by the right vagus nerve and the right side of the sympathetic innervation. The SA node contains the actual pacemaker cells (P cells). The pacemaking cells have membrane potentials which slowly drift to the threshold level after each impulse. The action potentials are largely due to influx of calcium ions through the slower-opening calcium channels, with little contribution from sodium ion influx.

9.4 A E

See also question 9.1. Due to the slow drift of the membrane potential to the firing level after each impulse, the cells in the SA node discharge spontaneously. Stimulation of the vagus nerve releases acetylcholine, which acts via the muscarinic receptors to slow the opening of the calcium channels, and hence to decrease the firing rate and slow its conduction rate. Conversely, noradrenaline (norepinephrine) stimulates the β_1-adrenergic receptors, increases the firing rate and speeds up its conduction rate. The depolarisation initiated from the SA node spreads through the atria and converges on the AV node, before it is conducted through the bundle of His to the Purkinje system. The spontaneous rate of conduction in the SA node is about 70 beats per minute, and is faster than any other location in the heart. Otherwise, the other locations may take over as pacemakers. Diseases affecting the SA node may lead to marked bradycardia as the rate of spontaneous discharge from the AV node is slower (about 45 beats per minute). This is known as the sick sinus syndrome, and patients may complain of dizziness and fainting.

9.5 A B D

The P and QRS complexes are due to atrial and ventricular contractions respectively. Hence the PR interval represents the time taken for the impulse to travel from the SA node to the ventricles. The rate of conduction is increased by sympathetic stimulation (via adrenaline (epinephrine)) and reduced by parasympathetic stimulation (via acetylcholine). Increased rate of conduction may be seen in people with an additional abnormal conducting pathway (e.g. in Wolff–Parkinson–White syndrome). Supraventricular tachycardia (increased heart rate due to abnormality above the ventricles) results. Measures which reduce the rate of conduction (e.g. stimulation of vagus nerve, adenosine, calcium antagonist, disopyramide, digoxin) may alleviate the condition. Reduced rate of conduction results in heart block. If all the atrial impulses reach the ventricles, the PR interval is prolonged, and the condition is known as first-degree heart block. Second-degree heart block is said to occur if not all atrial impulses reach the ventricles. In third-degree (complete) heart block, the conduction of impulses is completely interrupted.

9.6 A D E

Atrial fibrillation is due to multiple circulating re-entrant excitation in the atria. This results in an irregular and fast atrial rate (up to 500 per minute). Hence the AV node also discharges at an irregular, but slower rate (about 90–150 beats per minutes). P waves cannot usually be detected on the ECG. There are many pathological causes for atrial fibrillation, which include myocardial ischaemia, stenosis of the mitral valve and thyrotoxicosis.

9.7 C E

Cardiac cells are dependent on calcium ions in two ways. Firstly, the pacemaker cells in the SA and AV nodes rely on the slow influx of calcium ions for their automaticity. Secondly, in phase two of the action potential in non-pacemaker cells, a fast influx of sodium ions is followed by a slow influx of calcium ions, which activate contraction of cardiac muscle. Hence calcium channel blockers have potentially two effects. Firstly, they slow the rate of

9

A

SYSTEM-BASED MEDICAL SCIENCES

The cardiovascular system

discharge at the SA and AV nodes. Conduction at the AV node is slowed, and the refractory period is prolonged. Thus they are effective in the treatment of supraventricular tachycardia. Secondly, they depress contractility (i.e. they are a negative inotrope).

9.8 B D E

Cardiac glycosides act via two mechanisms. Firstly, they enhance the vagal activity. Hence they reduce conduction through the AV node and are beneficial in supraventricular tachycardia and atrial fibrillation. Secondly, they inhibit the membrane-bound ATPase. ATPase supplies energy for the pump which transports sodium out of and potassium into contracting cells. Hence, inhibition of the enzyme results in an increase in intracellular sodium and a reduction in intracellular potassium. This is accompanied by an increase in extracellular calcium, which accounts for the positive inotropic effect.

9.9 A C

The heart rate is controlled by both sympathetic and parasympathetic nerves to the heart, and the baroreceptor-mediated reflexes. The heart rate is increased during exercise through sympathetic stimulation, and is decreased during sleep through parasympathetic stimulation. Propranolol slows the heart rate through blockage of the β_1-adrenergic receptors, and atropine increases the heart rate by blocking the muscarinic receptors. The heart rate normally varies with the phases of respiration: it increases during inspiration and decreases during expiration. This is due to normal variations in the parasympathetic output to the heart during respiration. In inspiration, impulses from the vagus nerve are decreased.

9.10 A

Ventricular systole follows atrial systole. The mitral and tricuspid valves close at the beginning of ventricular systole. The aortic and pulmonary valves open soon afterwards with the isovolumetric contraction of the ventricles. The P and R waves mark the beginning of the atrial and ventricular systole respectively. During ventricular systole, the left ventricular pressure increases from less than 10 mmHg to about 120 mmHg in the middle of ventricular systole.

9.11 A C

The mitral valve regulates the flow of blood from the left atrium to the left ventricle, and lies posterior to the sternum at the apex of the heart (at the level of the fourth costal cartilage). Whilst the tricuspid valve has three cusps, the mitral valve has two. Since the work done by the left ventricle far exceeds that done by the right ventricle, the associated papillary muscles are much larger

than those of the right ventricle. The first heart sound is caused by the vibrations set up by the sudden closure of the mitral valve (and the tricuspid valve to a lesser extent), whilst the second heart sound is associated with the closure of the aortic and pulmonary valves.

9.12 A E

The left atrium forms most of the base, as well as the superior part of the left border of the heart. It receives blood oxygenated during its passage in the lungs from four pulmonary veins. The pulmonary veins enter the left atrium in its posterior wall. Embryologically, a large proportion of the left atrium develops from the primitive pulmonary vein. Hence, a significant proportion of the interior of the left atrium is smooth, apart from the muscular ridges in the auricle.

9.13 A C D E

Cardiac output is the amount of blood pumped out of each ventricle per unit time, whilst the stroke volume is the amount of blood pumped out per beat. Hence cardiac output equals the product of the stroke volume and the heart rate. Traditionally, it may be measured by the Fick method or the indicator dilution method. In the Fick method, oxygen consumption per unit time is measured, and the difference in oxygen concentration in the arterial and venous blood is measured via a cardiac catheter. Cardiac output can be calculated from the equation

$$\text{Cardiac output} = \text{Oxygen consumption per unit time}/$$
$$(\text{Arterial oxygen concentration} - \text{Venous}$$
$$\text{oxygen concentration})$$

In the indicator dilution method, a dye is injected into the vein, and the log of the arterial concentration of the dye is plotted against time. Cardiac output can be calculated from the amount of dye injected and the instantaneous concentration of the indicator in the arterial blood.

In clinical practice, cardiac output can be calculated more easily by estimating the velocity and volume of blood passing through heart valves. These parameters can be measured using echocardiography and Doppler techniques.

9.14 B C D

Cardiac output is equal to the product of heart rate and stroke volume. Hence either an increase in heart rate or an increase in stroke volume would result in an increase in cardiac output. Stimulation of the sympathetic nervous system results in an increase in both the stroke volume and the heart rate. According to Starling's law, the energy of contraction of a cardiac muscle fibre is proportional to its initial length (the preload). For the heart, the length of the muscle fibres is proportional to the end-diastolic volume. Hence the stroke volume increases with the ventricular end-diastolic volume. In the abnormal heart, however, the stroke volume may decrease with increasing ventricular end-diastolic volume above a certain threshold. The arterial pressure is equal to the product of the peripheral resistance and the cardiac output. Standing motionless increases venous pooling of the blood in the legs, and hence reduces the venous return. This reduces the end-diastolic volume and the stroke volume.

9.15   A D E
During exercise, cardiac output may increase up to seven-fold. This is brought about by an increase in both stroke volume and heart rate. The heart rate increases rapidly due to stimulation of the sympathetic nervous system, and the stimulatory effect of the increased carbon dioxide on the medulla. The enhanced activity of the muscle pumps increases the venous return, which contributes to the increase in cardiac output. The arterioles in the muscles dilate due to local mechanisms (fall in local oxygen, and increase in carbon dioxide and other metabolites). This greatly reduces the peripheral resistance. Hence, whilst the systolic pressure may rise slightly during exercise, the diastolic pressure remains constant or falls slightly.

9.16   B C D E
Cardiac failure is said to occur when the heart is unable to pump blood from the ventricles at a rate required for the metabolism of the body. This is often due to reduced capacity of the heart to pump blood (low output failure). However, it may also be caused by increased demands of the body for blood (e.g. in the presence of severe anaemia or pregnancy). Hence cardiac failure may occur in spite of a normal cardiac output, and the condition is known as high output failure. In the early stages of heart failure, the heart may pump sufficient blood by its compensating mechanisms (e.g. by increasing ventricular end-diastolic volume, according to Starling's law). However, in later stages, this may be ineffective, and cardiac output may decrease with an increase in ventricular end-diastolic volume on exercise. If the heart failure exists for some time, the heart may attempt to cope with the demand by ventricular hypertrophy. Ventricular dilatation may result from the extra workload. However, a consequence of the law of Laplace is that the tension in a distensible object to create a given pressure is proportional to its radius. Hence, even more work is needed from the dilated ventricles.

9.17   A B C E
Although the failure of one ventricle may result in the failure of the other, often only one ventricle is failing in the early stages. The commonest causes of left ventricular failure are ischaemic heart disease (e.g. acute myocardial infarct), systemic hypertension and valvular diseases.

Ischaemic heart disease affects the ability of the heart to pump blood, whilst systemic hypertension and some valvular disease (e.g. aortic stenosis) provide extra workload on the ventricles. Cardiomyopathy represents cardiac diseases not caused by the above aetiologies or congenital heart diseases. Chronic obstructive airways disease may cause right heart failure.

9.18   D E
Drugs may relieve cardiac failure by reducing the venous return and ventricular filling pressure (preload), reducing the peripheral resistance (afterload), or increasing the contractility of the myocardium (positive inotropic effect). Diuretics increase salt and water loss from the body and reduce venous return, hence their main mechanism of action is to reduce preload. Nitrates dilate the smooth muscle of venous capacitance vessels and so reduce the ventricular filling pressure. They also act by reducing preload. Hydralazine relaxes the arterial smooth muscle and reduces peripheral resistance, hence it reduces afterload. ACE prevents the conversion of angiotensin I to the active component angiotensin II, which is a strong arterioconstrictor. This also prevents the formation of aldosterone, which promotes retention of sodium and water. Therefore ACE inhibitor has the effect of reducing afterload (by reducing arterioconstriction) and preload (by reducing sodium and water retention). Cardiac glycosides (e.g. digoxin) stimulate cardiac contractility by inhibiting membrane-bound ATPase.

9.19   A B D E
Cardiac failure results in congestion of the pulmonary veins and an increase in pulmonary venous pressure. This results in pulmonary oedema, and patients often complain of breathlessness especially while lying flat, and at night. When the patient lies flat, there is increased venous return. The kidneys often attempt to compensate for cardiac failure by retaining sodium and fluid. As a result, there is widespread systemic venous congestion. The liver is often congested and enlarged. The ventricles may dilate, but this increases the workload of the heart further (see question 9.15).

9.20   B C E
The arch of the aorta is developed from the embryological fourth aortic arch on the left side. On the right side, the embryological fourth aortic arch becomes the proximal part of the right subclavian artery. The embryological sixth aortic arch becomes the ductus arteriosus, which joins the left pulmonary artery with the arch of the aorta. The left recurrent laryngeal nerve, which is the nerve of the sixth pharyngeal arch on the left side, hooks around the arch of the aorta and the ligamentum arteriosum. The coronary arteries are branches of the ascending aorta. The branches

of the arch of aorta are the brachiocephalic artery (which divides to right common carotid and right subclavian arteries), left common carotid artery and left subclavian artery.

9.21 A C D E
The pericardium is a double-walled sac which encloses the heart and the roots of the great vessels. It consists of the fibrous and serous pericardium. The fibrous pericardium is inelastic. The serous pericardium consists of the parietal and the visceral layers. The visceral layer is the continuation of the external layer of the epicardium, the external layer of the heart wall. The pericardial cavity is the space between the visceral and parietal layers of the serous pericardium. It contains a small quantity of clear fluid which minimises friction during the cardiac cycle. Inflammation of the pericardium is called pericarditis, and is commonly caused by viral infection. The characteristic symptom is precordial pain. As the surfaces of the pericardium are rough, a friction rub may be heard with a stethoscope. Extensive fluid in the pericardial cavity may be caused by stab wounds to the heart causing the pericardial cavity to be filled with blood. This may seriously restrict the movement of the heart (cardiac tamponade) and cause circulation failure.

9.22 B C E
Compared to arterial walls, the arteriolar walls contain a lower proportion of elastic tissues but a higher proportion of smooth muscle. The smooth muscle is constricted by stimulation of the noradrenergic nerve fibres. Hence the arterioles contribute significantly to the total peripheral resistance, and a small change in the diameter of the vessels results in a large change in the peripheral resistance. The arterioles only contain about 1% of the blood volume. The major capacitor of blood is the venous system.

9.23 A C D
The arterial pressure is the product of cardiac output and peripheral resistance. Peripheral resistance decreases with vasodilatation. Hence the arterial pressure decreases with vasodilatation. Cardiac output is equal to the product of heart rate and stroke volume (the volume of blood pumped by the left ventricle per contraction). Hence an increase in the heart rate or stroke volume increases the arterial blood pressure in the absence of other regulatory mechanisms.

9.24 B D
The arterial pressure in any vessel becomes higher the lower the vessel is vertically. This is due to the effect of gravity. If the sphygmomanometer method is used, the recorded blood pressure would appear lower if the mercury column is raised. If a narrow cuff is used to measure blood pressure in an obese person, the fatty tissue dissipates some of the cuff pressure, and the recording would be abnormally high. For the same reason, the blood pressure recorded would be inappropriately high if the same cuff is used over the legs. The palpation method with the sphygmomanometer usually underestimates the blood pressure, as it is difficult to determine exactly when the first beat is felt.

9.25 C D
There is no universal definition of clinical hypertension, and it should not be diagnosed on a single blood pressure reading, as the high reading may be due to anxiety. Hypertension is more common with increasing age, and there is an inherited component. As blood pressure is equal to the product of cardiac output and peripheral resistance, increase of either cardiac output or peripheral resistance will cause an increase in arterial blood pressure. Clinically, however, sustained hypertension is almost always due to abnormally high peripheral resistance.

9.26 A D E
In over 90% of cases of hypertension, no obvious causes are found (i.e. essential hypertension). The known causes for hypertension include renal disease (e.g. chronic renal failure, acute glomerulonephritis, renal artery stenosis), endocrine diseases (e.g. Cushing's disease, Conn's syndrome with excessive aldosterone secretion), coarctation of the aorta and drug treatment (e.g. corticosteroid therapy). Aortic stenosis is associated with a narrow pulse pressure, but not arterial hypertension.

9.27 A B C D E
Although benign hypertension may be symptomless, patients are at risk of developing atherosclerosis and consequently ischaemic heart disease. Also, they have increased risk for intracerebral haemorrhage, aortic dissection and subarachnoid haemorrhage (from rupture of berry aneurysms). Hence benign hypertension is a serious condition needing prompt treatment.

9.28 B C D
Antihypertensives may act by depleting body sodium and reducing plasma volume (e.g. diuretics); reducing cardiac output by reducing heart rate and/or myocardial contractility (e.g. β-adrenergic blockers); reducing peripheral resistance by dilating arterioles (e.g. calcium blockers, ACE inhibitors); or dilating venous capacitance vessels to reduce venous return (e.g. nitrates, some calcium blockers).

9.29 B C D E
Atherosclerosis affects large and medium-sized arteries. Lesions often begin as fatty streaks. In those who are

predisposed to arteriosclerosis, they may progress to fibrolipid plaques. Haemorrhage and thrombi may occur in the plaques. This may lead to total occlusion of the blood supply to important organs such as the coronary arteries.

9.30 A B E
Risk factors for increased atherosclerosis include increased age, hypertension, male sex, high LDL-cholesterol level, obesity and diabetes mellitus. Other less important factors include lack of exercise and low social class. A high level of HDL-cholesterol appears to protect against atherosclerosis.

9.31 –
The oxygen consumed by the heart is directly proportional to the work done by the heart. The work done by the heart is proportional to the product of the heart rate, the stroke volume, and the arterial pressure. By the law of Laplace, the tension in the wall of the heart to sustain a given pressure is proportional to its radius. Hence dilatation of the ventricles results in an increase in work done and oxygen consumed. Sympathetic stimulation results in an increase in stroke volume, heart rate and peripheral resistance. Hence the oxygen consumed is increased.

9.32 A B D
The heart is particularly susceptible to ischaemia, and it is particularly important to match coronary blood flow with the oxygen consumption by the heart. Coronary blood flow depends on three factors: the pressure gradient, chemical factors and neural factors. Probably several chemical factors are involved. Hypoxia, acidosis and an increase in lactic acid and adenosine cause coronary vasodilatation and consequent increased coronary blood flow. As these factors are normally associated with increased metabolic demand on the heart, a balance between supply and demand for oxygenation can be achieved. Neural factors include α-adrenergic receptors (stimulus of which causes coronary vasoconstriction) and β-adrenergic receptors (stimulation of which causes coronary vasodilatation).

9.33 A D E
Both the right and left coronary arteries arise from the ascending aorta just above the aortic valve. Obstruction of the right coronary artery results in inferior myocardial infarction. The right coronary artery gives off the right marginal artery at the inferior border of the heart, which supplies the right ventricle. Obstruction of this branch is unlikely to result in significant myocardial infarct. The most important branch of the right coronary artery is the posterior descending artery, which supplies both ventricles. The left coronary artery has two major branches: the left anterior descending artery, which supplies both ventricles

and the interventricular septum, and the circumflex branch, which supplies the left atrium and left ventricle. Obstruction of the left anterior descending artery results in anterior infarction, whilst obstruction of the circumflex artery results in lateral infarction.

9.34 A B C D
Most ischaemic symptoms of the heart are caused by atherosclerosis, either via stenosis of the coronary artery or atherosclerosis with superimposed thrombi. Occasionally, angina symptoms may be experienced by those with no minimal atherosclerosis, and their symptoms may be due to coronary artery spasm. Rarely, severe aortic stenosis may cause ischaemic symptoms by impairing coronary blood flow. Whilst pericarditis may cause precordial pain, the pain is secondary to inflammation and not ischaemia.

9.35 A E
The size of a myocardial infarct is likely to be significant if a major branch of the coronary artery is obstructed, the degree of obstruction is large, and there is a lack of anastomosis between the obstructed artery with the rest of the coronary circulation. Administration of intravenous streptokinase and oral aspirin immediately after a myocardial infarct has been proven to reduce the size of the infarct. Continuous exercise in spite of ischaemic symptoms increases the oxygen demand of the heart, and is liable to increase the size of the infarct.

9.36 A B E
The three established classes of anti-anginal drugs are organic nitrates, β-adrenergic blockers and calcium channel blockers. Organic nitrates act mainly by dilating the capacitance veins (reducing the preload) and dilating the main coronary arteries. The β-adrenergic blockers block the β-adrenergic receptors, and therefore slow the heart rate, reduce the mechanical contractility of the heart and reduce the peripheral resistance. Calcium channel blockers act by dilating the arterioles (reducing the peripheral resistance), dilating the coronary arteries and reducing the contractility of the heart.

9.37 A B C
The histological changes of myocardial infarcts follow a predictable sequence. No changes are usually seen in the first 18 h. Acute inflammatory response occurs between the first and second day. Necrosis occurs between the third and fourth day. Granulation tissue starts to develop after the first week and fibrosis occurs after about two weeks of infarct. Between the first 24–48 h the affected cardiac muscle may appear pale and oedematous and acute inflammatory changes may be seen microscopically. This may be associated with a transient increase in white cell count. The immediate ECG changes are ST elevation due

9 **A**

SYSTEM-BASED MEDICAL SCIENCES

The cardiovascular system

to delayed depolarisation of the infarcted cells. Q waves are due to failure of the infarcted cardiac muscles to contribute to the positivity of the QRS complex, and usually appear at least a few days later.

9.38 C
Although less than 5% of the circulating blood is in the capillaries, the capillary circulation plays an important role in the delivery of oxygen and nutrients to the tissue, as well as the removal of carbon dioxide and other waste products from the tissue. Capillary hydrostatic pressures differ according to the tissues, but capillary pressures at the arteriole and venule end are typically about 30 and 15 mmHg respectively. The osmotic pressure gradient across the capillary wall is roughly constant along the capillary. The rate of filtration at any point along the capillary depends on the balance of hydrostatic and osmotic pressure gradients (Starling forces), and differs according to the tissues. For example, fluid moves out of the capillaries along almost their entire length in the renal glomerulus, but into the capillaries along almost their entire length in the intestines. Over 80% of the filtered fluid in the capillaries is returned to the circulation via reabsorption and the rest via the lymphatics.

9.39 A C
See question 9.38 above. Albumin molecules are too large to diffuse across the capillary wall.

9.40 A E
The pathway for circulation of blood in the adult heart is as follows:
* Deoxygenated blood enters the right atrium via the superior and inferior vena cava
* Deoxygenated blood enters the right ventricle from the right atrium
* Deoxygenated blood is ejected to the lungs by the right ventricle via the pulmonary arteries
* Oxygenated blood is returned from the lungs to the left atrium via the pulmonary veins
* Oxygenated blood enters the left ventricle from the left atrium
* Oxygenated blood is ejected into the aorta by the left ventricle

9.41 B D
Deoxygenated blood from the body returns to the heart via the superior and inferior vena cava. It enters the right atrium and is directed to the right ventricle via the tricuspid valve. It is ejected by the right ventricle through the pulmonary valve into the pulmonary arteries, where it enters the lung capillaries to be reoxygenated. The oxygenated blood leaves the lung via the pulmonary veins and enters the left atrium, where it is directed to the left

ventricle through the mitral valve. The oxygenated blood is then ejected by the left ventricle through the aortic valve into the aorta.

9.42 B E
The correct pathways for the flow of oxygenated blood entering the fetal circulation from the placenta are:
* Blood enters through the umbilical veins towards the liver
* Blood flows directly through the ductus venosus into the inferior vena cava, bypassing the liver
* Blood enters the right atrium
* Blood is shunted across the left atrium through the foramen ovale
* Blood enters the left ventricle
* Blood is ejected into the ascending aorta, and supplies the brain and heart

9.43 B
The correct pathways for the flow of deoxygenated blood returned from the fetal head and neck are:
* Blood enters the right atrium via the superior vena cava
* Blood enters the right ventricle via the tricuspid valve
* Blood enters the pulmonary artery, and is shunted across to the descending aorta via the ductus arteriosus
* Blood is returned to the placenta via the umbilical arteries

9.44 B C
See questions 9.42 and 9.43 above for the pathways of the oxygenated and deoxygenated blood. Oxygenated blood mixes with deoxygenated blood at several sites: the inferior vena cava, the right atrium, the left atrium, and at the entrance of the ductus arteriosus into the descending aorta. However, blood in the inferior vena cava and ascending aorta are mostly well oxygenated, whilst blood in the superior vena cava, pulmonary veins and descending aorta are mostly deoxygenated.

9.45 B D
It is important to note the following general points about systolic pressure:
* The ventricles have much higher systolic pressure than the corresponding atria
* The right ventricle and pulmonary arteries have equal systolic pressures
* The left ventricle and the aorta have equal systolic pressures
* The left side of the heart has much higher systolic pressure than the right
The approximate normal systolic pressures are:
* Right atrium – 8 mmHg
* Right ventricle (= pulmonary artery) – 25 mmHg

- Left atrium – 10 mmHg
- Left ventricle (= aorta) – 120 mmHg

9.46   A B E

The usual primary cause of cardiac failure is reduced myocardial contractility. This causes reduced effective arterial blood volume. In order to maintain the blood pressure, both the sympathetic nervous system and the renin–angiotensin system are stimulated. The stimulation of the sympathetic nervous system explains why sweatiness and tachycardia are common in cardiac failure. The activation of the sympathetic nervous system and renin–angiotensin system results in renal vasoconstriction, reduction in glomerular filtration rate, and increased tubular reabsorption of sodium and water. Increased secretion of aldosterone also increases tubular reabsorption of sodium and water. Hence the urinary excretion of sodium and water is reduced, and oedema results.

9.47   B C D

Whilst most peripheral pulses can be used to assess the pulse rate and rhythm, the pulse character (e.g. volume, the rate of rise and decline) is best assessed at an accessible large artery close to the heart. At a small peripheral artery far away from the heart, the pulse may be 'damped'. Clinically, the brachial, carotid and femoral pulses are the best sites for assessing pulse character.

9.48   C D

Central cyanosis causes blue lips and tongue, and is due to a reduction in the oxygen saturation of arterial blood. Central cyanosis may be caused by heart or lung diseases. Blue hands and feet may be due to either central cyanosis or poor circulation to the limbs. If a patient's hands were blue, but the lips and tongue were of normal colour, the cause cannot be central cyanosis, but due to poor circulation to the limbs (peripheral cyanosis). Causes include cold weather, Raynaud's phenomenon or a low cardiac output.

9.49   D

Blood from the internal jugular vein enters the right atrium via the superior vena cava without passing through any valves. This is why the jugular venous pulse gives valuable information about the haemodynamics of the right atrium. The internal jugular vein is more reliable than the external jugular vein in this respect, as the latter may be kinked. The internal jugular vein lies deep to both the sternal and clavicular heads of the sternomastoid muscle. Hence, examination of the jugular venous pulse is easier if the neck muscles are relaxed. Unlike arterial pulses, venous pulses cannot be palpated. They can only be seen.

9.50   D

The jugular venous pressure is the *vertical height* (in centimetres) of the jugular venous pulse from the sternal angle. In a healthy subject, the jugular venous pressure is less than 2 cm. Hence the venous pressure would not be visible in the upright position. If a healthy subject were to lie horizontally, the internal jugular vein would be completely extended, and the jugular venous pulse could not be seen. Hence the pulse is examined with the subject lying at 45° to the horizontal. The subject should be examined with the head turned slightly to the left. Turning the head as far as possible to the left would tense the right sternomastoid muscle and obscure the jugular venous pulse. If the jugular venous pressure is extremely high, the jugular venous pulse may be above the level of the earlobe and therefore could not be seen.

9.51   C D E

The jugular venous pulse mainly reflects the haemodynamics in the right atrium. The correct causes for the phases of the jugular venous pressures are:
- 'a' wave – atrial systole
- 'c' wave – transmission of pressure to atrium from onset of ventricular systole
- 'a–x' descent – atrial relaxation
- 'x–v' ascent – filling of blood from venae cavae
- 'v–y' descent – emptying of blood from right atrium into right ventricle
- 'y–a' ascent – filling of blood from venae cavae until next cycle begins

9.52   B

The correct associations between the heart conditions and their associated jugular venous pulse abnormalities are:
- Atrial fibrillation – absent 'a' waves (due to ineffective atrial contractions)
- Complete heart block – cannon waves (due to occasional contraction of the right atrium against a closed tricuspid valve)
- Superior vena caval obstruction – raised venous pressure with little or no pulsation
- Tricuspid stenosis – slow 'v–y' descent (slow emptying of blood from right atrium into right ventricle)
- Tricuspid incompetence – giant 'v' wave

9.53   B E

The apex beat is defined as the furthest point laterally and inferiorly on the left side of the precordium at which a cardiac impulse is palpable. In healthy subjects, the apex beat lies at the left fifth intercostal space on the mid-clavicular line. A laterally displaced apex beat may be due to left ventricular enlargement, or a right-sided space-occupying lesion (e.g. right-sided pneumothorax).

9

A

The cardiovascular system

9.54 C E
Cardiac thrills are palpable vibrations synchronous with certain phases of the cardiac cycle. Like cardiac murmurs, they are caused by turbulent blood flow. In fact, cardiac thrills can be regarded as murmurs which are so loud that they are palpable. Whilst soft systolic murmurs may be innocent, cardiac thrills are always pathological.

9.55 A
The first heart sound occurs at the beginning of the ventricular systole, and is caused by the closure of the mitral and the tricuspid valves. Hence it is louder at the apex of the heart. The first heart sound has a lower pitch and a longer duration than the second because the mitral and tricuspid valves close more gradually than the pulmonary and aortic valves.

9.56 B D E
The second heart sound is caused by the brisk closure of the aortic and pulmonary valves at the end of diastole. Hence it is better heard at the base than the apex of the heart. Since it has a high pitch, it is best heard with the diaphragm of the stethoscope, as the diaphragm filters out low-pitched sounds and helps to identify the high-pitched sounds. Closure of the aortic valve usually precedes the pulmonary valve. As the difference is more pronounced in inspiration than expiration, the second heart sound usually appears single on expiration, but is split during inspiration.

9.57 A C
The types of second heart sound abnormalities can be deduced by the facts that closure of the aortic heart valve usually precedes the pulmonary valve, and that the difference is more pronounced in inspiration than expiration. The correct types of second heart sound abnormalities are:
- Aortic stenosis – soft aortic component
- Pulmonary hypertension – loud pulmonary component
- Right bundle branch block – wide splitting (as the pulmonary component is delayed)
- Left ventricular outflow obstruction – reverse splitting
- Pulmonary stenosis – wide splitting
(Fixed splitting occurs in atrial septal defect as the pressure of left and right atria is equal throughout the cardiac cycle.)

9.58 A C
If one remembers that murmurs radiate in the direction of the blood flow which causes the murmur, then the sites of radiation of murmur can be deduced. The sites of radiation are:
- Aortic stenosis – upper right sternal edge and neck
- Aortic regurgitation – down left sternal edge

- Mitral stenosis – apex of the heart
- Pulmonary regurgitation – left sternal border
- Ventricular septal defect – lower sternal edge

9.59
A
Cardiac output is the amount of blood pumped out of each ventricle per unit time. Cardiac failure is due to the inability of the heart to maintain a cardiac output to satisfy the body's metabolic requirements.

B
- Increase in heart rate caused by sympathetic stimulation.
- Increase in myocardial contractility resulting from an increase in end-diastolic volume (Starling's Law) caused by an increased venous return.
- Increase in myocardial contractility resulting from an increase in catecholamines caused by sympathetic stimulation.

C
i As a result of excessive sympathetic stimulation.
ii Because failure of the left ventricle to increase its output leads to an increase in pulmonary venous pressure. This causes pulmonary congestion.

D
This may be due to reduced myocardial contractility (e.g. ischaemic heart disease, myocarditis, cardiomyopathy) or increased metabolic demands (e.g. anaemia, thyrotoxicosis).

E
Digoxin inhibits membrane-bound Na^+, K^+-ATPase → increase in intracellular sodium → decrease in sodium concentration gradient across membrane → reduction of $Na^+ - Ca^{2+}$ exchange at the cell membrane → increase in intracellular Ca^{2+} → increase in myocardial contractility → increase in cardiac output.

F
- Diuretics: reduce sodium and water retention.
- Arterial vasodilators: reduce afterload.
- Venodilators: reduce preload.
- Angiotensin-converting enzyme: reduces formation of angiotensin II (which is a vasoconstrictor) and aldosterone (which promotes sodium and water retention).

9.60
A
See Fig. 9.3.

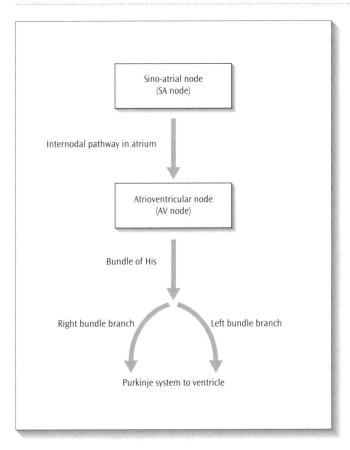

Fig. 9.3 Main structures and pathways for normal conduction of electrical impulses in the heart.

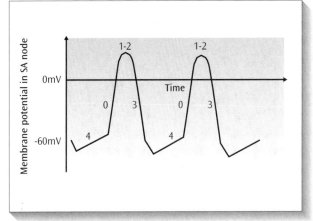

Fig. 9.4 Variation of membrane potential of the cardiac pacemaker with time (see text for description of phases).

- phase 2–3: Increase in K^+ current
- end of phase 3: decay of K^+ current.

(*Note* In contrast to other cardiac cells, Na^+ contributes very little to the action potential. This explains the slow rise in depolarisation spike.)

Phase 4 accounts for the 'pacemaker' role.

E
Generally speaking, the right vagus nerve supplies the embryological right heart, and the left vagus nerve supplies the embryological left heart. Hence, the SA node is mainly supplied by the right vagus nerve, and the AV node is mainly supplied by the left vagus nerve.

F
In the experiment, the right vagus nerve was stimulated. Since the right vagus nerve supplies mainly the SA node, the SA node was inhibited. This occurred because the acetylcholine released at the nerve endings acted on the M_2 muscarinic receptors, which in turn open a special set of K^+ channels via G protein. This slowed the decay of potassium current (I_K) and reduced the pacemaker rate.

G
See Fig. 9.5. The student would be expected to be still in sinus rhythm after vagal stimulation, as the heart beats at a rate set by the pacemaker.

H
Atropine acts exactly opposite to vagal stimulation, as it acts as an antagonist at the muscarinic receptor. It may be used as a temporary measure in the treatment of sinus bradycardia.

B
The sino-atrial (SA) node is located at the junction of the superior vena cava and the right atrium. It has characteristic histological features but no macroscopic features that indicate its position. The atrioventricular (AV) node is also a small mass of specialised myocardial cells situated in the right atrium on the interatrial septum, above the attachment of the septal cusp of the tricuspid valve and to the left of the opening of the coronary sinus.

C
The cardiac pacemaker is normally in the SA node.

D
See Fig. 9.4. The ionic conductance associated with the phases is:
- phase 4: prepotential – transient increase in Ca^{2+} current ($I_{Ca}T$)
- phase 0: long-lasting increase in Ca^{2+} current ($I_{Ca}L$)
- phase 1–2: decay of Ca^{2+} current

The cardiovascular system

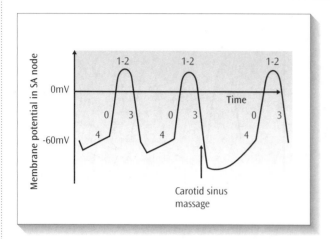

Fig. 9.5 Effect of vagal stimulation (see Fig. 9.4).

9.61
A

The QRS complex of the ECG corresponds to ventricular depolarisation. (*Note* The P wave corresponds to atrial depolarisation and the ST interval corresponds to ventricular repolarisation.)

B

Ventricular tachycardia is caused by a series of rapid regular ventricular depolarisations, usually the result of a damaged area of ventricular myocardium that conducts in one direction only. This allows a continuous circulation of impulse to occur (so-called 'circus movement') in the ventricles. In this patient, the initial damage to the ventricular myocardium was likely to have been caused by ischaemia.

C

Ventricular fibrillation occurs when the ventricular muscle fibres contract in a totally uncoordinated manner due to rapid multiple ventricular discharges or circus movement. It is a serious condition because the fibrillating ventricles cannot pump blood efficiently and there is virtually no cardiac output. Electrical defibrillation might be effective in treating this condition because it might simultaneously depolarise all ventricular muscle fibres and put them into a refractory state. This allows the cardiac pacemaker to retake control of the beating of the heart.

D

Lidocaine (lignocaine) is class 1b antidysrhythmic drug in Vaughan Williams' classification. It acts by binding and dissociating rapidly to open sodium channels during phase 0 of the action potential. For normal heartbeat,

dissociation would have occurred for the next action potential. For premature beat, however, the sodium channels are still blocked and hence action potential is aborted.

9.62
A

P waves on the ECG correspond to atrial depolarisation. In atrial fibrillation, the atria beat very rapidly (more than 300 beats per minute) and irregularly. Since the AV node discharges irregularly, the ventricles beat at an irregular pace; individual P waves cannot be detected, and the QRS complexes are irregular.

B

The pulse reflects the rate and rhythm of the left ventricular output. Since the ventricular rhythm is irregular, it accounts for the patient's irregular pulse rate.

C

The atrial rate could have been 300–500 beats per minute, while the ventricular rate was 100 beats per minute.

D

Atrial fibrillation could be due to damaged atrial myocardium causing multiple concurrent circulating currents in the atria. This causes the atria to beat in a rapid, completely irregular and disorganised manner.

E

Digoxin acts by reducing AV conduction and increasing vagal activity. This tends to slow the ventricular rate in rapid atrial fibrillation.

F

Amiodarone (a class III antidysrhythmic drug) may be useful for atrial fibrillation. It acts by increasing both the action potential duration and effective refractory period. The exact mechanism is still unclear.

9.63
A

It can be argued that the cause of tachycardia in atrial fibrillation is 'above the ventricles' and is therefore a type of supraventricular tachycardia. However, supraventricular tachycardia is usually used to indicate tachycardia originating from the AV node. In atrial fibrillation, there is a lack of P waves and the ventricular rate is irregular. In nodal tachycardia, P waves may be present and the ventricular rate is regular.

B

Ventricular tachycardia is caused by circus movement in the ventricles. Hence, in supraventricular tachycardia, the QRS complex is normal (narrow, less than 120 ms or three small squares). In ventricular tachycardia, the QRS complex is abnormally wide (more than 120 ms).

C

Carotid sinus massage (i.e. directly stimulating the vagus nerves) or the Valsalva manoeuvre might be effective in treating supraventricular tachycardia.

D

Adenosine is normally produced in the body. Intravenous adenosine acts as agonist on the A_1 receptors in the AV node. These G protein-coupled A_1 receptors are linked to the same cardiac K^+ channels that are activated by acetylcholine via the M_2 muscarinic receptors. Hence, stimulation of the A_1 receptors makes the action potential in the cardiac conducting tissue more negative (i.e. hyperpolarises the cardiac pacemaker) and slows the rate of rise of the prepotential. Hence, it might be effective in the treatment of supraventricular tachycardia.

E

Adenosine may cause bronchoconstriction and symptoms of wheezing. This is caused by a combination of direct effects on A_1 receptors and by release of mediators from mast cells via its effects on A_3 receptors.

F

The effect of intravenous adenosine is short-lived (about 20–30 s), as it is taken up by a specific nucleotide transporter by red blood cells and metabolised by enzymes on vascular endothelium; hence, intravenous adenosine is safe.

9.64

A

In first-degree heart block, all the atrial impulses reach the ventricles, but the time taken is longer than normal. In second-degree heart block, some but not all atrial impulses reach the ventricles. In third-degree (complete) heart block, the conduction from atria to the ventricles is completely blocked and no atrial impulses reach the ventricles.

B

In first-degree heart block, the PR interval is abnormally long, but there is a QRS complex after every P wave. In second-degree heart block, a QRS complex occurs only for a proportion of P waves. This may appear as a 2:1 or 3:1 block, or the PR interval may lengthen progressively until

a ventricular beat is dropped. In third-degree heart block, the QRS complex occurs at a rate of 15–50 beats per minute independent of P waves, while P waves occur regularly, and much faster (e.g. 60–110 per minute).

C

Isoprenaline is a non-selective β-agonist. In the heart, it stimulates $β_1$ receptors to increase both the heart rate (chronotropic effect) and the force of contraction (inotropic effect). Stimulation of the $β_1$ receptors causes the membrane potential to fall more rapidly, and hence more rapid spontaneous discharges.

D

The slow heart rate in this patient results in reduced cardiac output and reduced blood supply to the brain. This is likely to be the cause of this patient's falls. It is also known as a Stokes–Adams attack.

9.65

A

According to the Fick principle, the amount of a substance taken up by an organ per unit time is equal to the difference between the arterial and venous concentration times the rate of blood flow:

$$\text{Amount taken up} = A - V \text{ difference in concentration} \times \text{blood flow}$$

B

Applying the Fick principle to this laboratory subject:

$$\text{amount of oxygen taken up} = A - V \text{ difference in oxygen concentration} \times \text{blood flow}$$

Now,

$$\text{amount of oxygen consumed} = 1000\,\text{ml/min} \\ \text{(at standard pressure and temperature)}$$

$$\text{arterial concentration of oxygen} = 200\,\text{ml/l}$$

$$\text{venous concentration of oxygen} = 150\,\text{ml/l}$$

Substituting into the above formula gives:

$$1000\,\text{ml/min} = (200\,\text{ml/l} - 150\,\text{ml/l}) \times \text{blood flow (l/min)}$$

Hence,

$$\text{cardiac output} = \text{blood flow (litres)} = 1000/(200 - 150) \\ = 20\,\text{l/min}$$

9.66

A

Stroke volume is the amount of blood pumped out of each ventricle per beat. The relationship between cardiac output, stroke volume and heart rate is:

$$\text{Cardiac output} = \text{stroke volume} \times \text{heart rate}$$

The cardiovascular system

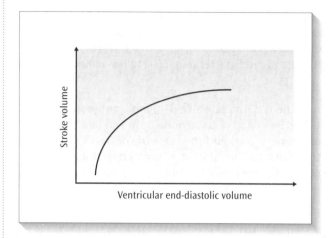

Fig. 9.6 Diagram to illustrate Starling's law of the heart.

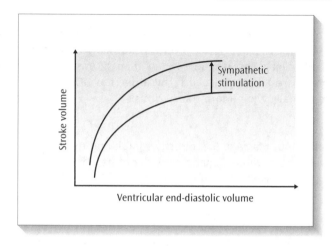

Fig. 9.7 Effect of increased contractility (see Fig. 9.6).

B

Exercise increases the heart rate. Just before and during exercise, the sympathetic nervous system is stimulated and the concentration of circulating adrenaline (epinephrine) and noradrenaline (norepinephrine) is increased. They increase the heart rate by stimulating β_1 receptors.

C

The stroke volume is determined by the degree of myocardial fibre shortening and left ventricular size. Greater myocardial fibre shortening is caused by increased myocardial contractility, increased preload and reduced afterload.

D

According to the Starling's law of the heart, the energy of contraction is proportional to the initial length of the cardiac muscle fibre (which is proportional to the end-diastolic volume). See Fig. 9.6.

E

From Fig. 9.6, stroke volume may be increased by increasing the ventricular end-diastolic volume. The end-diastolic volume can be increased during exercise. First, muscular activity increases the pumping action of skeletal muscle and increases the venous return. Second, the increased negative intrathoracic pressure due to increased respiratory effort during exercise increases the pressure gradient along which blood flows to the heart.

F

i   Preload is the degree to which the myocardium is stretched before it contracts. Afterload is the resistance against which blood is expelled.
ii Exercise increases the contractility of the myocardium via the positive inotropic effects of sympathetic

nervous stimulation and circulating catecholamines. The catecholamines exert their effect on cardiac β-adrenergic receptors, with resulting activation of adenyl cyclase and increase in intracellular cAMP.

G

See Fig. 9.7.

H

Afterload decreases during exercise. It depends mainly on the resistance from arterioles and small arteries (resistance vessels). During exercise, the vessels in the muscle dilate (via the effect of the sympathetic nervous system) and peripheral resistance falls. The myocardial fibre shortening increases, the stroke volume increases and the cardiac output increases.

I

The increased oxygen requirements of the heart are met by coronary vasodilatation. This occurs as a result of chemical factors such as hypoxia, increased local concentration of carbon dioxide and H^+.

J

There are several mechanisms for increasing blood flow to the skeletal muscles during exercise. First, blood flow increases dramatically between contractions in rhythmically contacting muscles. Second, stimulation of the sympathetic nervous system and increase in circulating catecholamines result in skeletal muscle vasodilatation. Third, a fall in tissue oxygen, a rise in tissue carbon dioxide and accumulation of H^+ may all cause vasodilatation and an increase in blood flow to the skeletal muscles.

9.67

A

The normal aortic pressure would be the same as the normal blood pressure. The systolic pressure is about 120 mmHg and the diastolic pressure is about 80 mmHg.

B

The normal left ventricular systolic pressure is the same as the arterial systolic pressure (i.e. about 120 mmHg); the normal diastolic left ventricular diastolic pressure is 0 mmHg. The low diastolic pressure allows blood to flow from the left atrium to the left ventricle in diastole.

C

The normal right ventricular systolic pressure (about 20–25 mmHg) is much lower than the corresponding pressure in the left ventricle. The normal right ventricular diastolic pressure is 0 mmHg.

D

i   The normal difference in pressure between the aorta and left ventricle in systole is 0 mmHg. The normal difference in pressure in diastole is about 80 mmHg.

ii The normal difference in pressure between the aorta and the right ventricle in systole is about 100 mmHg. The normal difference in pressure in diastole is about 80 mmHg.

E

For the left ventricle, blood can flow from the aorta via a coronary artery to the left ventricle only during systole. In the right ventricle, blood can flow throughout both systole and diastole. Hence, the left ventricle is more liable to myocardial ischaemia.

F

If the aortic valve is narrowed (aortic stenosis), the systolic pressure in the left ventricle is much higher than in the aorta. Hence, the branches of coronary arteries supplying the left ventricle are actually compressed during systole and the blood supply decreases further.

G

Applying the general formula that:

$$\text{work done} = \text{pressure} \times \text{volume of blood moved}$$

the relationship between the oxygen consumption per beat of the ventricle, the stroke volume and the intraventricular pressure is:

$$\text{oxygen consumption per beat} = \text{stroke volume} \times \text{left intraventricular pressure}$$

H

In aortic stenosis, the left intraventricular pressure increases. Hence, the oxygen consumption per beat increases.

I

Since the work done by the left ventricle increases, left ventricular hypertrophy (thickening of the ventricular muscular wall) occurs. Hypertrophy is an increase in size without an increase in the number of cells. Furthermore, the left ventricle expends more energy in expelling blood against the narrowed aortic valve. Hence, the oxygen requirement increases.

9.68

A

i   In the auscultatory method, the cuff is inflated well above the systolic pressure in the brachial artery. No sound can be heard with the stethoscope over the artery because the artery is occluded. The cuff pressure is gradually lowered. At the point when the systolic pressure is just above the cuff pressure a tapping sound is heard with each beat. This is the measured systolic arterial pressure. When the cuff pressure is lowered further, the tapping sound becomes muffled and then disappears. The diastolic pressure is usually taken as the reading when the sound disappears (for adults).

ii The 'sounds of Korotkoff' are the tapping sound heard with the stethoscope in the auscultatory method of blood pressure measurement. They are caused by turbulent flow of blood in the artery. Turbulent flow occurs when blood flows through a narrowed artery (e.g. caused by cuff compression). When blood flows through a normal artery, the flow is streamlined (laminar) and no sounds are produced. When the artery is constricted, the velocity increases; when the blood flow exceeds a certain critical velocity, turbulent flow occurs and the sounds of Korotkoff can be heard.

iii There are two important precautions in using the ascultatory method for measuring blood pressure:

1. The mercury manometer must be at the same level as the patient's heart.

2. A wide cuff should be used in obese individuals, as a proportion of the cuff pressure may be dissipated through the fat.

B

In patients with essential hypertension, the main factor is an increase in peripheral resistance.

$$\text{Blood pressure} = \text{cardiac output} \times \text{peripheral resistance.}$$

The cardiovascular system

C

The exact aetiology of essential hypertension is still not fully understood. The following are some of the current hypotheses.

i *Sodium homeostasis*. Impaired sodium excretion by the kidney may cause sodium retention. This causes an increase in blood volume and hence an increase in cardiac output (Starling's law). To regulate the amount of blood to various organs, increase in peripheral vascular resistance may occur as a result of peripheral autoregulation. This may lead to essential hypertension. It has been postulated that a circulating substance may inhibit sodium transport in the kidney, but the nature of this substance is unknown.

ii *Sympathetic nervous system*. Subjects with essential hypertension may either have a higher level of circulating catecholamines or be highly sensitive to catecholamines. Blood pressure is the product of cardiac output and peripheral resistance, and catecholamines may increase both.

iii *Renin–angiotensin–aldosterone system*. Many patients with essential hypertension respond to angiotensin converting enzyme (ACE) inhibitors, and angiotensin can stimulate sympathetic nervous system centrally. It is postulated that abnormal angiotensinogen, ACE and receptors for angiotensin II may be the cause of essential hypertension.

D

Hypertension represents an increase in the afterload of the left ventricle: the left ventricular workload increases and the left ventricle responds by hypertrophy. However, the increase in the mass of heart muscle increases the demand for oxygen even more. Applying the law of Laplace to the heart, the pressure is proportional to the tension in the ventricle but inversely proportional to its radius (pressure = tension/radius). As the heart dilates, the tension must increase to maintain the same pressure: the dilated heart must do more work. Initially, the increase in end-diastolic volume increases cardiac output by an increase in the strength of contraction of the heart, according to Starling's law. However, the ability of the heart to keep up with an increase in cardiac output may finally be exceeded.

E

Hypertension accelerates atherosclerosis in larger arteries. It also causes thickening of the media of muscular arteries as a result of hyperplasia of smooth muscle cells and collagen deposition in the internal elastic laminae in smaller arteries and arterioles.

F

There are several drugs that may be used to treat hypertension. Thiazide diuretics act on the distal convoluted tubule, decreasing active reabsorption of sodium and chloride ions by binding to the chloride site of the Na^+/Cl^- cotransport system. This increases the excretion of sodium by the kidneys.

9.69

A

The two coronary arteries arise from the aortic sinuses at the beginning of the ascending aorta. The right coronary artery arises from the anterior aortic sinus, the left coronary artery arises from the left posterior aortic sinus behind the pulmonary trunk.

B

There are two coronary arteries:
- Right coronary artery – the main branches are right marginal and posterior interventricular branches.
- Left coronary artery – the main branches are circumflex branch and left anterior descending branch.

The three main sites for coronary occlusion are: left anterior descending artery, right coronary artery and circumflex artery. This patient suffered an anterior myocardial infarct. The artery likely to have been involved is the left anterior descending artery.

C

The main factors are:
- the site of coronary artery obstruction
- the degree of coronary artery obstruction
- the anatomical pattern of blood supply
- the presence or otherwise of anastomotic circulation.

Rapid onset of obstruction is likely to result in a larger infarct as there is no time to develop anastomotic circulation.

D

The common cause for coronary artery obstruction is thrombosis occurring in an atheromatous plaque.

E

i Atherosclerosis occurs particularly in large- and medium-sized arteries.

ii Atherosclerotic lesions include fatty streaks, fibrolipid plaques and complicated lesions. Fatty streaks are usually linear elevations composed of lipid-filled histiocytes. In susceptible individuals, they may progress to fibrolipid plaques or complicated lesions. Fibrolipid plaques contain a mixture of macrophages, T-lymphocytes and smooth muscle cells, covered by a layer of fibrous tissue. Complicated lesions include thrombus formation on atheromatous plaques, plaque rupture or fissuring, aneurysm formation, and embolism of atheromatous debris.

iii • Old age.

Table 9.1

Time from infarct	Histological features	Macroscopic features
Less than 1 day	None	None
1–2 days	Oedema, necrosis of muscle cells, acute inflammatory cell infiltration	Pale oedematous muscle
2–4 days	Marked necrosis and inflammation	Yellow centre with haemorrhagic border
1–3 weeks	Granulation tissue progressing to fibrous tissue	Pale and thin infarcted muscle
3–6 weeks	Marked fibrosis	White fibrous scar

- Male gender.
- Smoking.
- Hypertension.
- Diabetes.
- Increase in LDL-cholesterol level.

F

The patient died 4 days after the initial myocardial infarct. Macroscopically, the expected appearance of the left ventricles would be yellow with a haemorragic border. Microscopically, there would be evidence of necrosis and inflammation, and early granulation tissue formation. If the death had occurred 2–3 weeks later, the infarct area would be expected to be pale and thin. Microscopically, there may be evidence of both granulation and fibrosis. The macroscopic and histological features of myocardial infarct are summarised in Table 9.1.

9.70

A

Isosorbide mononitrate is an organic nitrate. It acts by releasing nitric oxide (NO), which in turn activates a soluble cytosolic form of guanylate cyclase in vascular smooth muscle. Hence, cGMP production is increased, causing an increase in the degree of phosphorylation of various smooth muscle proteins and dephosphorylation of the myosin light chain. This causes relaxation of the coronary vessels: the coronary blood flow is increased.

B

Organic nitrates also causes dilatation of venules with resultant reduction in the central venous pressure. This tends to cause venous pooling in the legs. Moreover, organic nitrates also cause arteriolar dilatation with resultant reduction in peripheral resistance and blood pressure. The blood pressure may drop considerably when the subject stands up (postural hypotension).

C

Atenolol may be beneficial in relieving angina symptoms by reducing the heart's oxygen consumption. This is achieved by its negative inotropic and chonotropic effects via its antagonism at β-adrenergic receptors.

D

Diltiazem is a calcium antagonist. There is a spectrum of calcium antagonists. Some (e.g. verapamil) mainly affect the heart; others (e.g. nifedipine) mainly act on smooth muscle. Diltiazem is intermediate in its effects. It relaxes vascular smooth muscles, causes arteriolar dilatation and reduces peripheral resistance. It also has a negative inotropic effect by inhibiting the slow inward current during the action potential plateau.

9.71

A

In its early development, the 'heart tube' differentiates into four cavities. In the cephalocaudal direction, they are the bulb, ventricle, atrium and sinus venosus. The upper part of the bulb becomes most of the right ventricle; the original ventricle becomes most of the left ventricle. In the floor of the original ventricle, a partition grows upwards to form the muscular (lower) part of the interventricular septum. The truncus arteriosus developed from the bulb, which later forms the ascending aorta and the pulmonary trunk, becomes separated by two internal swellings called bulbar ridges. The lower ends of the bulbar ridges become the fibrous part of the interventricular septum. A ventricular septal defect results from abnormalities of these processes. Most ventricular septal defects are in the fibrous part.

B

See Fig. 9.8.

C

In a normal adult, the systolic pressures in the left and right ventricles are 120 and 80 mmHg respectively. The corresponding normal pressures in a child are about 80 and 55 mmHg. Blood flows from the left to the right ventricle in systole in the presence of a ventricular septal defect (see Fig. 9.8). In diastole, the pressures in both

The cardiovascular system

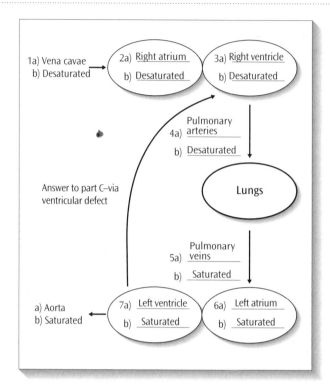

Fig. 9.8 Adult circulation from the vena cavae to the aorta.

ventricles are close to 0 mmHg: there is no blood flow across the defect.

D

Heart murmurs are abnormal sounds resulting from turbulent blood flow as a result of blood flowing through a constriction above a certain critical velocity. In this child, the murmur occurs in systole when there is abnormal flow of blood across the septal defect.

E

The child would not be cyanosed. This is because the flow of blood via the defect results from the flow of oxygenated blood in the left ventricle with deoxygenated blood in the right ventricle. Although the left ventricle has to work much harder, the blood delivered to the aorta via the left ventricle is saturated. If blood were to flow from the right ventricle to left ventricle (as in a child with long-standing untreated defects), then the blood in the left ventricle would be desaturated and the child would be cyanosed.

9.72

A

The ductus arteriosus is a thick artery joining the left branch of the pulmonary trunk to the aorta, distal to the origin of the three branches of the aortic arch. Before

birth, it allows deoxygenated blood from the superior vena cava, passing through the right atrium and right ventricle into the pulmonary trunk, to bypass the airless lung to enter the aorta, so that it can enter the umbilical arteries to be reoxygenated in the placenta. The left recurrent laryngeal nerve (branch of the vagus nerve) hooks around the ductus arteriosus. The ductus arteriosus usually closes to become the ligamentum arteriosum.

B

Embryologically, the ductus arteriosus is developed from the dorsal part of the left sixth branchial arch artery. It is connected to the left fourth branchial arch artery and the pulmonary trunk. After birth, the ductus arteriosus becomes the ligamentum arteriosum and the left fourth branchial artery becomes the arch of the aorta. The recurrent laryngeal nerves represent the nerves of the sixth arch. Hence, the left recurrent laryngeal nerve hooks around the liagmentum arteriosum. On the right side, the embryological sixth arch artery disappears. Hence, the right recurrent laryngeal nerve hooks around the subclavian artery, which is developed embryologically from the fourth arch artery.

C

After birth, the pulmonary pressure drops. Blood would therefore flow from the aorta to the pulmonary trunk in this infant.

9.73

A

See Fig. 9.9.

B

Structures (8) and (9) are the ductus arteriosus and foramen ovale, respectively.

C

Placenta → umbilical vein → ductus venosus → inferior vena cava (1b) → right atrium (2) → (through foramen ovale (9)) → left atrium (6) → left ventricle (7) → aorta to supply head. The blood is oxygenated.

D

Deoxygenated blood from body → superior vena cava (1a) → right atrium (2) → right ventricle (3) → (through pulmonary trunks (4)) → (through ductus arteriosus (8)) → aorta → umbilical arteries → placenta (to be re-oxygenated). The blood is deoxygenated.

E

Little blood passes through the lungs and pulmonary veins because in the fetus the lungs are airless and the pulmonary pressure is very high.

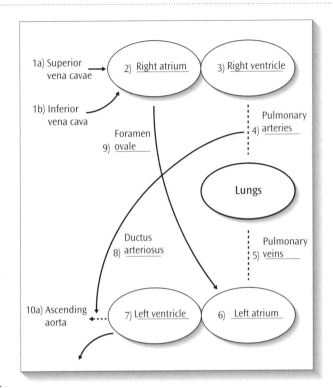

Fig. 9.9

9.74

A

The mitral valve separates the left atrium and the left ventricle.

B

There are two cusps in the mitral valve: the anterior and posterior. The cusps are flat and their edges are serrated. The two papillary muscles (anterior and posterior) are connected by chordae tendinae to each valve cusp.

C

The mitral valve opens at the beginning of diastole and closes at the beginning of ventricular systole.

D

During mitral closure in systole, the mitral valve is kept competent by active contraction of the papillary muscles, which pull on the chordae. The centrally attached chordae restrict the degree of ballooning of the cusps towards the atrium. The pull of the marginal chordae prevents eversion of the free edges into the cavity of the atrium.

E

Since blood flow occurs in diastole, the murmur occurs in diastole (especially mid-diastole).

F

The first heart sound is caused by the closure of the mitral and tricuspid valves; the second heart sound is caused by the closure of the pulmonary and aortic valves. In mitral stenosis, the first heart sound may be abnormally loud.

9.75

A

'Shock' describes the clinical state caused by inadequate tissue perfusion with insufficient cardiac output. Hypovolaemic shock refers to such a clinical state caused by there being inadequate fluid in the vascular system to fill it. It is characterised by hypotension and may be caused by internal or external haemorrhage, or generalised increased vascular dilatation.

B

In hypovolaemic shock, the blood volume and venous return are decreased. Hence, there are reduced discharges from the arterial baroreceptors. This results in reflex tachycardia and vasoconstriction. Furthermore, the sympathetic nervous system is stimulated and the patient is cold, pale and has a fast heart rate.

C

i   Stimulation of the sympathetic nervous system probably explains the restlessness associated in patients

131

The cardiovascular system

with hypovolaemic shock. The restlessness may help to increase muscular pumping of venous blood, increasing the venous return.

ii Rapid breathing may help to increase thoracic pumping of venous blood, increasing the venous return.

iii The efferent renal arterioles are constricted: renal plasma flow is reduced. There may be shunting of blood through the medullary portion of the kidneys.

Vasopressin (antidiuretic hormone) levels increase. These mechanisms (together with increased aldosterone) result in reduction of urine formation and sodium and water retention. This helps to maintain blood volume.

iv Increased renin activity during haemorrhage causes thirst. Increased renin and angiotensin levels also increases aldosterone levels and cause sodium retention. This helps to conserve sodium and water.

The respiratory system

10.1 The following are present in the respiratory bronchioles:
A Cartilage
B Cilia
C Smooth muscle
D Muscarinic receptors
E β-Adrenergic receptors

10.2 Gas exchange may occur across the walls of:
A The alveoli
B The bronchi
C The respiratory bronchioles
D The acini
E The terminal bronchioles

10.3 Surfactant:
A Is secreted by type I pneumocytes in the alveoli
B Increases the surface tension of the fluid lining the alveoli
C Increases the compliance of the lungs
D Increases the work of breathing
E Is a carbohydrate

10.4 The right main bronchus:
A Is wider than the left main bronchus
B Is longer than the left main bronchus
C Divides into two secondary bronchi
D Is more likely to be entered into by a foreign body than the left main bronchus
E Is circulated by a complete ring of cartilage

10.5 The following statements about lung volumes are true:
A The vital capacity is the amount of air that moves into the lungs on maximal inspiration after maximal expiratory effort
B The residual volume is the volume of air in the lungs at the end of passive expiration
C The tidal volume is the amount of air that moves into the lungs on maximal inspiratory effort after passive expiration
D The expiratory reserve volume is the amount of air left in the lungs after passive expiration
E The inspiratory reserve volume is the amount of air that moves into the lungs on maximal inspiratory effort after normal inspiration

10.6 The following statements about respiratory dead spaces are true:
A The anatomical dead space never exceeds the physiological dead space
B The anatomical dead space may be significantly increased by pulmonary emboli
C The physiological dead space may be significantly increased by pulmonary emboli
D The anatomical dead space may be significantly increased by breathing through a long tube
E The physiological dead space may be significantly increased by breathing through a long tube

10.7 The following statements about lung ventilation and perfusion are true:
A Perfusion at the apices of the lungs is higher than at the bases of upright normal lungs
B Ventilation at the apices of the lungs is higher than at the bases of upright normal lungs
C The ventilation/perfusion ratio at the apices is higher than at the bases of upright normal lungs
D Cyanosis may result if there is widespread ventilation–perfusion mismatch
E A reduced level of carbon dioxide in the blood may result from widespread ventilation–perfusion mismatch

10.8 The following parameters of respiratory function tests are significantly lower than normal in fibrosis of the lungs:
A Peak expiratory flow rate
B Forced expiratory volume in 1 s (FEV_1)
C Vital capacity (VC)
D Forced expiratory ratio (FEV_1/VC)
E Carbon monoxide transfer (T_{CO})

10.9 The following parameters of respiratory function tests are significantly lower than normal in bronchial asthma:
A Peak expiratory flow rate
B FEV_1
C VC
D FEV_1/VC
E T_{CO}

10.10 The following statements about haemoglobin are true:
A It is a globular protein
B It consists of six subunits
C There is one haem moiety per haemoglobin molecule
D The haem moiety contains ferric iron (Fe^{3+})
E In normal human adults, all haemoglobin molecules are of the same type

10.11 The following statements about the reaction of haemoglobin and oxygen are true:
A Haemoglobin increases the oxygen-carrying capacity of the blood by about two-fold

10 **Q**

The respiratory system

B The globin molecules bind to the oxygen molecules

C Each haemoglobin molecule is capable of binding up to four oxygen molecules

D Binding of the haemoglobin with the first oxygen molecule reduces the affinity for binding to a second oxygen molecule

E Binding to an oxygen molecule increases the likelihood of the haem moieties assuming a tense (T) state

10.12 When the oxygen–haemoglobin dissociation curve is shifted to the right:

A A higher partial pressure of oxygen is required for haemoglobin to bind to a given amount of oxygen

B It becomes easier to oxygenate the blood in the pulmonary capillaries

C The oxygen saturation of haemoglobin is higher for a given partial pressure of oxygen

D It becomes easier for the blood in the capillaries to deliver oxygen to the tissues

E It is almost always clinically undesirable

10.13 The following factors shift the oxygen–haemoglobin dissociation curve to the right:

A Increase in temperature

B Increase in pH

C Increase in 2,3-diphosphoglycerate (2,3-DPG)

D Living at high altitude

E Exercise

10.14 Myoglobin:

A Is mainly found in skeletal muscles

B Can bind up to four oxygen molecules per molecule of myoglobin

C Has a sigmoid oxygen–haemoglobin dissociation curve

D Has an oxygen dissociation curve to the right of the haemoglobin curve

E Can easily deliver oxygen to haemoglobin in the blood

10.15 The following statements about the transport of carbon dioxide in blood are true:

A A higher proportion of oxygen than carbon dioxide is dissolved in the plasma

B Most of the carbon dioxide is transported by forming carbamino compounds with haemoglobin

C Oxygenated blood carries more carbon dioxide than deoxygenated blood

D Carbonic anhydrase facilitates the formation of carbamino-haemoglobin

E The role of the red blood cells in carbon dioxide transport is insignificant

10.16 Compared to the red blood cells in the arterial blood, those in the venous blood:

A Contain more bicarbonate ions

B Contain more chloride ions

C Contain more hydrogen ions

D Contain more oxygen

E Are larger

10.17 The following may occur in the airways of patients with extrinsic asthma:

A The bronchi are hyperreactive to common stimuli

B Excessive histamine is released from mast cells

C Oedema occurs in the mucosa of the bronchioles

D There is excessive mucus secretion from the bronchioles

E An excess of IgM is produced

10.18 The following types of drugs are useful in the treatment or prevention of asthma owing at least partly to the mechanism stated:

A Corticosteroids – reduction in bronchial hyperreactivity

B Sodium cromoglicate – prevents the release of mediators from mast cells

C β_1-Adrenoceptor agonists – dilate narrowed bronchioles

D Methylxanthines (e.g. theophylline) – adenosine agonists

E Antimuscarinic agents (e.g. ipratropium) – reduction in bronchial hyperreactivity

10.19 The following statements about neural control of breathing are true:

A The neural control of respiration always overrides chemical control mechanisms

B The neural system for voluntary control of respiration is located at the pons

C The neural system for automatic control of respiration is located at the medulla oblongata

D The expiratory and inspiratory muscles are generally reciprocally innervated

E Diseases which interfere with the automatic control of respiration always disrupt voluntary control as well

10.20 The following changes will result in a significant increase in respiratory minute volume in a normal subject under normal conditions:

A Decrease in arterial pH from 7.31 to 7.15

B Increase in inspired carbon dioxide level by 20%

C Decrease in inspired carbon dioxide level by 20%

D Increase in inspired oxygen by 20%
E Decrease in inspired oxygen by 20%

10.21 The following factors significantly contribute to the increase of ventilation rate immediately before and during vigorous exercise:
A Psychic stimuli
B Afferent impulses from muscle and joint proprioceptors
C Reduced sensitivity of chemoreceptors to carbon dioxide
D Fluctuations in arterial carbon dioxide level
E Increased production of lactic acid

10.22 Causes of oxygen deficiency at the tissue level include:
A Ventilation–perfusion mismatch
B Anaemia
C Carbon monoxide poisoning
D Stagnation at the tissue
E Cyanide poisoning

10.23 Respiratory failure may result from:
A Severe muscle diseases
B Lung fibrosis
C Ventilation–perfusion mismatch
D Shunt of blood from the venous to the arterial circulation through a defect in the ventricular septum
E Severe kyphoscoliosis (abnormal curvature of the spine)

10.24 Significant clinical improvement can be expected from administering 100% oxygen for hypoxia due to the following conditions:
A Shunting of blood from the venous to the arterial circulation due to congenital abnormalities of the heart
B Severe chronic obstructive airway disease with chronic carbon dioxide retention
C Acute asthmatic attack
D Fibrosis of the lung
E Pneumonia

10.25 The long-term consequences of reduced ventilation may include an increase in:
A Arterial partial pressure of oxygen
B Arterial partial pressure of carbon dioxide
C Plasma pH
D Plasma HCO_3^-
E Renal reabsorption of HCO_3^-

10.26 The following statements about chronic respiratory alkalosis are true:

A Loss of acid by vomiting is a cause
B Hysterical hyperventilation is a cause
C The arterial partial pressure of CO_2 is characteristically raised
D The plasma pH is characteristically raised
E The plasma HCO^- is characteristically raised

10.27 The following statements about cough are true:
A It is usually initiated by irritation of the lining of the trachea or larynx
B It is usually preceded by a deep inspiration
C Expiration is forced against a closed glottis
D It is important in expelling foreign bodies from the respiratory tract
E It always serves a useful purpose

10.28 The following statements about neural control of cough are true:
A It is under substantial voluntary control
B Stimuli to the trachea or larynx are the main afferent inputs of the cough reflex
C The main centre for the autonomic control of the cough reflex is located in the pons
D The cough centre in the brain stem receives inputs from the cerebral cortex
E Increased partial pressure of carbon dioxide in the arterial blood stimulates the cough reflex

10.29 The following measures may be effective in relieving cough:
A Ceasing smoking
B Staying in a dry atmosphere
C Oral administration of a thick syrup with no active pharmacological ingredient
D Oral codeine
E Water inhalation as an aerosol

10.30 Potential sources of pulmonary emboli include thrombi from:
A The leg veins
B The pulmonary veins
C The pelvic veins
D The femoral arteries
E The brachial arteries

10.31 Significant risk factors for pulmonary embolism include:
A Frequent physical exercise
B Pregnancy
C Taking oral contraceptive pills
D High cholesterol level
E Recovery from a major operation

10.32 Possible sequelae of pulmonary emboli include:
A Pulmonary infarct of a lung segment

10

Q

SYSTEM-BASED MEDICAL SCIENCES

The respiratory system

B Pulmonary hypertension
C Arterial hypertension
D Pulmonary oedema
E Sudden death

10.33 Causes of pulmonary arterial hypertension include:
A Pulmonary emboli
B Chronic obstructive airway disease
C Myocardial infarction
D Mitral stenosis
E Ventricular septal defect

10.34 Causes of pulmonary oedema include:
A Left ventricular failure
B Mitral stenosis
C Low plasma albumin level
D Pulmonary stenosis
E Bronchial carcinoma

10.35 The following muscles are active during forced inspiration:
A The diaphragm
B Internal intercostal muscles
C External intercostal muscles
D Sternocleidomastoid muscles
E Anterior abdominal wall muscles

10.36 The following statements about emphysema are true:
A The disease is usually localised to a few bronchopulmonary segments of the lungs
B It is defined clinically as productive cough for three months in two consecutive years
C The air spaces distal to the terminal bronchioles are permanently enlarged
D The elastin in the walls of the airspaces is thickened
E It occurs much more commonly in people with α_1-antitrypsin deficiency

10.37 Risk factors for bronchial carcinoma include:
A Passive cigarette smoke
B Exposure to asbestos
C Excess alcohol intake
D Increased exposure to radon
E Low-fibre diet

10.38 The following statements about an open pneumothorax are true:
A Air is accumulated between the layers of parietal pleura and visceral pleura
B It may result from penetrating wound to the parietal pleura
C The lung on the affected side expands

D The intrapleural pressure on the affected side is lower than the other side
E Air enters the pleural cavity during expiration

10.39 Squamous cell bronchial carcinomas:
A Are usually peripheral
B Arise from squamous metaplasia
C Metastasise early to distant sites
D Usually secrete ectopic ADH
E Are the commonest histological type of bronchial carcinoma

10.40 The vocal folds:
A Are wide open during speech production
B Are longer in females than in males
C Are adducted by the posterior cricoarytenoid muscles
D Are paralysed when the recurrent laryngeal nerves are damaged
E Are controlled by the actions of the extrinsic laryngeal muscles

10.41 The trachea is palpable:
A Above the hyoid bone
B Above the suprasternoid notch
C Throughout its entire course
D In all subjects
E Only on swallowing

10.42 The following lesions cause deviation of the trachea to the opposite side:
A Lymphoma in the mediastinum
B Collapse of the upper lobe of the lung
C Enlarged thyroid gland
D Fibrosis of the upper lobe of the lung
E Asthma

10.43 The following observations in the adult may suggest respiratory diseases:
A The anteroposterior diameter of the chest measures half that the lateral diameter
B A respiratory rate of 15 breaths per minute
C Maximum chest expansion of about 2 cm
D Contraction of sternomastoid and scaleni muscles on normal inspiration
E Pursed lips on expiration

10.44 Causes of dullness to percussion over an area of the lung field include:
A Pulmonary collapse
B Pulmonary effusion
C Pneumothorax
D Pulmonary emphysema
E Pulmonary consolidation

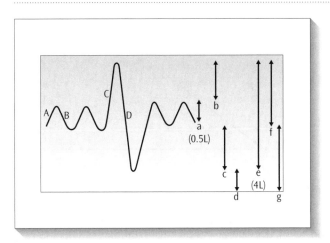

Fig. 10.1 Respiratory capacity in a normal subject.

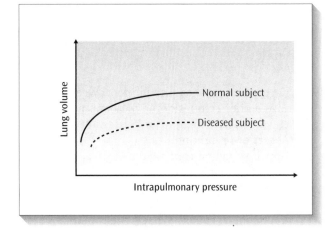

Fig. 10.2 Relationship between lung volume and intrapulmonary pressure in a normal subject (solid line) and a diseased subject (dotted line).

10.45 Bronchial breath sounds:
  A Resemble sounds produced at the larynx
  B Indicate that the relevant major bronchus is completely obstructed
  C May be heard even when the vocal resonance is reduced
  D Are usually heard more loudly during inspiration than expiration
  E Are continuous between the end of inspiration and the beginning of expiration

10.46 Figure 10.1 shows the excursions of a spirometer, for a 'normal' medical student, plotted against time. After two normal breaths, the student took a deep breath in with maximum effort and then breathed out with maximum effort. This was followed by two normal breaths. For this particular student, the lung volume labelled 'a' and 'e' measured 0.5 litres and 4 litres, respectively. The respiratory rate was 12 breaths per minute.
  A For the following phases of respiration, which muscles or group of muscles (if any) are active? Explain how these phases of respiration occur and the changes that occur in intrapleural pressures during these phases.
    i Phase A.
    ii Phase B.
    iii Phase C.
    iv Phase D.
  B Give the terms for the lung volumes labelled (a)–(g) in the diagram.
  C Explain what the lung volume labelled 'd' consists of.
  D Calculate the respiratory volume at rest per minute.

10.47 Figure 10.2 shows the relationship between lung volume and intrapulmonary pressure in a normal subject and a diseased subject during expiration.
  A What quality of the lungs do the slopes of these curves represent? Explain.
  B What is the main factor affecting this quality of the lung?
  C i What substance produced by the lung considerably alters this quality of the lung?
    ii Briefly explain how this substance alters this quality of the lung, using the law of Laplace.
    iii Briefly explain the composition of this substance and where this substance is produced.
  D How is the work of breathing related to the volume and pressure? What is the effect of the lack of this substance on the work of breathing? Explain.
  E Give a condition in which the production of this substance is abnormally low.
  F What condition might the diseased person, represented by the dotted curve, be suffering from?

10.48 Compare the respiration of two subjects. The first subject breathes at a rate of 12 breaths per minute with a tidal volume of 500 ml. The second subject breathes rapidly at a rate of 24 breaths per minute with a tidal volume of 250 ml. Assume the total dead space for both subjects is 150 ml.
  A What is meant by the total dead space? Explain what the components of the total dead space are?
  B Calculate the minute volume of the two subjects.

137

10

Q

SYSTEM-BASED MEDICAL SCIENCES

The respiratory system

C Calculate the alveolar ventilation of the two subjects.

D From your results in (C), who is breathing more effectively?

10.49 A 50-year-old man had a cough for 3 weeks.

A Give a brief account of the mechanism of coughing, describing what happens at various phases of respiration.

B How is coughing controlled by the central nervous system?

C In general terms, what may cause a cough?

D What type of drugs may be effective for the treatment of cough? What is their mechanism of action?

10.50 In a physiology experiment, the time for which a medical student could voluntarily hold her breath was 45 s. The experiment was repeated after a minute of voluntary hyperventilation. The medical student was then able to hold her breath for 70 s.

A Briefly describe how respiration is normally controlled.

B In the first part of the experiment, explain the physiological mechanisms by which the medical student became unable to hold her breath for longer than 45 s.

C Explain why the student was able to hold her breath longer after a period of hyperventilation.

10.51 A 65-year-old man suffered from moderately severe chronic obstructive airways disease.

A How are chronic bronchitis and emphysema defined?

B What is the most important aetiology for chronic bronchitis?

C Which lung structures are affected in chronic bronchitis? Describe the morphology in this disease.

D How do alveolar oxygen and carbon dioxide levels in a person with chronic bronchitis compare with those in a normal subject?

Figure 10.3 shows the ventilation at different alveolar carbon dioxide partial pressures, but with alveolar oxygen held constant at 50 mmHg, in a *normal* subject.

E Sketch the corresponding curve for an alveolar Po_2 of 100 mmHg in this normal subject.

F Sketch the corresponding curves for a person with severe chronic bronchitis (for alveolar Po_2 of 50 and 100 mmHg).

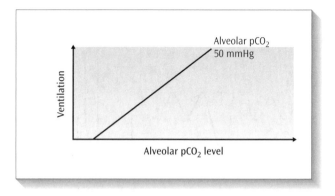

Fig. 10.3 Relationship between ventilation and alveolar carbon dioxide level, with alveolar oxygen held constant at 50 mmHg.

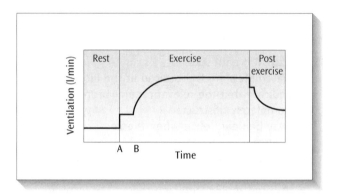

Fig. 10.4 Ventilation before, during and after a period of exercise.

G Is it advisable to administer a high concentration of oxygen to a person suffering from chronic bronchitis? Explain. (*Note* At a very high arterial level of carbon dioxide this may cause coma.)

10.52 Figure 10.4 illustrates an athlete's ventilation (in l/min) just before and during a race.

A What is the mechanism for the increase in ventilation at A?

B What are the possible mechanisms for the increase in ventilation at B?

C After exercise, ventilation did not immediately return to the basal level.

i What is the mechanism for maintaining this higher level of ventilation?

ii Why is it necessary to maintain ventilation above basal level for some time after exercise?

10.53 Most of the oxygen in the blood is carried by haemoglobin; myoglobin is present in skeletal muscle.

A Describe the structure of haemoglobin.

Table 10.1

	Trachea	Bronchi	Bronchioles	Respiratory bronchioles	Alveoli
Presence of cartilage					
Presence of smooth muscle					
Presence of cilia					
Presence of mucous glands					
Gas exchange					
Lined by pneumocyte					

B Sketch the curve showing the relationship between oxygen saturation and partial pressure of oxygen in the blood.

C How can this curve be explained by the way oxygen molecules bind to haem moieties.

D Sketch the corresponding curve for myoglobin.

E What is the advantage of myoglobin over haemoglobin as the oxygen-carrying agent in skeletal muscle?

10.54 A student ascended quickly from sea level (barometric pressure 750 mmHg) to 4000 metres (barometric pressure 500 mmHg). He suffered from headache, breathlessness and nausea for the first 2 days. After 3 weeks, his haemoglobin level rose from 12 g/dl to 15 g/dl.

A Assuming the partial pressure of oxygen at sea level is 125 mmHg, give a rough estimation of the corresponding partial pressure of oxygen at 3000 m.

B Explain why the student suffered from a headache.

C Give two possible explanations as to why the student became breathless after the ascent.

D Would you expect the alveolar oxygen pressure to fall by an amount more or less than a third? Explain.

E Describe the acid–base balance immediately after ascent. How would the alveolar carbon dioxide and arterial bicarbonate ion levels compare with normal?

F What is the effect of acid–base changes on the oxygen–haemoglobin dissociation curve? What other factor opposes this effect?

G Why did the student become less breathless a week after ascent?

H Explain why his haemoglobin level rose.

10.55 A 20-year-old man suffered from asthma, with episodes of wheezing.

A Compare the structures of the various air passages by completing Table 10.1.

B What airway structures are mainly affected in asthma? Describe how they are affected.

C Which of the following pulmonary function tests would you expect to be abnormal in a mild attack of asthma: forced expiratory volume in 1 s (FEV_1); ratio of forced expiratory to vital capacity (FEV_1/VC)? Explain.

D Describe the mechanisms by which allergens may cause bronchoconstriction in allergic asthma.

E What type of drug (other than bronchodilators) are effective in preventing attacks of allergic asthma? What are their mechanisms of action?

10.56 A patient suffered from recurrent attacks of asthma and was prescribed a salbutamol inhaler, ipratropium inhaler, oral theophylline and oral prednisolone (a glucocorticoid). Give the mechanism of action of these drugs in the treatment of asthma.

A Salbutamol

B Ipratropium

C Theophylline

D Prednisolone

10.57 A 66-year-old man was diagnosed to have bronchial carcinoma.

A What is the most important aetiological factor for the disease?

B Name three occupational hazards for developing the disease.

C Which histological types are usually hilar?

D Which histological type is associated with ectopic ACTH and ADH secretion?

E Which histological type has the worst prognosis? Explain.

139

10

Q

SYSTEM-BASED MEDICAL SCIENCES

The respiratory system

10.58 A singer waited for her musical entry and sang with different intensity, pitch and quality. Afterwards, she whispered to her accompanist.
  A What muscles abduct and adduct the vocal folds? Which nerve supplies these muscles?
  B Describe the state of the vocal folds while she waited for her musical entry.
  C Describe how a sound is produced. Describe the state of the vocal folds.
  D What were the mechanisms for changing the intensity, pitch and quality of her singing?
  E Describe the mechanism for whispering.

10.59 A teenager who inhaled a peanut developed lobar pneumonia (infection) in the right middle lobe of his lung. The doctor heard bronchial breath sounds over the area.
  A Explain why the right lung is more often affected than other lobes of the lungs by aspirated foreign bodies.

  B Describe the surface anatomy of the right middle lobe.
  C Explain why bronchial breath sounds were heard.

10.60 A 66-year-old bed-ridden woman suddenly developed chest pain and was diagnosed to have pulmonary emboli.
  A What are the most common sources for such emboli?
  B What factor in this patient may have contributed to the development of pulmonary emboli?
  C What is the likely outcome if a small embolus is lodged in a peripheral pulmonary artery?
  D What is the likely outcome if a massive coiled embolus is lodged in the main pulmonary artery?
  E What type of drugs, if given previously, might have been effective in prevention? Describe the mechanism of action.
  F What type of drugs might have been effective in treating major pulmonary emboli? Describe the mechanism of action.

The respiratory system

10.1 B C D E
Cartilage protects against collapse of the respiratory passages, and is present in the walls of the trachea and bronchi only. Cilia are present from the trachea down to the respiratory bronchioles, and are important in protecting the lungs from microorganisms. Smooth muscle is present in all the bronchioles. Contraction of the smooth muscle results in bronchospasm and wheezing. The epithelium of both the bronchi and bronchioles is innervated by both muscarinic receptors and β_2-receptors, which mediate bronchoconstriction and bronchodilation respectively. This is important clinically, as muscarinic antagonists (e.g. ipratropium) and β_2-adrenoceptor agonists (e.g. salbutamol) are effective in the treatment of bronchospasm due to asthma.

10.2 A C D
As bronchioles branch, those which are less than 2 mm in diameter are called terminal bronchioles. The terminal bronchioles branch into respiratory bronchioles. The alveoli have flat walls. The respiratory system distal to the terminal bronchioles is comprised of acini, where gas exchange occurs.

10.3 C
Surfactant is secreted by type II pneumocytes in the alveoli, and is essentially a mixture of lipids and proteins, the major component being dipalmitoylphosphatidylcholine. Its main action is to lower the alveolar surface tension, which is an important factor in determining the stretchability (or compliance) of the lung. Stiff lungs have low compliance. Compliance is formally defined as the change in lung volume per unit change in airway pressure. The energy expended on inflating a compliant lung is much less than that of a stiff lung.

10.4 A B D
The right main bronchus is wider, longer and more vertical than the left main bronchus. This is clinically important, as, foreign bodies are more likely to enter the right than the left main bronchus. The right main bronchus divides into three secondary (lobar) bronchi, whereas the left main bronchus divides into two secondary bronchi. Each of these secondary bronchi correspond to a lobe of the lung: the superior lobe, the middle lobe (right lung only) and the inferior lobe.

10.5 E
The amount of air which moves into the lungs with each inspiration is the tidal volume. The amount of air which moves into the lungs with maximal inspiratory effort at the end of a normal inspiration is the inspiratory reserve volume. Similarly, the amount of air which moves out of the lungs with maximal expiration after passive expiration is the expiratory reserve volume. The inspiratory capacity is equal to the sum of the tidal volume and inspiratory reserve volume. Similarly, the expiratory capacity is equal to the sum of the tidal volume and expiratory reserve volume. The vital capacity is the amount of air that moves into the lungs with maximal inspiratory effort after passive expiration. The residual volume is the volume of air left in the lungs on maximal expiration. Hence the total lung capacity is equal to the sum of the vital capacity and the residual volume.

10.6 A C D E
The anatomical dead space is the volume of respiratory system from the mouth and nose to the terminal bronchioles. The gas in this space is not involved in gas exchange, and measures about 150 ml. The physiological dead space is the volume of gas which is not involved in gas exchange. For normal lungs, the two spaces are almost identical. However, if some alveoli are not perfused by capillaries, or if there is excessive air in alveoli necessary to oxygenate the alveolar capillaries, this also contributes to the physiological dead space. Pulmonary emboli may cause ventilation–perfusion mismatch, and hence may increase the physiological dead space, but not anatomical dead space. However, breathing through a long tube increases both the anatomical and the physiological dead space, since the air in the tube is not involved in gas exchange.

10.7 C D E
In the upright normal lungs, both perfusion and ventilation decline linearly from the bases to the apices of the lungs. However, the rate of decline is greater for perfusion, and the ventilation/perfusion ratio is higher in the apices than in the bases of the lungs. Widespread ventilation–perfusion mismatch would result in the failure of the blood in the lung capillaries to be reoxygenated, and cyanosis may occur. Severe ventilation–perfusion mismatch results in carbon dioxide retention.

10.8 B C E
Lung diseases may be categorised into obstructive or restrictive defects, or a mixture of the two types of defects. The vital capacity is the amount of air that moves into the lungs with maximal inspiratory effort after passive expiration. Hence it is usually normal in pure obstructive defects, but is reduced in the presence of restrictive defects such as lung fibrosis, oedema or chest wall deformities. The forced expiratory volume (FEV_1) is the maximum volume of air expelled from the lungs within the first second after maximal inspiration. It depends both on the vital capacity as well as the degree of airway obstruction. Hence it is reduced both in restrictive and obstructive defects. However, the FEV_1/VC ratio depends

The respiratory system

mainly on the airway obstruction, and is low in obstructive defects but normal or even high in restrictive defects. The transfer factor for carbon monoxide (T_{CO}) is the amount of carbon monoxide absorbed when air containing a known concentration of carbon monoxide is inhaled and the breath is held for 15 s before exhalation. It is a measure of pulmonary gas exchange. Hence it is reduced in restrictive defects but is normal in pure obstructive defects.

10.9 A B D
See question 10.8 above.

10.10 A
The haemoglobin molecule plays an important role in carrying oxygen in the red blood cells. It is a globular protein made up of four subunits. In normal human adults, most haemoglobin is of the type haemoglobin A, which consists of four polypeptide chains: two α chains and two β chains. However, a small proportion of the haemoglobin is haemoglobin A_2, which consists of two α chains and two δ chains. This is clinically important, as the proportion of haemoglobin A_2 increases in diseases with defective β chain production. There is a haem moiety conjugated to each polypeptide chain. The haem moiety is a porphyrin derivative containing ferrous iron, and is responsible for binding to oxygen molecules. When exposed to various oxidising drugs, the ferrous iron may be converted to ferric iron, forming methaemoglobin. Methaemoglobin is dark-coloured, and may give rise to bluish discoloration of the skin resembling cyanosis.

10.11 C
Haemoglobin increases the oxygen-carrying capacity of the blood by about 70-fold. The haem moiety binds to the oxygen molecules. Since there are four haem moieties per haemoglobin molecule, up to four oxygen molecules may bind to one haemoglobin molecule. The haem moieties may assume either a relaxed (R) or tense (T) state, depending on the distance between the two β chains. Binding to an oxygen molecule increases the likelihood of an R state, which favours further oxygen binding. Hence, binding to an oxygen molecule increases the affinity for binding to a second oxygen molecule. This explains the sigmoid-shaped oxygen–haemoglobin dissociation curve.

10.12 A B
In the oxygen–haemoglobin dissociation curve, the partial pressure of oxygen is represented on the horizontal axis, whilst the percentage oxygen saturation is represented on the vertical axis. If the curve is shifted to the right, the oxygen saturation of haemoglobin is lower for a given partial pressure of oxygen. Conversely, a higher partial pressure of oxygen is required for haemoglobin to bind to a given amount of oxygen. In other words, the

haemoglobin molecule holds less tightly to the oxygen molecules. The venous blood haemoglobin oxygen saturation is about 75%, whilst the arterial blood haemoglobin oxygen saturation is about 97%. Since the oxygen dissociation curve for haemoglobin is sigmoid, the oxygen–haemoglobin dissociation curve is steeper at the 75% than the 97% oxygen saturation point. Hence, if the oxygen–haemoglobin dissociation curve is shifted to the right, it is becomes easier to oxygenate the oxygen in the pulmonary capillaries, but more difficult for the blood in the capillaries to deliver oxygen to the tissues. Hence it may be clinically desirable to shift the oxygen–haemoglobin dissociation curve in the tissues to the right.

10.13 A C D E
Shifts of the oxygen–haemoglobin dissociation curve are important mechanisms to ensure oxygen is effectively delivered to the tissues. Increase in temperature, reduction in pH and increase in 2,3-DPG shift the oxygen–haemoglobin dissociation curve to the right, reduce the affinity of haemoglobin for oxygen, and ease the delivery of oxygen to the tissues. Living at high altitude usually triggers an increase in 2,3-DPG. During exercise, a combination of a temperature increase, a reduction in pH and an increase in 2,3-DPG shifts the oxygen–haemoglobin dissociation curve to the right. Furthermore, the steep part of the curve is in operation as partial pressure of oxygen is low. Hence more oxygen is released to the tissues for the given oxygen gradient.

10.14 A
Myoglobin is mainly found in the skeletal muscle. Its function is to extract oxygen from haemoglobin in the blood and deliver it to the exercising skeletal muscles. Each myoglobin molecule can only bind to one oxygen molecule, and thus has a hyperbolic oxygen–haemoglobin dissociation curve. The oxygen dissociation curve of myoglobin is well to the left of the haemoglobin curve, and it is therefore efficient in extracting oxygen from haemoglobin.

10.15 –
Several mechanisms are responsible for carbon dioxide transport, and there are significant roles for both the plasma and the red cells. Almost 90% of the carbon dioxide is transported as bicarbonate ions, about 5% is dissolved, and about 5% is transported as carbamino-haemoglobin. A negligible amount of oxygen is dissolved, but carbon dioxide is about 20 times more soluble than oxygen. Deoxygenated blood carries more carbon dioxide than oxygenated blood (Haldane effect), and this facilitates the uptake of carbon dioxide from the tissues and its delivery to the pulmonary capillaries. Most carbon

dioxide is transported as bicarbonate ions. Carbon dioxide enters the red blood cell, and is hydrated to H_2CO_3. This process depends on the enzyme carbonic anhydrase. H_2CO_3 is then dissociated into hydrogen and bicarbonate ions. About 70% of the bicarbonate ions enters the plasma by exchanging with a chloride ion.

10.16 A B C E
See also question 10.15 above. Carbon dioxide enters the red blood cell, and is converted to H_2CO_3 with the action of carbonic anhydrase. It is then dissociated into hydrogen and bicarbonate ions. Hence venous blood contains more bicarbonate and hydrogen ions. About 70% of the excess bicarbonate ions move out of the red blood cells and are exchanged for chloride ions. Hence, there are more chloride ions in the red blood cells in the venous than the arterial blood. Since the red cell in the venous blood contains extra osmotically active particles (chloride or bicarbonate ions), the cells swell.

10.17 A B C D
Asthma is defined as hypersensitivity of the bronchial tree with intermittent narrowing of the airways. Extrinsic (atopic) asthma may be triggered by common stimuli such as food, house dust mites and pets. Narrowing of the airways is mediated by release of histamine and slow-reacting substance of anaphylaxis (SRS-A) from inflammatory cells such as mast cells via type I hypersensitivity reaction. Excess IgE may be produced. The hypersensitivy reaction may lead to bronchial obstruction, mucus plugging of the bronchi and mucosal oedema of the bronchioles.

10.18 A B
Anti-asthmatic drugs may act by reducing bronchial hyperreactivity, reducing bronchial inflammation, and dilatation of the narrowed bronchi. Corticosteroids act by generally reducing bronchial hyperreactivity, and they may also inhibit the release of mediators from inflammatory cells. Sodium cromoglicate was thought to act mainly by preventing the release of mediators from mast cells, but it may also act on other inflammatory cells or on local axon reflexes. The adrenoceptors in the bronchi are mainly of the β_2 type, and agonists to these receptors act by dilating narrowed bronchioles. Methylxanthines have two modes of action: adenosine receptor antagonists and phosphodiesterase inhibitors. Antimuscarinic agents act as competitive inhibitors of muscarinic receptors, and induce dilatation of narrowed bronchioles.

10.19 C D
Respiration is controlled by both neural and chemical mechanisms. The neural control is usually moderated by chemical control. However, chemical control may override

neural control in some situations. An example is that chemical control may initiate inspiration if the breath is voluntarily held for a prolonged period of time. The voluntary and automatic neural control mechanisms are entirely separate. The voluntary system is located in the cerebral cortex and sends impulses to the respiratory motor neurones in the medulla via the corticospinal tract, whilst the automatic neural system is located in the medulla. This may be clinically important. For example, diseases which affect the medulla may result in the loss of automatic control without affecting the voluntary control (Ondine's curse). To coordinate the breathing movements, motor neurones supplying the inspiratory muscles are inhibited whilst those supplying the expiratory muscles are activated, and vice versa.

10.20 A B
The chemoreceptors which mediate the chemical control of respiration are situated at the medulla oblongata near the respiratory centre. The carotid and aortic bodies (situated at the carotid bifurcation and near the arch of the aorta respectively) are sensitive to hypoxia. In general, chemical control tends to restore the arterial blood gases to their normal levels. Hence, a reduction in pH, an increase in carbon dioxide and a reduction in oxygen tend to result in an increase in ventilatory response. However, under normal conditions, the control of carbon dioxide is more sensitive than oxygen. With a normal level of carbon dioxide, the ventilatory response to hypoxia is slight when the partial pressure of oxygen of the inspired air is over 60 mmHg (a reduction of over 40% below normal). One reason for this is that a slight increase in ventilatory response results in a reduction in carbon dioxide and pH. However, when the partial pressure of oxygen of the inspired air is below 60 mmHg, a marked increase in ventilatory response occurs.

This usual respiratory drive by carbon dioxide is of clinical importance, as a high concentration of oxygen may be given to a patient with intact chemical control of respiration for acute hypoxia (e.g. acute asthma) without seriously reducing the respiratory drive.

10.21 A B D E
Several factors contribute to the increased ventilation rate immediately before and during exercise. Immediately before exercise, psychic stimuli and afferent impulses from muscle and joint proprioceptors to the respiratory centre may increase the ventilation rate. During moderate exercise, the arterial oxygen, carbon dioxide and pH do not change much. However, the chemoreceptors may become more sensitive to fluctuations in carbon dioxide levels, which results in an increase in ventilation rate during exercise. In vigorous exercise, pH drops as a result of excessive lactate production. Arterial carbon dioxide

The respiratory system

SYSTEM-BASED MEDICAL SCIENCES

may rise and arterial oxygen may drop slightly. All these factors may result in stimulation of the chemoreceptors in the medulla and cause an increase in ventilation rate.

10.22   A B C D E
Oxygen deficiency at the tissue level is known as hypoxia. This may be caused by a low oxygen partial pressure in the arterial blood (hypoxic hypoxia), lack of oxygen-carrying capacity of the blood (anaemic hypoxia), inadequate blood flow to the tissues (ischaemic hypoxia) or inability of the tissue to make use of the available oxygen (histotoxic hypoxia). Causes of hypoxic hypoxia include lung diseases and shunting of blood from the venous to the arterial circulation. Anaemic hypoxia may be caused by either anaemia or carbon monoxide poisoning. Carbon monoxide combines with haemoglobin to form a compound (carbonmonoxyhaemoglobin) which cannot bind to oxygen. Histotoxic hypoxia may be caused by cyanide poisoning, which inhibits enzymes (e.g. cytochrome oxidase) involved in the tissue oxidative processes.

10.23   A B C E
Respiratory failure occurs when hypoxia and carbon dioxide retention occur as a result of ineffective gas exchange between the alveoli and the pulmonary capillaries. This may be caused by ventilation defects, perfusion defects or defects of gas exchange. Causes of ventilation defects include mechanical factors (e.g. obesity, severe abnormal curvature of the spine), muscle weakness (e.g. due to muscular dystrophy or motor neurone disease) or loss of lung volume (e.g. collapse of the lobe of a lung). Ventilation – perfusion mismatch may be caused by multiple pulmonary emboli. Defects of gas exchange may be caused by pulmonary fibrosis or emphysema. Whilst shunting of blood from the venous to the arterial circulation can cause hypoxia, it is not a cause of respiratory failure.

10.24   C D E
100% oxygen therapy increases the alveolar partial pressure of oxygen, and is useful in hypoxia caused by ventilation defects or gas-exchange defects. Hence it is effective for pneumonia and fibrosis of the lung. It is also partially effective in treating hypoxia due to ventilation–perfusion mismatch. However, increasing the alveolar partial pressure of oxygen will have no effect on the shunting of blood from the venous to the arterial circulation. 100% oxygen is effective and safe in acute asthma, as the chemoreceptors at the medulla are driven by increased carbon dioxide level. However, in a patient with severe chronic obstructive airway disease and chronic carbon dioxide retention, the chemoreceptors at the medulla may not be sensitive to carbon dioxide level. Instead, respiration is driven by hypoxia. Therefore

administering 100% oxygen may be dangerous as it may depress the respiratory drive and cause respiratory arrest.

10.25   B D E
Reduced ventilation immediately results in a rise in the arterial partial pressure of carbon dioxide, and a reduction in the arterial partial pressure of oxygen. Since carbon dioxide equilibrates with H_2CO_3, which is in turn in equilibrium with H^+ and HCO_3^-, the pH decreases. This is uncompensated respiratory acidosis. In the long term, the respiratory acidosis is compensated, though only partially, by increased renal secretion of H^+ and reabsorption of HCO_3^-. Hence the plasma HCO_3^- is raised in the compensated respiratory acidotic state.

10.26   B D
Respiratory alkalosis is caused by excessive ventilation as in hysterical hyperventilation. Excessive carbon dioxide is washed out from the lungs, and the arterial partial pressure of carbon dioxide decreases. As a result, the pH increases. In chronic respiratory alkalosis, the kidneys attempt to compensate for the alkalosis by reduced secretion of H^+ and reduced reabsorption of HCO_3^-. Hence the plasma HCO_3^- level decreases.

10.27   A B C D
Cough may be valuable in expelling foreign bodies and secretions from the respiratory tract. However, cough unproductive of sputum sometimes serves no useful clinical purpose. Cough is usually initiated by irritation of the lining of the trachea, larynx or pharynx. During coughing, expiration is forced against a closed glottis, and it is usually preceded by a deep inspiration.

10.28   A B D
Like most other autonomic reflexes, the main centre for the autonomic control of the cough reflex is located in the medulla oblongata. The main afferent inputs are from stimuli to the trachea, larynx or pharynx. However, it also receives neural inputs from the cerebral cortex, and cough is under substantial voluntary control. Changes in the partial pressure of carbon dioxide are monitored by the chemoreceptors which regulate respiratory drive, but do not affect the cough reflex.

10.29   A C D E
In the treatment of cough, the causes of the cough (e.g. infection, tumour) must be diagnosed and appropriately treated. If the cough still persists and is unproductive, it may be treated by measures which reduce the peripheral stimuli for the cough reflex or act on the central nervous system. Measures which would reduce the peripheral stimuli include ceasing smoking, staying in a warm, moist environment, the use of water inhalation as an aerosol, or

the oral administration of a demulcent which coats and soothes the pharynx (e.g. simple linctus). Drugs which act centrally are mostly opioids (e.g. codeine, pholcodine).

10.30   A C
Emboli which reach the lung originate from the venous circulation and the right side of the heart. The commonest source of pulmonary emboli is venous thrombosis from the leg veins. The rest usually originate from pelvic veins.

10.31   B C E
Pulmonary emboli frequently originate from venous thrombi in the leg veins. Most venous thrombi are initiated at the venous valves, as they tend to encourage turbulent blood flow. The venous flow of blood from the legs depends on calf muscle contraction. Hence immobilisation is a major risk factor for pulmonary emboli. During a surgical operation, blood pressure may fall, and stasis may occur in the leg veins. Hence, the risk of pulmonary emboli is increased in the immediate post-operative period after a major operation. Other risk factors include malignancy (which may increase blood viscosity), oral contraceptive pills (which increase the risk for both arterial and venous thrombi) and pregnancy. High cholesterol level is a risk factor for atherosclerosis and arterial thrombosis.

10.32   A B E
The sequelae of pulmonary emboli depend on the size of the emboli and where they are lodged. A large pulmonary embolus lodged at the bifurcation of the pulmonary artery (saddle embolus) will significantly deprive both lungs of their blood supply. It is a frequent cause of sudden death. Alternatively, the patient may complain of severe chest pain with intense breathlessness, cyanosis and shock. If an embolus is lodged at a lobar or segmental artery, it may lead to the infarction of a lobe or segment. If there are multiple small pulmonary emboli, this will lead to gradual blockage of the pulmonary arterioles and pulmonary arterial hypertension. Pulmonary oedema may be caused by increased pulmonary venous hydrostatic pressure.

10.33   A B C D E
Pulmonary arterial hypertension may be classified according to the site of the pathology in relation to the pulmonary capillaries: pre-capillary, capillary or post-capillary. 'Pre-capillary' causes include multiple pulmonary emboli and shunt of blood from the left to the right side of the heart as in ventricular septal defects. 'Capillary' causes are primary lung diseases, and include lung fibrosis and chronic obstructive airway disease. 'Post-capillary' causes are due to high pressure in the pulmonary venous system resulting in back-pressure in the pulmonary arterial system. Examples are any causes of left ventricular failure and mitral stenosis.

10.34   A B C
The general causes of pulmonary oedema include increased pulmonary venous hydrostatic pressure, reduced plasma oncotic pressure, increased permeability of the alveolar capillary wall and blockage of the lymphatic drainage. The commonest cause of pulmonary oedema is increased pulmonary venous hydrostatic pressure due to left ventricular failure. Other causes of increased pulmonary venous hydrostatic pressure are mitral stenosis and severe aortic stenosis. A low plasma albumin level results in reduced plasma oncotic pressure. Increased permeability of the alveolar capillary wall may be caused by toxic fumes.

10.35   A C D
The diaphragm is the most important inspiratory muscle, and accounts for over three-quarters of the increase in intrathoracic volume during inspiration. The accessory inspiratory muscles (scalene and sternocleidomastoid muscles) lift the thoracic cage to increase the intrathoracic volume in laboured respiration. These muscles are clinically important, as they may be seen to contract actively in the presence of moderately severe respiratory diseases, as in an acute asthmatic attack. Another group of inspiratory muscles are the external intercostal muscles, which run obliquely downwards and forwards from one rib to the rib below. Contraction of these muscles increases the anteroposterior diameter of the chest. The main group of expiratory muscles are the internal intercostal muscles, which run obliquely downwards and backwards from one rib to the rib below. Contractions of these muscles pull the rib cage downwards and decrease the intrathoracic volume. Expiration may also be assisted by contraction of the muscles of the anterior abdominal wall, which both increases the intra-abdominal pressure and pulls the rib cage downwards.

10.36   C E
Chronic bronchitis and emphysema usually coexist. Both are diffuse diseases usually affecting all lobes of the lungs to some extent. Whilst chronic bronchitis is defined clinically as productive cough for three months in two consecutive years, emphysema is defined anatomically as enlargement of the air spaces in the alveoli due to destruction of elastin in their walls. In emphysema, the air spaces distal to the terminal bronchioles are permanently enlarged. Both chronic bronchitis and emphysema usually occur in smokers. The majority of people with deficiency of the enzyme α_1-antitrypsin also develop this disease. α_1-Antitrypsin is an acute-phase protein which inhibits the enzyme elastase as well as other protein-denaturing

SYSTEM-BASED MEDICAL SCIENCES

The respiratory system

enzymes. This may explain why elastin in the walls of the alveoli is destroyed in these patients.

10.37 A B D
Known risk factors for bronchial carcinoma include cigarette smoking, passive cigarette smoke, occupational exposure to asbestos and chromate, and exposure to excessive radiation. Radon is a radioactive gas. There is no evidence that excessive alcohol or low-fibre diet is associated with bronchial carcinoma.

10.38 A B
The pleural cavities are potential spaces between the layers of parietal pleura and visceral pleura. Normally, the pressure in the pleural cavities is below atmospheric pressure. Air may enter the pleural cavities either if a lung ruptures or a hole is created on the parietal pleura by a penetrating wound. The lung on the affected side collapses due to elastic recoil. The intrapleural pressure on the affected side becomes atmospheric, which is higher than the other side. Thus the mediastinum is shifted towards the normal side. The intrapleural pressure usually decreases normally during inspiration to allow lung expansion and increases during expiration. Hence air enters the pleural cavity during inspiration.

10.39 B E
Just over half of all bronchial carcinomas are of the squamous cell type. About 30% are small cell carcinomas, and just over 10% are adenocarcinoma. Large cell carcinomas are rare. Squamous cell carcinomas arise from squamous metaplasia, and usually arise at the hilum. They tend to metastasise locally to hilar lymph nodes, and distant metastases are rare. Whilst small cell carcinomas are prone to produce ectopic ADH and ACTH, squamous cell carcinomas usually produce ectopic PTH.

10.40 D
The vocal folds control sound production. They consist of elastic tissues derived from the cricothyroid ligaments, and the vocalis muscles. They are wide open during forced inspiration, half-open during normal inspiration, and approximate each other during speech production. The pitch of the voice is controlled by alteration of the length of the vocal folds. They are shorter in women than in men, which accounts for the higher pitch of a woman's voice. Whilst the extrinsic muscles of the larynx control the movement of the larynx as a whole, the length of the vocal folds is indirectly controlled by the intrinsic muscles of the larynx. The posterior and the lateral cricoarytenoid muscles are the main abductors and adductors of the vocal folds respectively. All the intrinsic muscles of the larynx except the cricothyroid are supplied by the recurrent laryngeal nerve. Hence paralysis of the vocal folds may

result if it is damaged during surgery, and the patient may present with hoarseness or aphonia.

10.41 B
The trachea is palpable only for the upper 5 cm below the cricoid cartilage and above the suprasternal notch. To find the trachea clinically, the forefinger should be introduced just above the suprasternal notch. It may not be palpable in some subjects, especially the obese.

10.42 A C
Displacement of the trachea may be caused by thyroid, mediastinal and intrathoracic lesions. Mediastinal lesions may include lymphoma or carcinoma. Lesions affecting the upper parts of the lungs are especially likely to cause tracheal deviation. However, in collapse or fibrosis of the upper lobe of the lung, the trachea is deviated to the opposite side.

10.43 D E
The anteroposterior diameter of the chest is usually between 50% and 70% that of the lateral diameter. An increase in the anteroposterior diameter (i.e. barrel chest) may indicate respiratory diseases such as emphysema. The normal respiratory rate in adults is about 12–15 breaths per minute. The maximum chest expansion should be above 5 cm. The intercostal muscles and the diaphragm are usually sufficient for normal respiration. Use of accessory respiratory muscles such as sternomastoids and scaleni may indicate respiratory diseases. Pursed lips during expiration is characteristic of patients with diseases associated with air trapping in the alveoli such as emphysema. This is because the manoeuvre increases the pressure inside the bronchi, and hence delays the collapse of the bronchial wall.

10.44 A B E
Normal lung resonance is due to air in the lung tissues. Dullness to percussion may be due to separation of the chest wall from the underlying lung tissues by pleural fluid (i.e. pleural effusion) or thickened pleural tissue. Alternatively, it may be due to loss of air in the lung tissues (e.g. in consolidation of fibrosis). Pneumothorax or emphysema is associated with hyperresonance.

10.45 A
Normal vesicular breath sounds are caused by the change in the quality of the breath sounds at the larynx on its passage through the normal lung tissues to the stethoscope over the chest wall. Bronchial sounds are heard if the lung tissues become more solid and conduct sound more effectively, and they resemble the sounds produced at the larynx. Hence, the presence of bronchial breathing indicates that the relevant bronchi are patent,

and that the consistency of the lung tissues has become more solid (e.g. in consolidation). Bronchial sounds are equally loud and long during inspiration and expiration, and there is a pause between the end of inspiration and the beginning of expiration. Since the presence of bronchial sounds indicates that the underlying lung tissues conduct sounds better than normally, the vocal resonance is always increased.

10.46

A

i   Phase A (quiet inspiration). The fibres of the diaphragm contract so that only the domes descend. The external intercostal muscles are active in inspiration, but are important only for stiffening the chest wall to prevent paradoxical movement of the interspaces. The intrathoracic volume increases and the intrapleural pressure at the base of the lung decreases from −2.5 mmHg to −6 mmHg. The pressure in the airway also becomes negative, so air flows into the lungs.

ii   Phase B (quiet expiration). The internal intercostal muscles are active in expiration but the main expiratory effort is the elastic recoil of the lungs assisted by contraction of the muscles of the abdominal wall, which makes the relaxed diaphragm regain its domed form. The intrathoracic volume decreases and the intrapleural pressure increases.

iii   Phase C (forced inspiration). The external intercostal muscles are active, as in quiet inspiration. In addition, the scalene muscles and the sternocleidomastoid elevate the first rib and the manubrium. The erector spinae extend the spine, and pectoralis major contributes to chest expansion. Contraction of the diaphragm may evert the ribs of the costal margin in a 'bucket-handle'-like movement with widening of the subcostal angle.

iv   Phase D (forced expiration). The internal intercostal muscles are active as in quiet expiration. In addition, latissimus dorsi contracts to compress the lower ribs. The diaphragm is wholly passive.

B

(a)   Tidal volume.
(b)   Inspiratory reserve volume.
(c)   Expiratory reserve volume.
(d)   Residual volume.
(e)   Vital capacity.
(f)   Inspiratory capacity.
(g)   Functional residual capacity.

C

The residual volume is the volume of air left in the lungs after a maximal expiratory effort. This consists of air in the conducting zone of the airways.

D

Respiratory volume at rest per minute = tidal volume × respiratory rate per minute = 0.5 litres × 12 = 6 l/min.

10.47

A

The slope of these curves measures the compliance (stretchability) of the lungs (compliance = $\Delta P/\Delta V$). The lung expansion per unit increase in intrapulmonary pressure is smaller in stiff lungs compared with elastic lungs.

B

The main factor affecting the compliance of the lungs is the surface tension of the film of fluid that lines the alveoli. A reduction in surface tension is associated with lower compliance.

C

i   Lung compliance is lowered by the presence of surfactant lining the alveoli.

ii   By the law of Laplace, in spherical structures like the alveoli the required distending pressure equals twice the tension divided by the radius ($P = 2T/r$). If the radius is small and the tension is large, the required distending pressure would be too large and the alveoli would collapse. By reducing the surface tension, surfactant lining the alveoli increases the compliance of the lungs.

iii   Surfactant is composed of a mixture of dipalmitoylphosphatidylcholine (DPCC), other lipids and protein. Lamellar bodies are secreted from type II alveolar epithelial cells and converted to tubular myelin. This is the source of phospholipid surface film.

D

The work of breathing has the same dimensions as pressure × volume; it can be estimated from the relaxation pressure curve (a plot of lung volume against (intrapulmonary pressure − intrapleural pressure)). The lack of surfactant would necessitate a larger increase in pressure to sustain a given tidal volume. Hence, the work of breathing increases with a lack of surfactant.

E

Surfactant is abnormally low in respiratory distress syndrome (hyaline membrane disease) in very premature infants. Surfactant synthesis is not fully functional until about 36 weeks of gestation. Affected infants often have very stiff lungs requiring high-pressure ventilation.

F

The lung compliance is lower than normal. This may represent a range of conditions, such as lung fibrosis and pulmonary oedema.

SYSTEM-BASED MEDICAL SCIENCES

The respiratory system

10.48

A

Total dead space is the physiological dead space. It is the volume of gas not equilibrating with blood (i.e. ventilation which does not contribute to blood oxygenation). It is made up of the anatomical dead space (air in the conducting system from the naso-oral pharynx to the terminal bronchioles, which does not engage in gas exchange) and physiological dead space (alveolar air that does not engage in gas exchange owing either to non-perfused alveoli or overdistended alveoli).

B

> For the first subject, minute volume = tidal volume × respiratory rate (per minute) = 0.5 litres × 12 = 6 l/min
> For the second subject, minute volume = tidal volume × respiratory rate (per minute) = 0.25 litres × 24 = 6 l/min

C

> For the first subject, alveolar ventilation per minute
> = (tidal volume − dead space) × respiratory rate (per minute)
> = (0.5 − 0.15) litres × 12
> = 4.2 l/min
> For the second subject, alveolar ventilation per minute
> = (tidal volume − dead space) × respiratory rate (per minute)
> = (0.25 − 0.15) litres × 24
> = 2.4 l/min

D

The alveolar ventilation of the first subject is larger than the second. Hence, the first subject is breathing more effectively. The second subject spends proportionally more energy in shifting air in and out of the anatomical dead space.

10.49

A

Coughing is usually initiated by irritation in the trachea or oropharynx. It begins with a deep inspiration followed by forced expiration against a closed glottis. This greatly increases the intrapleural pressure. The glottis suddenly opens, resulting in an explosive and rapid outflow of air.

B

Coughing is controlled by centres in the medulla oblongata. Currently, the 'cough centre' is ill defined and ill understood.

C

In general terms, cough is initiated by the presence of mucus, exudate, tumour or foreign material in the trachea or oropharynx.

D

Drugs effective in the treatment of cough are largely opiates. They include codeine and pholcodine. They act by depressing the cough centres in the medulla oblongata.

10.50

A

There are two separate neural mechanisms for controlling respiration: voluntary control and automatic control. The voluntary system resides in the cerebral cortex and sends impulses in the respiratory motor neurones via the corticospinal tracts. The automatic control resides in the respiratory centres in the medulla. The respiratory centre is controlled by chemical stimuli from the carotid bodies (near the carotid bifurcation) and aortic bodies. There are also chemoreceptors in the medulla oblongata, separate from the respiratory centre, which respond to a high arterial carbon dioxide level.

B

The student initially held her breath by voluntary inhibition. After a while, her arterial carbon dioxide level rose and arterial oxygen level fell. This stimulates the carotid bodies, which send impulses to the respiratory centre. At a certain point (breaking point), the respiratory centre overrides the voluntary inhibition and the student could no longer hold her breath.

C

After a period of voluntary hyperventilation, the carbon dioxide in the lungs is washed out and the arterial carbon dioxide is lowered. Since she started off with a lower arterial carbon dioxide level, it took longer for the arterial carbon dioxide level to reach the breaking point and she could therefore hold her breath voluntarily for a longer period.

10.51

A

Chronic bronchitis is defined clinically as cough and sputum for 3 months in 2 consecutive years. Emphysema is defined anatomically as enlargement of alveolar airspace with destruction of elastin in the walls.

B

Cigarette smoking is by far the most important aetiology for chronic bronchitis.

C

Chronic bronchitis first affects bronchi and bronchioles. Initially, there is respiratory bronchiolitis affecting airways less than about 2 mm in diameter. This leads to destruction of their walls and surrounding elastin. Mucous plugging may occur. There is excessive mucous secretion in the bronchi and bronchoconstriction, causing chronic cough and sputum.

D

Patients with chronic bronchitis usually have a large element of bronchiolar obstruction and fall into the 'blue bloaters' spectrum of chronic obstructive airways disease. The arterial oxygen level is low and the carbon dioxide level is high.

E

See Fig. 10.5.

F

See Fig. 10.6.

G

Since a high arterial level of carbon dioxide results in coma or death, there is a maximum level of alveolar carbon dioxide clinically possible. It can be seen from Fig. 10.6 that patients with severe chronic bronchitis depend on a

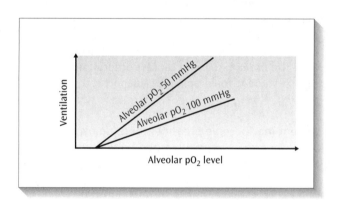

Fig. 10.5 Relationship between ventilation and alveolar carbon dioxide level, with alveolar oxygen held constant at 100 mmHg.

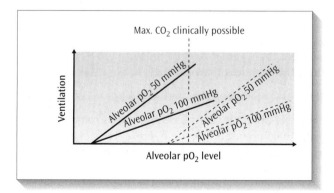

Fig. 10.6 Effect of severe chronic bronchitis (dotted line) on the normal relationship (solid line) between ventilation and alveolar carbon dioxide pressure.

low alveolar oxygen level to drive their respiration. Hence, it is inadvisable to administer a high concentration of oxygen level to such patients.

10.52

A

There was a stepwise increase in ventilation just before exercise. This increase was likely to be due to psychic stimuli and impulses from proprioceptors in muscles and tendons to the respiratory centre. This may cause an increase in the depth of respiration.

B

The increase in ventilation during exercise is proportional to the oxygen consumption. However, the mechanisms are not altogether clear and it may be caused by a combination of many factors. Exercise may be accompanied by an increase in K^+, which may stimulate peripheral chemoreceptors. The sensitivity of the respiratory centre to carbon dioxide may be increased. Arterial oxygen level may play a part.

C

i   Ventilation was above the basal level for a considerable period of time after exercise. This can be explained by the accumulation of lactic acid during exercise. This metabolic acidosis stimulates the carotid bodies, which increases ventilation.

ii To repay the 'oxygen debt'. During exercise, aerobic respiration via the citric acid cycle is insufficiently fast to generate the energy required. The extra energy is derived from anaerobic respiration. Hence, extra oxygen is required after exercise to remove the excess lactic acid and to replenish the ATP store.

10.53

A

Haemoglobin is a globular protein made up of four subunits. Each subunit consists of a haem (iron-containing porphyrin derivative) moiety conjugated to a polypeptide. The polypeptides are called the globin portion of the haemoglobin. In the normal adult human haemoglobin, there are two α chains and two β chains.

B

See Fig. 10.7, the oxygen dissociation curve. It has a characteristic sigmoid shape.

C

A haemoglobin molecule consists of four haemoglobin units; it can be represented by Hb_4. It reacts to 4 molecules of oxygen to form Hb_4O_8 in four rapid steps:

1. $Hb_4 + O_2 \rightleftharpoons Hb_4O_2$
2. $Hb_4O_2 + O_2 \rightleftharpoons Hb_4O_4$

The respiratory system

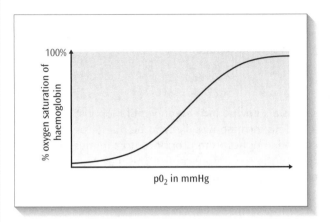

Fig. 10.7 Relationship between haemoglobin oxygen saturation and partial pressure (oxygen dissociation curve).

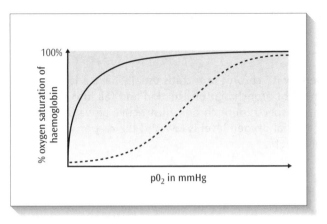

Fig. 10.8 The myoglobin (solid line) and haemoglobin (dotted line) oxygen dissociation curves.

3. $Hb_4O_4 + O_2 \rightleftharpoons Hb_4O_6$
4. $Hb_4O_6 + O_2 \rightleftharpoons Hb_4O_8$.

The haem moieties exist in either relaxed (R) or tense (T) state. The affinity of the haem moieties for oxygen is higher in the relaxed state than in the tense state. When haemoglobin takes up an oxygen molecule, the two β chains move closer together, favouring the relaxed state. Hence, the uptake of an oxygen molecule by the haemoglobin favours further binding to oxygen (cooperativity). This explains the sigmoid shape of the oxygen dissociation curve.

D
See Fig. 10.8. The solid line shows the myoglobin oxygen dissociation curve; the dotted line shows the corresponding curve for haemoglobin. The myoglobin oxygen dissociation curve is rectangular hyperbolic. This is because there is only a single unit in the myoglobin molecule.

E
From the curves in (D) above, haemoglobin is better at extracting oxygen to the arterial blood from the air in the lungs, where the partial pressure for oxygen is high. Myoglobin is better in delivering oxygen to the mitochondria of skeletal muscles, where the partial pressure for oxygen is low.

10.54
A
As a rough estimate, the partial pressure of oxygen is proportional to the barometric pressure. Hence, the partial pressure of oxygen at 3000 m is: 125 mmHg × (500/750) = 83 mmHg.

B
From (A) above, the partial pressure of oxygen at 3000 m is considerably lower than at sea level. Although cerebral autoregulation tends partially to offset the effect of this hypoxia on the brain, the hypoxia cannot compensate fully. Hence, the hypoxia may cause cerebral arteriolar dilatation. This may result in increased transudation of fluid into the brain tissue and causes cerebral oedema, causing the student to complain of headache.

C
The student may become breathless because hypoxia stimulates the chemoreceptor carotid bodies, which send impulses to the respiratory centre to increase ventilation. There is also a steady increase in ventilation over the next 4 days because of active transport of H^+ into the cerebrospinal fluid. This reduction in pH results in stimulation of respiratory drive.

D
If there is no increased ventilation as a result of the hypoxia, the alveolar oxygen pressure would be reduced by a third; however, since there is compensatory increased ventilation, the alveolar oxygen pressure would be reduced by much less than a third.

E
Immediately after the ascent, ventilation increases in an attempt to compensate for the hypoxia. Hence, there is respiratory alkalosis. The alveolar carbon dioxide level would decrease. Initially, in the uncompensated state, the bicarbonate level is normal. However, the kidneys soon attempt to compensate for the reduction in carbon dioxide by shifting the equilibrium

$$HCO_3^- + H^+ \rightleftharpoons H_2CO_3 \rightleftharpoons H_2O + CO_2$$

Table 10.2

	Trachea	Bronchi	Bronchioles	Respiratory bronchioles	Alveoli
Presence of cartilage	Yes	Yes	No	No	No
Presence of smooth muscle	Transverse trachealis muscle	Yes	Yes	Yes	No
Presence of cilia	Yes	Yes	Yes	Yes	No
Presence of mucous glands	Yes	Yes	No	No	No
Gas exchange	No	No	No	Yes	Yes
Lined by pneumocyte	No	No	No	No	Yes

to the right. Hence, the bicarbonate ion level is decreased in the compensated state.

F
Alkalosis shifts the haemoglobin oxygen dissociation curve to the left. This is compensated by an increase in 2,3-DPG level, which tends to shift the dissociation curve to the right.

G
The student became less breathless after a week because there had been a gradual desensitisation of the stimulatory effects of hypoxia.

H
His haemoglobin level rose because hypoxia stimulates erythropoietin secretion. This may occur 2–3 days after ascent.

10.55
A
See Table 10.2.

B
There is increased irritability of the bronchial tree. There may be mucous plugs in the bronchi.

C
Restrictive and obstructive defects are the two major types of pulmonary defect, although they may coexist. Asthma is the classical disease causing airway obstruction. FEV_1 is the maximum volume of air blown from the lungs within the first second and is mainly dependent on the state of the trachea and bronchi. Hence, it is low in asthma. Vital capacity is abnormal in restrictive but not obstructive lung defects. Hence, it is normal in asthma. The ratio FEV_1/VC is abnormally low in asthma.

D
In allergic asthma, inhaled antigens cause degranulation of mast cells bearing specific IgE molecules. Vasoactive substances such as histamine, slow-releasing substance A (SRS-A) and platelet activation factor are released. They may cause bronchoconstriction, bronchial oedema and hypersecretion of mucus.

E
Drugs that may be effective include glucocorticoids and sodium cromoglicate. Both are anti-inflammatory agents. Cromoglicate probably acts by depressing the exaggerated neuronal reflexes that are triggered by stimulation of the irritant receptors. Glucocorticoids probably act by reducing the formation of cytokines by inhibition of transcription of the relevant genes.

10.56
A
Salbutamol is a β_2-adrenoceptor agonist. It acts on the β_2-adrenoceptors on the smooth muscle to dilate the bronchi. They may also facilitate clearance of mucus by an action on cilia.

B
Ipratropium is a muscarinic receptor antagonist. It acts by binding to all muscarinic receptor subtypes (M_1, M_2 and M_3). It relieves bronchospasm due to parasympathetic nervous stimulation. It may also facilitate clearance of mucus.

C
Theophylline is one of the xanthine drugs. Traditionally, it is thought to act by inhibiting phophodiesterase, which results in an increase in cyclic AMP. This may cause bronchodilatation. However, it is now suspected that it may act by inhibiting a subtype of cyclic GMP phosphodiesterase.

10 **A**

SYSTEM-BASED MEDICAL SCIENCES

The respiratory system

D

Again, glucocorticoids probably act by reducing the formation of cytokines by inhibition of transcription of the relevant genes.

10.57

A

The most important aetiological factor for bronchial carcinoma is cigarette smoking.

B

Occupational hazards for developing the disease include exposure to:
- asbestos
- haematite (e.g. miners)
- radioactive gases
- nickel, coal-tar distillates.

C

Squamous cell carcinoma and small cell (oat cell) carcinoma are usually hilar. Adenocarcinomas are usually peripheral, and large cell undifferentiated carcinomas are usually central.

D

Ectopic ACTH and ADH secretion is characteristically associated with small cell lung carcinoma; ectopic PTH secretion is usually associated with squamous cell carcinoma.

E

Small (oat) cell carcinomas have the worst prognosis. As they usually arise from a hilar bronchus, they metastasise early.

10.58

A

The posterior cricoarytenoid is the only muscle that abducts the vocal folds. It arises from the back of the lamina of the cricoid and converges on the back of the ipsilateral arytenoid. Most of the other intrinsic laryngeal muscles adduct the vocal folds. They include transverse arytenoid, oblique arytenoids and lateral cricoarytenoid. All the muscles of the larynx are supplied by the recurrent laryngeal nerve, except cricothyroid which is supplied by the external laryngeal nerve.

B

While she was waiting for her musical entry, the vocal folds were separated.

C

A sound is produced by emitting a series of rapid discrete jets of air from the lungs while apposing the vocal folds.

The apposed vocal folds are slightly separated by the jet of air, and elastic recoil returns them to their original position. Repetition of these movements results in vibration of the vocal folds, giving rise to sound waves.

D

- The *intensity* of the sound varies with the pressure of the air forced through the vocal folds.
- The *pitch* of the sound varies with the length and tension of the vocal folds, which are in turn controlled by the intrinsic muscles of the larynx.
- The *quality* (timbre) of the voice depends on the resonating chambers above the vocal folds (e.g. the pharynx, the mouth, the nose and the paranasal sinuses). The shape and volume of these chambers can be varied by changing the position of the soft palate, tongue and the larynx (e.g. depression of the larynx results in an increase in the volume of the resonating chamber).

E

In whispering, the vocal folds are separated. A constant stream of air from the lungs set up vibrations in the vocal folds.

10.59

A

The right lung is more often affected by inhaled foreign bodies than other lobes of the lungs because at the point where the trachea bifurcates into the two bronchi, the right is slightly shorter and more vertical than the left.

B

The surface marking of the right middle lobe, bounded by the transverse fissure superiorly and the oblique fissure inferiorly, is on the anterior surface of the chest. The transverse fissure can be approximated by the level of the fourth costal cartilage. The oblique fissure is approximately at the level of the sixth rib in the mid-clavicular line, and meets the transverse fissure at the mid-axillary line.

C

Normal vesicular breath sounds are caused by the change in the quality of the breath sounds at the larynx on their passage through the normal lung tissues to the stethoscope over the chest wall. Bronchial breath sounds are heard if the lung tissues become more solid and conduct sound more effectively, and they resemble the sounds produced at the larynx. In lobar pneumonia, the relevant bronchi are patent and the consistency of the lung tissues has become more solid. Hence, bronchial breath sounds are heard.

10.60

A

Deep pelvic veins or the deep veins of the calf.

B

Immobilisation may have contributed to the development of deep venous thrombi and pulmonary emboli. Immobilisation causes stasis, one of the Virchow triad.

C

If a small embolus is lodged in a peripheral pulmonary artery, pulmonary infarct of the relevant lobule of the lung may occur. The patient may complain of chest pain.

D

If a massive coiled embolus is lodged in the main pulmonary artery, sudden death is the most likely outcome.

E

Anticoagulants may be effective in the prevention of pulmonary emboli. Heparin is a cofactor for antithrombin III. It inhibits the enzyme cascade associated with the intrinsic pathway (which begins with Hageman factor adhering to a negatively charged surface and converging on the final pathway of fibrin formation). Warfarin acts by inhibiting the synthesis of vitamin K-dependent clotting factors (factors II, VII, IX and X).

F

Fibrinolytic drugs (e.g. streptokinase, tissue plasminogen activators (tPA)) may be effective in treating major pulmonary emboli. They act by promoting the formation of plasmin from its precursor plasminogen.

The gastrointestinal system

11.1 The actions of the following muscles of mastication are correctly matched:
- A Masseter – elevation of mandible
- B Temporalis (anterior fibres) – depression of mandible
- C Temporalis (posterior fibres) – retraction of mandible
- D Medial pterygoid – depression and protrusion of mandible
- E Lateral pterygoid – elevation and protrusion of mandible

11.2 The functions of saliva include:
- A Lubricating food and facilitating swallowing
- B The breakdown of proteins into amino acids
- C Increasing the acidity of the gastric juice
- D The breakdown of nucleic acids into nucleotides
- E The breakdown of starch into oligosaccharides

11.3 Salivary secretion is increased under the following conditions:
- A The smell of food
- B Stimulation of sympathetic fibres at the lower end of the oesophagus
- C Stimulation of vagal fibres at the lower end of the oesophagus
- D Oral atropine
- E The passage of food through the pylorus of the stomach

11.4 The following structures and their secretion are correctly matched:
- A Parietal (oxyntic) cells – mucin
- B Parietal (oxyntic) cells – intrinsic factor
- C Chief (peptic) cells – hydrochloric acid
- D G cells in the antrum – gastrin
- E Glands in the cardia of the stomach – pepsinogen

11.5 The following gastric secretions and their main functions are correctly matched:
- A Mucin – neutralisation of acid
- B Intrinsic factor – facilitates breakdown of proteins
- C Gastrin – facilitates breakdown of fats
- D Pepsinogen – facilitates breakdown of carbohydrates
- E Hydrochloric acid – bactericidal actions

11.6 Gastric acid secretion is increased by stimulation of the following receptors:
- A Histamine H_1 receptors
- B Noradrenaline (norepinephrine) receptors
- C Dopamine receptors
- D Gastrin receptors
- E Muscarinic receptors

11.7 Gastric acid secretion is increased by the following:
- A Stimulation of the vagus nerve
- B The presence of food in the stomach
- C The presence of fat and acid in the duodenum
- D The smell of food
- E High blood glucose level

11.8 The following significantly predispose to peptic ulcers:
- A *Helicobacter pylori* infection
- B Oral treatment with non-steroidal anti-inflammatory drugs
- C Excess secretion of gastrin
- D Excess alcohol intake
- E Excessive peristalsis of the intestines

11.9 The following drugs are correctly paired with their mechanisms of action, and are effective in the treatment of peptic ulcers:
- A Magnesium trisilicate – reduction of gastric acid secretion
- B Ranitidine – muscarinic receptor antagonist
- C Bismuth – enhances mucosal resistance
- D Omeprazole – inhibition of the H^+, K^+-ATPase
- E Chlorpheniramine – histamine H_2 antagonist

11.10 Complications of duodenal ulcers include:
- A Haemorrhage
- B Obstruction due to fibrous stricture
- C Bacterial infection
- D Peritonitis due to perforation
- E Malignancy

11.11 Carcinomas of the stomach:
- A Are commoner in the United Kingdom than in the Far East
- B Have increased in incidence in the last 50 years
- C Are predisposed to by chronic gastritis
- D Are mostly of the squamous type
- E Usually present before they spread beyond the stomach wall

11.12 The following statements about the intestines are true:
- A Both circular and longitudinal muscles are present in the walls
- B The venous blood is drained into the inferior vena cava
- C The outer myenteric plexus mainly mediates the secretion of gastrointestinal hormones
- D Both sympathetic and parasympathetic nervous systems supply the intestinal walls
- E They receive arterial blood supply from branches of the external iliac arteries

11.13 The area of small intestinal mucosa available for absorption is increased by:
A Villi
B Crypts
C Microvilli
D Peyer's patches
E The length of the intestine

11.14 Malabsorption may result from:
A Pancreatic disease
B Poor dietary intake
C Coeliac disease
D Surgical resection of small bowel
E Diverticulitis affecting the sigmoid colon

11.15 The following gastrointestinal hormones and their actions are appropriately paired:
A Gastrin – reduces gastrointestinal mobility
B Secretin – increase volume and alkalinity of pancreatic juice
C Vasoactive intestinal polypeptide (VIP) – inhibits intestinal secretion
D Substance P – increases intestinal motility
E Cholecystokinin – pancreozymin (CCK-PZ) – increases pancreatic secretion

11.16 The vomiting centre receives significant neural input from the following sources:
A The chemoreceptor trigger zone (CTZ)
B The acoustic system
C The vestibular system
D The peripheral organs such as the heart and biliary tree
E The cerebellum

11.17 The following types of drugs are potentially effective in alleviating vomiting:
A Muscarinic receptor agonists
B Dopamine receptor antagonists
C Histamine H_2 receptor antagonists
D Serotonin receptor agonists
E Nicotinic receptor antagonists

11.18 The following measures may reduce symptoms of gastro-oesophageal reflux:
A Lying down after a meal
B Avoid being overweight
C Antacids
D Antimuscarinic drugs
E Metoclopramide

11.19 A large proportion of the following substances are absorbed in the colon:
A Water

B Amino acids
C Carbohydrates
D Fats
E Sodium

11.20 Disaccharides include:
A Glucose
B Sucrose
C Lactose
D Starch
E Fructose

11.21 Amylase:
A Is secreted by the salivary glands
B Is secreted by the small intestine
C Is secreted by the pancreas
D Functions optimally when the pH is 3
E Breaks down disaccharides into monosaccharides

11.22 The following statements about carbohydrate digestion are correct:
A Starch is broken down into glucose in the stomach
B Sucrose is broken down into glucose and fructose in the lumen of the small intestine
C Lactose is broken down into glucose and galactose at the brush border of the small intestinal mucosa
D Maltose is broken down into fructose and galactose at the brush border of the small intestinal mucosa
E Deficiency in intestinal lactase may result in diarrhoea

11.23 The following enzymes play significant roles in the digestion of lipids:
A Lingual lipase
B Stomach lipase
C Pancreatic lipase
D Jejunal lipase
E Ileal lipase

11.24 The following statements about fat absorption are true:
A Lipid is delivered to the intestinal mucosa in the form of micelles
B Most of the lipids are absorbed in the terminal part of the ileum
C Lipid is transported into intestinal mucosa cells as triglycerides
D Triglycerides leave the intestinal mucosa and enter the portal vein
E About 50% of all ingested lipids are absorbed

11.25 The following enzymes play significant roles in the digestion of proteins:

155

SYSTEM-BASED MEDICAL SCIENCES Q

11

The gastrointestinal system

A Lingual pepsin
B Stomach pepsin
C Stomach trypsin
D Pancreatic chymotrypsin
E Pancreatic carboxypeptidase

11.26 Coeliac disease:
A Occurs in one in every 2 million people in the United Kingdom
B Results from sensitivity to gliaden in gluten
C Has a strong association with HLA-B8
D Is more common in those with a positive family history
E Affects the duodenum more severely than the ileum

11.27 Coeliac disease is associated with:
A Villous atrophy
B Crypt atrophy
C Reduced surface area for absorption
D Normal absorption of amino acids
E Long-term development of malignant lymphoma

11.28 Microorganisms which may cause gastroenteritis include:
A *Salmonella*
B *Campylobacter*
C *Staphylococcus*
D *Escherichia coli*
E Small round structured viruses

11.29 Stimulant laxatives:
A Include lactulose
B Include senna
C May cause abdominal cramps
D Act by increasing the number of osmotically active particles in the stool
E Swell rapidly with water

11.30 Bulk laxatives:
A Include methylcellulose
B Include bran
C Increase the volume of intestinal contents
D Increase the pressure within the intestinal lumen
E Are useful in irritable bowel syndrome

11.31 Crohn's disease characteristically:
A Causes skip lesions
B Spares the terminal ileum
C Causes diffuse mucosal inflammation
D Affects all layers of the bowel
E Causes deep fissures

11.32 The indirect inguinal hernia:
A Is caused by a weakened posterior wall of the inguinal canal
B Can be controlled by finger pressure just above the midpoint of the inguinal ligament
C May extend to the testis
D Is palpable below the pubic tubercle
E Is palpable medial to the pubic tubercle

11.33 A healthy subject chewed a piece of buttered toast and swallowed it.
A What joints are involved in chewing? When the mouth is closed, what structures stabilise the mandible from (1) forward movement, and (2) backward movement? Are the joints more or less stable when the mouth is opened? Explain.
B i What are the main sets of jaw movements in chewing?
   ii For each set of jaw movements, name the muscles responsible.
C What is the nerve supply to these muscles? Trace the nerve supply from the brainstem.
D Explain how chewing might help in the subsequent digestion of food?
E i What are the components of saliva and what is their function?
   ii List five possible functions of saliva.
F Explain the control of the secretion of saliva. What type of drugs might cause a dry mouth? Explain.
G Name the salivary glands. What are their nerve supplies?
H List the steps in the swallowing mechanism.

11.34 A patient suffered from a duodenal ulcer and had been treated with antacids, ranitidine and omeprazole intermittently. He had also received a course of combined antibiotics and bismuth chelate in an attempt to eradicate *Helicobacter* infection.
A Where is hydrochloric acid produced in the stomach?
B Draw a simple diagram of the acid-secreting cell in the stomach and explain how hydrochloric acid is secreted. Indicate which of the steps involve energy expenditure.
C Draw another diagram of an acid-secreting cell and outline how the secretion of hydrochloric acid in the stomach is controlled. Indicate which surface receptors and second messengers are involved.
D What substances protect the stomach mucosal wall from damage by hydrochloric acid?
E What substances other than hydrochloric acid are secreted into the gastric juice?

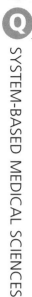
F What factors cause peptic ulcer?

G Why does aspirin ingestion predispose to peptic ulcer?

H Explain the mechanisms of action for the following drugs in the treatment of peptic ulcer.
  i Antacids
  ii Ranitidine
  iii Omeprazole
  iv Bismuth

11.35 A healthy subject consumes a bowl of rice, which consists mainly of starch. Consider its digestion and absorption.

A Describe the structure of starch.

B To what extent (if at all) is rice digested at the following sites? For each of these sites, state the enzymes involved and to what form the starch is digested.
  i Mouth
  ii Stomach
  iii Small intestine

C Where does absorption take place? Explain the mechanism for absorption. Is energy required for this process?

11.36 A healthy subject consumes food that consists mainly of triglycerides. Consider their digestion and absorption.

A Describe the structure of triglycerides.

B To what extent (if at all) are triglycerides digested at the following sites? For each of these sites, state the enzymes involved and to what form the lipids are digested.
  i Mouth
  ii Stomach
  iii Small intestine

C Where does absorption take place? Explain the mechanism for absorption.

D From first principles, what are the possible reasons for malabsorption of fat? Give one disease associated with each cause.

11.37 A healthy subject consumes food that consists mainly of protein. Consider its digestion and absorption.

A What are proteins made up of?

B To what extent (if at all) are proteins digested at the following sites? For each of these sites, state the enzymes involved and to what form the proteins are digested.
  i Mouth
  ii Stomach
  iii Small intestine

C Where does absorption take place? Explain the mechanism for absorption. Is energy required for this process?

11.38 A Describe the physiological mechanisms associated with vomiting.

B How is vomiting controlled?

C What is the mechanism of action for the following antiemetic drugs?
  i Cyclizine
  ii Hyoscine
  iii Metoclopramide
  iv Ondansetron

11.39 A Draw a simple cross-sectional diagram of the intestine showing the muscle layers and the nerve plexus.

B Compare the structure of the small intestine and the large intestine in terms of the following.
  i Diameter
  ii Structure of mucosa
  iii External appearance
  iv Organisation of the external muscle layer

C i What are the extrinsic nerve supplies of the intestine?
  ii Explain the function of the two nerve plexuses.
  iii Name five mediators secreted by neurones in the enteric nervous system of the gastrointestinal tract.

D Explain the term peristalsis. What initiates peristalsis? What controls the rate of peristalsis?

E Explain the mechanism of action for the following purgatives.
  i Methylcellulose
  ii Lactulose
  iii Senna
  iv Docusate sodium

11.40 A 6-year-old boy was malnourished due to coeliac disease.

A Give a brief account of the absorptive surface of the normal small intestine. List the features that increase its absorptive capacity.

B What is the aetiology of coeliac disease? Who is more likely to have the disease?

C Which part of the gastrointestinal tract does coeliac disease affect most? Give the abnormal morphological features.

D What other disease are patients with coeliac disease more prone to later on in life?

11.41 Compare and contrast the pathology of ulcerative colitis and Crohn's disease by completing Table 11.1.

11

Q

SYSTEM-BASED MEDICAL SCIENCES

The gastrointestinal system

Table 11.1

	Ulcerative colitis	Crohn's disease
Distribution		
Affected lumen (dilated or narrowed?)		
Extent of gut wall affected		
Histological appearance		
Skipped lesions		
Fistulae present		
Fissures present		
Granulomas present		
Cancer risk		
Malabsorption		

11.42 A 60-year-old man was found to have a hernia in the groin.
   A Describe the anatomy of the inguinal canal.
   B What structures pass through the deep inguinal ring?
   C Describe the anatomy of the femoral canal.
   D How might one distinguish between a femoral hernia and an inguinal hernia?
   E How might one distinguish between a direct and an indirect inguinal hernia?

11.43 An 8-year-old boy developed a central abdominal pain which later settled in the right iliac fossa. A diagnosis of appendicitis was made.
   A Describe the anatomy of the appendix. What forms the longitudinal muscle layer of the appendix?
   B What is the surface anatomy of the appendix?
   C Describe the development of the gut from the sixth week.
   D From your answer to (C), explain why the child developed central abdominal pain initially, although the appendix is found in the right side of the abdomen.
   E What might predispose to acute inflammation of the appendix?

The gastrointestinal system 11

11.1 A C
The correct actions of the muscles of mastication are:
- Masseter – elevation of mandible
- Temporalis (anterior fibres) – elevation of mandible
- Temporalis (posterior fibres) – retraction of mandible
- Medial pterygoid – elevation and protrusion of mandible
- Lateral pterygoid – depression and protrusion of mandible

11.2 A E
Saliva performs a number of functions. It contains the digestive enzymes salivary α-amylase (which breaks starch down into oligosaccharides) and lingual lipase (which converts triglycerides into fatty acids). It contains mucins which help to lubricate food and facilitate swallowing. It is slightly alkaline and helps to neutralise the acid refluxed into the oesophagus. It also contains IgA, lysozyme and lactoferrin, which have antibacterial actions. Saliva does not facilitate the digestion of proteins or nucleic acids.

11.3 A C
Reflex secretion of saliva occurs at the sight or smell of food. Pavlov showed that reflex secretion can be conditioned to occur as a result of a stimulus (e.g. the sound of a bell) which immediately precedes the presentation of food. Stimulation of the parasympathetic supply to the salivary glands increases salivary production, and this may be achieved by food stimulating the vagal fibres at the lower end of the oesophagus. Anticholinergic drugs reduce salivary secretion and may cause dry mouth. Stimulus of the sympathetic nerve supply generally causes vasoconstriction of the salivary glands, and may explain the association of stress with dry mouth (e.g. during public speaking).

11.4 B D
Several substances are secreted in the stomach. Mucus (which contains mucin) is secreted by the glands in the cardia and pylorus of the stomach. This is important in protecting the gastric epithelium from damage by gastric acid. Parietal cells in the body of the stomach secrete hydrochloric acid and intrinsic factor. Hydrochloric acid is useful for its bactericidal activity; it helps to digest proteins and allows pepsin to function optimally. It also stimulates the flow of bile and pancreatic juice. Intrinsic factor is important in the absorption of vitamin B_{12}. The chief (peptic) cells secrete pepsinogens, which are the precursors of pepsins. Pepsins break down proteins and polypeptides into smaller polypeptides. The G cell in the antrum of the stomach produces gastrin. Gastrin stimulates gastric acid and pepsin secretion, as well as the growth of the mucosa of the stomach and the intestines.

11.5 E
See question 11.4 above.

11.6 D E
Gastric acid secretion by the parietal cells is increased by stimulation of the histamine H_2 receptors, the muscarinic M_3 receptors, the gastrin receptors and prostaglandin E_2 receptors. Intracellular calcium acts as the second messenger for gastrin and muscarinic receptors, whereas cAMP acts as the second messenger for the histamine H_2 and prostaglandin E_2 receptors. The hydrogen ions produced in the parietal cells are transported into the gastric lumen by H^+, K^+-ATPase.

11.7 A B D
Gastric acid secretion is regulated by cephalic factors, local factors in the stomach and intestinal factors. Cephalic factors include sight, smell and thought of food, low plasma glucose level, as well as other stimuli which are conditioned with the presence of food. These factors increase gastric acid secretion via vagal stimulation. Food in the stomach increases acid secretion via local reflex in the stomach wall. Intestinal factors, acids, fats and carbohydrates in the duodenum inhibit gastric acid secretion.

11.8 A B C D
The mucosal barrier of the stomach protects the gastric epithelium from damage by the acid. Hence, risk factors for peptic ulcers are those which increase acid secretion or reduce mucosal resistance. *Helicobacter pylori* infection and treatment with non-steroidal anti-inflammatory drugs both reduce mucosal resistance of the stomach to acid. High levels of gastrin and excess alcohol increase acid secretion.

11.9 C D
Drugs for peptic ulcers act either by neutralising excess acid secreted, reducing the secretion of acid, or enhancing the mucosal resistance of the stomach to acid. Antacids such as magnesium trisilicate neutralise excess acid in the stomach. Drugs which reduce acid secretion may act by blocking histamine H_2 receptors (e.g. cimetidine, ranitidine); blocking muscarinic receptors (e.g. pirenzepine); or inhibiting the enzyme H^+,K^+-ATPase, which catalyses the pump for the transport of H^+ out of the parietal cell in exchange for K^+ (e.g. omeprazole). Chlorpheniramine is an H_1 antagonist and cannot be used to treat peptic ulcers.

11.10 A B D
Duodenal ulcers may heal completely. Complications include penetration and erosion of adjacent organs such as the liver; haemorrhage, resulting in altered blood in stools

or blood in the vomit; perforation, resulting in severe chemical peritonitis as gastric contents enter the peritoneal cavity; and obstruction due to fibrous stricture. Malignancy occurs rarely following gastric ulcers, but duodenal ulcers are not predisposed to malignancy.

11.11   C
Carcinomas of the stomach are much commoner in the Far East than in the United Kingdom. The incidence has decreased over the past 50 years throughout the world, the reasons for which are not clear. Most carcinomas are adenocarcinomas, and may have progressed from epithelial metaplasia or dysplasia. Chronic atrophic gastritis is an important predisposing factor. As carcinomas of the stomach cause little or no symptoms in the early stages, most carcinomas present when they are clinically advanced with metastases.

11.12   A D
Although there are minor local differences, the structure of the walls of the gastrointestinal tract is broadly similar There are usually two longitudinal muscle layers with one layer of circular muscle layer in between. There are two major networks of nerve fibres: an outer myenteric plexus and an inner submucous plexus. In general, the inner submucous layer regulates the secretion of exocrine and endocrine secretion by cells, whilst the outer myenteric plexus regulates the control of peristaltic activity. These plexuses also receive extrinsic innervation from both sympathetic and parasympathetic nervous systems. The blood supply to the intestines is usually derived directly from branches of the abdominal aorta. The venous blood in drained via the portal vein to the liver. This is important clinically as orally administered drugs may undergo metabolism before reaching the systemic circulation.

11.13   A C E
The main functions of the small intestine are the digestion of food and absorption of nutrients. A large area of small intestinal mucosa is necessary for optimum absorption. This is achieved in several ways. Firstly, the small intestine is long (over 2.5 m). Secondly, the mucous membrane is thrown into fingerlike projections called villi. Thirdly, the edges of the cells (enterocytes) which make up the villi are themselves divided into smaller microvilli. As a result, the total area for absorption approaches 200 m². The enterocytes originate in the crypts, but migrate up the villi and ultimately shed into the intestinal lumen. Peyer's patches are dense aggregates of lymphoid tissue.

11.14   A C D
Malabsorption describes the failure of the intestines to absorb the nutrients available in the ingested food.

Digestion and absorption of food mainly occur in the small intestines, and digestion is dependent on the appropriate pancreatic enzymes. Hence, malabsorption may be due to deficiency of digestive enzymes (e.g. pancreatic disease or specific biochemical disorders) or small intestine diseases. The small intestine diseases may be due to a decrease in the length of the small bowel (e.g. following surgical resection), or due to a reduction in absorption surface (e.g. coeliac disease or giardiasis). Disorders affecting only the large bowel are unlikely to result in significant malabsorption.

11.15   B D E
Gastrointestinal hormones are polypeptides secreted in the gastrointestinal mucosa. Many gastrointestinal hormones have been identified, and their integrated actions are important in the regulation of gastrointestinal motility and secretion. The sight and smell of food, and the presence of food in the stomach, initiate gastrin secretion, which stimulate both acid secretion and increased motility. On the other hand, acid in the upper intestine stimulates the secretion of secretin, which increases the alkalinity and volume of pancreatic enzyme. This acts as negative feedback to neutralise the acid. VIP stimulates intestinal secretion, whilst substance P and somatostatin inhibit intestinal secretion. CCK-PZ is stimulated by food and acid in the duodenum, and its action is to increase pancreatic secretion and contract the gallbladder. Again, this serves to neutralise the acid. A number of polypeptides are involved in the coordination of a peristaltic movement. Acetylcholine and substance P are responsible for the contraction behind a stimulus, whereas NO and VIP are responsible for the relaxation in front.

11.16   A C D
Vomiting is controlled by the vomiting centre in the medulla oblongata. It coordinates the act of vomiting on receiving inputs from various sources. These include the chemoreceptor trigger zone (which is sensitive to the action of drugs and other chemicals), the periphery (e.g. the heart, biliary tree), cortical centres and the vestibular system (which initiates vomiting in motion sickness).

11.17   B
The vomiting centre in the medulla contains cholinergic (muscarinic) and histamine H_1 receptors. Hence antimuscarinics and histamine H_1 receptor antagonists are potential anti-emetics. Some drugs (e.g. cyclizine) have both antimuscarinic and antihistamine H_1 receptor activity. The chemoreceptor trigger zone (CTZ) contains dopamine D_2 receptors. Hence antagonists to these receptors are potentially good anti-emetics. Examples are metoclopramide and domperidone. However, these drugs also act peripherally on the gut by reducing the tone of

the oesophageal sphincter, relaxing the pyloric antrum and increasing peristalsis. Serotonin 5-HT$_3$ receptor antagonists (e.g. ondansetron) are also effective anti-emetics. They probably both act centrally on the CTZ and peripherally.

11.18   B C E
Normally, contraction of the lower oesophageal sphincter prevents reflux of gastric contents into the oesophagus. If the sphincter becomes incompetent, reflux of acid into the lower oesophagus occurs, and this causes symptoms of heartburn and oesophagitis. Lying down after a meal or bending would encourage reflux. Elevating the head of the bed may minimise reflux. Antacids, histamine H$_2$ antagonists or proton pump inhibitor (e.g. omperazole) reduce acid secretion and hence the symptoms. Metoclopramide increases the tone of the lower oesophageal sphincter and increases gastric emptying, and may alleviate symptoms. Antimuscarinics tend to relax the lower oesophageal sphincter and exacerbate the symptoms.

11.19   A E
The main functions of the colon are to absorb water and sodium. Amino acids, carbohydrates and fats are mostly absorbed in the small intestine.

11.20   B C
Starch is a glucose polymer and is a polysaccharide. Disaccharides include maltose (glucose–glucose), lactose (galactose–glucose) and sucrose (fructose–glucose). Glucose, galactose and fructose are monosaccharides.

11.21   A C
Amylase is an enzyme secreted by both the salivary gland and the pancreas. Its main action is to break down starch into the disaccharide maltose. This digestive action occurs both in the mouth and the small intestine. However, it does not occur in the stomach, as the enzyme functions optimally at a pH of between 6 and 7.

11.22   C E
Starch is broken down into disaccharides in the lumen by amylase. In general, oligosaccharides are broken down into monosaccharides in the brush border of the small intestinal epithelial cells. Different oligosaccharides are broken down by different enzymes. For example, maltose is broken down by maltase and sucrase, sucrose is broken down by sucrase, and lactose is broken down by lactase. Many negroes and orientals have a genetic lactase deficiency. Hence they are unable to digest lactose (which is present in milk). The osmotic pressure generated by these disaccharides may draw water into the bowel lumen and cause diarrhoea.

11.23   A C
The digestion of fats starts in the mouth by lingual lipase secreted by glands on the dorsal surface of the tongue, and accounts for about a quarter of fat digestion. Most fat digestion occurs in the duodenum by pancreatic lipases. There are at least two pancreatic lipases.

11.24   A
Lipids are emulsified in the small intestinal lumen by the detergent action of bile, and are delivered to the intestinal mucosa in aggregates called micelles. Lipids diffuse out of the micelles near the brush border of the small intestine, and most of the lipids are absorbed in the duodenum and jejunum. Fatty acids and monoglyceride enter the mucosal cell, in which triglycercide is synthesised. It is exocytosed into the extracellular space, from where it enters the lymphatic system. Over 90% of all ingested lipids are absorbed.

11.25   B D E
Protein digestion starts in the stomach, where stomach pepsins break down proteins into polypeptides. Pepsin no longer functions when it reaches the duodenum, as it requires an acidic pH to function optimally. In the intestines, the polypeptides are further broken down at the interior peptide bonds by endopeptidases such as trypsin, chymotrypsins and elastase. The pancreas also produces carboxypeptidases which act at the carboxy ends of the polypeptides.

11.26   B C D E
Coeliac disease occurs in one in every 2000 people in the United Kingdom, and is more prevalent in Ireland. It results from sensitivity to gliadin in gluten. However, genetic factors are also important. It is more likely to occur in those with a positive family history, and there is a strong association with HLA-B8. It affects the proximal small intestine most, probably due to a higher exposure to gliadin. Hence coeliac disease is often confirmed by histological examination of a jejunal biopsy.

11.27   A C E
Normally, cells are continually shed from the tips of the villi, and replaced by migration of cells from the crypts. In coeliac disease, the villous cells are lost at an increased rate, which often results in total villous atrophy. Hence malabsorption occurs for oligosaccharides, fatty acids and amino acids. The crypts attempt to compensate for this by hypertrophy and increased mitosis. Coeliac disease predisposes to the development of malignant lymphoma of the small bowel.

SYSTEM-BASED MEDICAL SCIENCES

The gastrointestinal system

11.28 A B C D E
Gastroenteritis can be caused by different microorganisms. Viruses are the commonest cause. Small round structured viruses commonly occur in winter, and may cause outbreaks of gastroenteritis in schools or nursing homes. Rotaviruses often occur in children. Bacterial infections may be associated with poor food hygiene, and are usually transmitted by infected meat. *Campylobacter* is the commonest bacterial gastroenteritis and is usually transmitted by infected poultry. A particular type of *Escherichia coli* may be associated with renal failure. *Staphylococcus aureus* can rarely caused fatal gastroenteritis.

11.29 B C
Stimulant laxatives include glycerol, senna and danthrons. They act by increasing the intestinal motility, and may directly stimulate the sensory endings in the lumen of the colon. Hence they may cause abdominal cramps, and should never by used when mechanical obstruction is a possibility. Osmotic diuretics such as lactulose increase the number of osmotically active particles in the stool. Bulk laxatives such as methlycellulose and ispahula husk swell rapidly with water.

11.30 A B C E
Bulk laxatives occur naturally as dietary fibres in vegetables and fruits. They also include bran, methycellulose and ispaghula husk. They act by increasing the volume of intestinal contents so that large soft bulky stool can be formed. It is important that the fluid intake is adequate for this to occur. As a result, the pressure within the intestinal lumen is reduced. Besides simple constipation, bulk laxatives are also useful in diverticulosis (partly caused by increased intestinal pressure) and irritable bowel syndrome.

11.31 A D E
About two-thirds of all Crohn's disease affects the small intestine only, and the terminal ileum is characteristically affected. Unlike ulcerative colitis, Crohn's disease is characterised by 'skip lesions' – segments of diseased bowel separated by segments of apparently normal bowel. Hence mucosal inflammation is usually patchy. Whilst ulcerative colitis generally affects the superficial layer of the bowel, Crohn's disease characteristically affect all layers of the bowel. It often causes deep fissures.

11.32 B C E
Both inguinal and femoral hernias occur near the groin. The femoral canal lies below the inguinal ligament. All inguinal hernias appear through the external inguinal ring, which lies above and medial to the pubic tubercle.

Hence inguinal hernia is palpable medially and above the pubic tubercle. An indirect inguinal hernia occurs due to persistence of the processus vaginalis. Hence it may extend to the testis. After reduction, it is controllable by pressure over the internal inguinal ring, which lies just above the mid-inguinal point. By contrast, direct inguinal hernia is caused by weakness of the posterior wall of the inguinal canal. Hence it is not controllable by pressure over the internal inguinal ring.

11.33
A
The temporomandibular joints. These are synovial joints between the head of the mandible and the mandibular fossa on the inferior surface of the squamous temporal bone. The two joints work as a single component. When the mouth is closed, the teeth are occluded and stabilise the mandible on the maxilla. Forward movement of the condyle of the mandible is minimised by the articular eminence and by the posterior fibres of the temporalis muscle. Backward movement is minimised by the fibres of the lateral pterygoid and the lateral ligament. The joints are much less stable when the mouth is opened because the condyles move forward on the slope of the articular eminence. Forward displacement is the most common form of dislocation.

B
i   • Opening and closing (i.e. depression and elevation).
    • Grinding movement (i.e. side-to-side).
    • Protraction and retraction.
ii • Opening: digastric, mylohyoid, geniohyoid.
    • Closing: masseters, medial pterygoids, temporalis.
    • Grinding (side-to-side): medial pterygoid on one side with lateral pterygoid on the contralateral side.
    • Protraction: both lateral and medial pterygoids.
    • Retraction: passive recoil and contraction of posterior fibres of temporalis and deep fibres of masseter.

C
The nerve supply for the muscles of mastication originate from the trigeminal nerve. For sensory innervation, the mandibular branch from the trigeminal ganglion lies in the middle cranial fossa lateral to the cavernous sinus. The motor root of the trigeminal nerve enters the foramen ovale and joins the sensory branch to form the mandibular nerve. The nerve to the medial pterygoid arises from the main branch of the mandibular nerve. The nerves for the temporalis, masseter and lateral pterygoid arise from the anterior division of the mandibular nerve.

D

Chewing helps in the digestion of food because large food particles are broken up and food is mixed with saliva. Mucins help to lubricate the food and subsequent digestion; salivary enzymes begin to digest the food.

E

i
- Salivary enzymes (e.g. salivary α-amylase for starch digestion, lingual lipase for lipid digestion)
- Mucins – lubricate the food and protect the oral mucosa
- IgA, lysozyme and lactoferrin – for their bacteriostatic function.

ii
- Keeping the mouth moist
- Facilitating swallowing
- Keeping the mouth and teeth clean
- Minimising infection
- Acting as a solvent for substances that stimulate taste buds.

F

Salivary secretion may be triggered by reflex, sympathetic and parasympathetic nervous control and by conditioning. Food in the mouth causes reflex salivary secretion. Stimulation of the parasympathetic innervation causes watery salivary secretion and marked vasodilatation in the gland, thought to be due to local release of vasoactive intestinal peptide (VIP). Stimulation of the sympathetic nervous supply causes vasoconstriction. Salivary secretion can occur after classical conditioning. Pavlov's experiments with dogs showed that the association of the sound of a bell followed by the presence of food led to salivary secretion initially. This salivary secretion persisted after the sound of the bell alone.

G

The parotid gland, the submandibular gland and the sublingual gland.

1. The parotid gland is supplied by parasympathetic and sympathetic fibres from the otic ganglion. The parasympathetic fibres originate from the inferior salivary nucleus and relate to the ganglion via the glossopharyngeal nerve. The sympathetic fibres originate from the superior cervical ganglion. From the otic ganglion, the fibres 'hitchhike' to the parotid gland via the auriculotemporal nerve.

2. The submandibular and sublingual glands are supplied by parasympathetic and sympathetic fibres from the submandibular ganglion. The parasympathetic fibres originate from the superior salivary nucleus in the pons, and travel to the submandibular ganglion via the nervus intermedius part of the facial nerve. The sympathetic fibres also originate from the superior cervical ganglion.

H

Swallowing is a reflex response with the following steps:

1. It is initially triggered by voluntarily collecting oral content in the mouth and pushing it backwards into the pharynx.
2. Afferent impulses are sent from trigeminal, glossopharyngeal and vagus nerves.
3. The impulses are integrated in the nucleus of tractus solitarus and the nucleus ambiguus.
4. The efferent impulses travel from these nuclei to the muscles of the pharynx and tongue via the trigeminal, facial and hypoglossal nerves.
5. These impulses trigger a wave of involuntary pharyngeal muscle contractions which propel the oral contents to the oesophagus.
6. The glottis is reflexly closed and respiration is temporarily inhibited.

11.34

A

Hydrochloric acid is secreted by parietal cells in the body of the stomach.

B

See Fig. 11.1. The transport systems shown in bold are active transport systems; the others are via either antiport or symport carriers. The main active transport system responsible for the secretion of hydrochloric acid is the proton pump, which pumps H^+ into the stomach lumen in exchange for K^+.

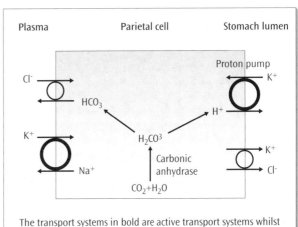

The transport systems in bold are active transport systems whilst others are via either antiport or symport carriers. The main active transport system responsible for the secretion of hydrochloric acid is the proton pump, which pumps H^+ into the stomach lumen in exchange for K^+.

Fig. 11.1 Secretion of hydrochloric acid from the stomach.

SYSTEM-BASED MEDICAL SCIENCES

11

The gastrointestinal system

C

See Fig. 11.2. Hydrochloric acid secretion in the parietal cell of the stomach is controlled by proton pump activity. Only the proton pump and the factors determining its activity are shown in the figure. Three main sets of factors influence acid secretion – conditioned responses, psychological influences and gastric/intestinal influences:

1. *Cephalic influences*. Food in the mouth, the sight and smell of food and prior conditioning may stimulate acid secretion. They are mediated via the vagus nerves. Stimulation of vagus nerve may both release acetylcholine or increase gastric secretion by release of gastrin-releasing peptide.
2. *Psychological influences*. Again, psychic stimuli are mediated via vagus innervation.
3. *Gastric/intestinal influences*. Stretch and chemical (e.g. amino acids) stimuli in the stomach cause both reflex secretion of acid or the secretion of gastrin.

D

Mucus is secreted by mucous cells in the body and fundus in the stomach. It forms a flexible gel that coats the mucosa. Surface mucous cells also produce HCO_3^- ions which are trapped in the mucous gel. Both mucous and bicarbonate ions protect the mucosa from damage by acid.

E

- Mucus
- Lipase
- Pepsinogen – precursor for pepsins
- Intrinsic factor.

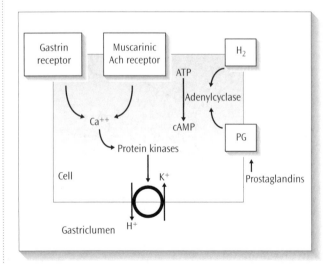

Fig. 11.2 Control of the secretion of hydrochloric acid in the stomach.

F

Generally speaking, peptic ulcer is caused by the breakdown of the barrier that normally prevents irritation and autodigestion of the mucosa by the acid. This may be contributed to by:

- excess secretion of acid
- infection with the bacterium *Helicobacter pylori*.

G

Aspirin inhibits prostaglandin synthesis. Prostaglandins usually:

- stimulate mucus secretion
- stimulate bicarbonate secretion
- decrease acid secretion (by inhibiting cAMP).

Hence, aspirin breaks down the barrier that normally prevents irritation and autodigestion of the stomach mucosa by acid.

H

i Antacids (e.g. magnesium trisilicate) act by neutralising gastric acid and raising the gastric pH. This inhibits peptic activity and allows the ulcers to heal.

ii Ranitidine is a H_2-receptor antagonist. It reduces acid secretion by decreasing cAMP production. It also reduces acetylcholine-induced acid production.

iii Omeprazole is a proton inhibitor and hence reduces acid production. Clinically, it is used for peptic ulcers resistant to H_2-receptor antagonists. It can also be used as a component of the combined therapy for *Helicobacter* infection.

iv Bismuth is most commonly used as one component of the combination therapy against *Helicobacter* infection. However, it may have the following anti-ulcer effects:
- coats the ulcer base and protects it against further damage by acid
- enhances local prostaglandin synthesis
- stimulates bicarbonate secretion.

11.35

A

Put simply, starch is a polymer of glucose with both $1:4\alpha$ and $1:6\alpha$ linkages.

B

i In the mouth, starch is partially digested by salivary α-amylase, which hydrolyses the $1:4\alpha$ linkages to produce oligosaccharides (e.g. maltose consists of 2 glucose molecules; maltotriose consists of 3 glucose molecules).

ii As the optimal pH for salivary α-amylase is about 6.5, further breakdown of the products is inhibited by the acidity in the stomach.

iii In the small intestine, both the salivary and pancreatic α-amylase break down starch into oligosaccharides of between 2 and 8 glucose molecules. These oligosaccharides are further broken down by the oligosaccharidases, in the outer portion of the brush border (i.e. microvilli) of the small intestine, into either glucose or shorter glucose chains.

C

Glucose is absorbed across the microvilli of the small intestine by facilitated diffusion. Glucose and Na^+ share the same cotransporter (symport). Since the intracellular Na^+ concentration is low in intestinal mucosal cells, Na^+ moves into the cell down its chemical gradient, and glucose also moves into the cell with Na^+. The energy is derived from the chemical gradient of sodium.

11.36

A

Triglycerides are basically made up of three fatty acids bound to glycerol. Fatty acids contains a terminal with —COOH. Fatty acids may be saturated (i.e. with no double bonds between carbon atoms) or unsaturated (with some double bonds between carbon atoms).

B

i Ebner's glands on the dorsal surface of the tongue secrete lingual lipase, which starts to break down triglycerides into fatty acids and 1,2-diacyglycerols.

ii A gastric lipase is secreted in the stomach and can break down triglycerides into fatty acids and glycerol. However, it is usually of little significance in a healthy subject.

iii Most of the fat digestion occur in the small intestine. The pancreas secretes a pancreatic lipase which flows into the duodenum. It hydrolyses the 1- and 3-bonds of the triglycerides to form free fatty acids and 2-monoglycerides. Pancreatic lipase is facilitated by colipase, which is also secreted by the pancreas. The bile salts discharged into the duodenum by the gallbladder emulsify fats to form micelles. This micellar formation makes lipid soluble and provides a transport mechanism to the brush border of the mucosal cells.

C

Absorption takes place in the enterocytes of the brush border of the mucosal cells of the small intestine. Lipids may enter either by passive diffusion or by carriers. For fatty acids containing less than about 12 carbon atoms, they pass directly into the portal blood. For longer fatty acids, they are re-esterified to triglycerides in the mucosal cells, coated with a layer of protein, cholesterol and phospholipid to form chylomicrons. They then leave the cell and enter the lymphatics.

D

From first principles, malabsorption of fats may occur if:
• the surface of brush border is reduced (e.g. coeliac disease)
• there is reduced secretion of pancreatic lipase (e.g. diseased pancreas in cystic fibrosis or after pancreatomy)
• there is reduced secretion of bile salts (e.g. gallbladder disease).

11.37

A

Proteins are made up of amino acids linked into chains by peptide bonds, which join the amino group of one amino acid to the carboxy group of another. The linear structure of this polypeptide chain is the primary structure of proteins. The way the polypeptide chains are folded is known as the secondary structure, and the arrangement of these twisted chains into layers or other 3-D structure is known as the tertiary structure.

B

i Proteins are not digested in the mouth.

ii The stomach secretes pepsinogen, the pepsin precursors. Pepsins hydrolyse the bonds between aromatic amino acids (e.g. tyrosine), so the products of peptic digestion are polypeptides of varying sizes. Pepsins have an optimal pH of about 1.5–3.0; hence, they are inactivated when the gastric contents are mixed with pancreatic juice in the duodenum.

iii The pancreatic juice and the intestinal mucosa contain powerful proteolytic enzymes: endopeptidases and exopeptidases. Endopeptidases (e.g. trypsin, chymotrypsins and elastase) act at the interior peptide bonds in the peptide molecules. Exopeptidases include carboxypeptidases of the pancreas, which hydrolyse the amino acids at the carboxy and amino ends of the polypeptides. Free amino acids, dipeptides and tripeptides are released in the intestinal lumen and at the brush border of the mucosal cells.

C

Amino acids in the intestinal lumen are cotransported into mucosal cells by different transport systems, with either Na^+ or Cl^-. These systems used the energy from the chemical gradients of Na^+ or Cl^-. Any short peptides still remaining in the lumen are actively transported into the intestinal cells and hydrolysed by the intracellular peptidases into amino acids. This process requires energy.

11.38

A

Vomiting may be initiated by a variety of stimuli such as irritation of the upper mucosa of the gastrointestinal tract,

11
A

The gastrointestinal system

emotion or travelling in vehicles. The following steps occur:

1. Reverse peristalsis empties material from the upper part of the intestine into the stomach.
2. The vocal cords close to prevent aspiration of the vomitus into the lungs. The breath is held in mid-inspiration.
3. The muscles of the abdominal wall then contract, which increases the intra-abdominal pressure.
4. The lower oesophageal sphincter relaxes.
5. The gastric contents are expelled from the stomach.

B

See Fig. 11.3. Vomiting is a reflex response integrated in the medulla oblongata. Stimuli may be sent to the vomiting centre from the intestinal mucosa, the labrinth (e.g. in motion sickness) or the limbic system (e.g. emotional stress). Impulses reach the reticular formation of the medulla via the nucleus of the solitary tract. In addition, vomiting may be initiated when the chemoreceptor cells in the medulla (chemoreceptor trigger zone) are stimulated by certain circulating chemical agents (e.g. morphine, digoxin). Dopamine D_2 and 5-HT$_3$ receptors are involved.

C

i Cyclizine is a histamine H_1 antagonist. It is effective in preventing motion sickness-induced vomiting by antagonising the H_1 receptors in the vestibular nuclei. It is also effective in preventing vomiting induced by substances acting locally in the stomach by antagonising the H_1 receptors in the nucleus of the solitary tract. It is not effective against substances that act directly on the chemoreceptor trigger zone.

ii Hyoscine is a muscarinic antagonist. It is effective in preventing vomiting triggered by motion sickness or substances that act locally in the stomach by antagonising the muscarinic receptors in the vestibular nuclei and the nucleus of the solitary tract, respectively. It is not effective against substances that act directly on the chemoreceptor trigger zone.

iii In normal dosage, metoclopramide has both central and peripheral actions. Centrally, metoclopramide is a dopamine-receptor antagonist. It acts by blocking the dopamine D_2 receptors on the chemoreceptor trigger zone. Peripherally, metoclopramide increases the motility of the stomach and intestine.

iv Ondansetron is a selective 5-HT$_3$ receptor antagonist. It may act both on the chemoreceptor trigger zone and to decrease afferents from local stimuli.

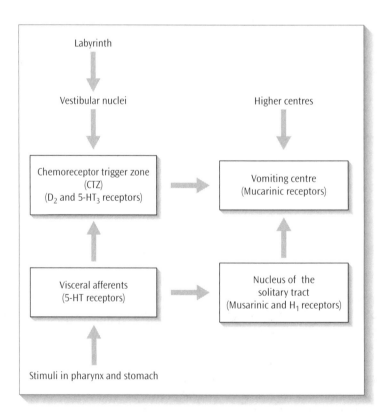

Fig. 11.3 Neurological pathway for vomiting.

11.39

A

See Fig. 11.4.

B

i Generally speaking, the diameter of the large intestine is larger than the small intestine.

ii The mucosa of the small intestine is organised into villi and microvilli. These are absent in the large intestine.

iii Haustra appear in the wall of the large intestine, but the wall of the small intestine is smooth. Haustra are outpouchings between the three taeniae coli.

iv The external muscle layer of the large intestine is collected into three longitudinal bands called the taeniae coli. In the small intestine, the external muscle layer is distributed uniformly.

C

i The intestine receives both sympathetic and parasympathetic nerve supplies. The parasympathetic nervous system increases the activity of the intestinal smooth muscle; the sympathetic nervous system decreases it and contracts the sphincters.

ii The two nerve plexus are connected. They contain:
- motor neurones that innervate the smooth muscle
- secretory neurones that regulate endocrine and exocrine secretions.

iii Mediators secreted by neurones in the enteric nervous system of the gastrointestinal tract include those connected with the motor function and those connected with the secretory function. Mediators connected with the motor function include those which contract intestinal smooth muscles (e.g. substance P) and those which relax intestinal smooth muscle (e.g. vasoactive intestinal peptide, neurotensin, encephalin). Mediators connected with the secretory function include somatostatin (which inhibits acid and intestinal secretion), gastrin-releasing polypeptide (GRP), as well as substance P and VIP.

D

Peristalsis is a reflex response of the intestine resulting in a wave of coordinated contraction that moves in an oral–caudal direction and propels the contents of the lumen forward. It is usually initiated by the stretch in the intestinal wall caused by the contents of the lumen. The rate of peristalsis is controlled by the sympathetic and parasympathetic input to the intestine. It is also controlled by the presence of bulk in the lumen of the gut.

E

i Methylcellulose is a bulk laxative. It consists of polysaccharide polymers which are not digested in the upper part of the gut; hence, they retain water in the gut lumen and promote peristalsis.

ii Lactulose is an osmotic laxative. It is a semisynthetic disaccharide converted by colonic bacteria to fructose and galactose. As these are poorly absorbed in the colon, they are fermented to form lactic acid and acetic acid and act as an osmotic laxative.

iii Senna contains glycosides. It passes unchanged into the colon where bacteria hydrolyse the glycosidic bond, releasing free anthracene derivatives. These stimulate the myenteric plexus, resulting in increased smooth muscle activity of the gut. Hence, senna is a stimulant purgative.

iv Docusate sodium is a faecal softener. It acts on the gut in a similar manner to detergent and produces softer faeces.

11.40

A

The absorptive surface of the normal small intestine is provided by the villous structure of the mucosa. Each villus is a fingerlike projection covered by a single layer of columnar epithelium and containing a network of capillaries and lymphatic vessels. The villi are covered by tightly packed enterocytes, which are specialised epithelial cells. These enterocytes themselves have microvilli on the luminal surface. The features that increase the absorptive surface are:
- the length of the small intestine
- deep villi
- microvilli.

B

Coeliac disease is due to an abnormal reaction to gliadin, the toxic component of gluten in cereals. This abnormal

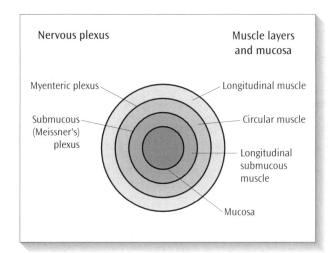

Fig. 11.4 Cross-sectional structure of the gut.

SYSTEM-BASED MEDICAL SCIENCES

11

A

The gastrointestinal system

reaction leads to tissue damage in the small intestine. Genetic factors are important. There is a strong association with HLA-B8; about 80% of patients with coeliac disease have this HLA.

C

Coeliac disease particularly affects the proximal small intestine (i.e. duodenum and proximal jejunum). The ileum is less affected. Normally, enterocytes are constantly shed from the tips of the villi and replaced by cells migrating up the villi from the crypts. Coeliac disease causes increased cell loss and is associated with villous atrophy. The crypts increase in size (crypt hyperplasia), with elongation and high mitotic activity.

D

Patients with coeliac disease are more likely to develop small bowel lymphomas (usually T-cell lymphoma). The reason for this is unclear.

11.41

See Table 11.2.

11.42

A

The inguinal canal is about 4 cm long and lies above the medial half of the inguinal ligament. It commences at the deep inguinal ring, which lies about 1.3 cm above the mid-inguinal point. The anterior wall is formed by the external oblique aponeurosis; the floor by the lower edge of the

inguinal ligament; the roof by the lower edge of the internal oblique and transversus muscle; and the posterior wall by the transversalis fascia and the strong conjoint tendon medially.

B

The deep inguinal ring transmits the spermatic cord and the ilioinguinal nerve in the male. The structures inside the spermatic cord include:

* the ductus deferens
* arteries – testicular artery, artery of the ductus, cremasteric artery
* veins – pampiniform plexus
* nerves – genital branch of the genitofemoral nerve
* the processus vaginalis – the remains of the peritoneal connection with the tunica vaginalis of the testis.

C

The femoral canal starts at the abdominal end as the femoral ring. Anterior to the femoral ring is the medial part of the inguinal ligament. Posteriorly lies the pectineal ligament, medially the crescentic edge of the lacunar ligament, and laterally the femoral vein. Hence, the femoral ring is below and lateral to the pubic tubercle.

D

The neck of an inguinal hernia (the superficial inguinal ring) lies above and medial to the pubic tubercle; the neck of a femoral hernia lies below and lateral to the pubic tubercle.

TAble 11.2

	Ulcerative colitis	Crohn's disease
Distribution	Usually colon and rectum	Anywhere from mouth to anus, but terminal ileum commonly affected
Affected lumen (dilated or narrowed?)	Dilated lumen	Narrowed lumen
Extent of gut wall affected	Mainly mucosal	Transmural
Histological appearance	Diffuse infiltration with mixed acute and chronic inflammatory cells	Presence of granulomas (epithelioid macrophages and giant cells)
Skipped lesions	Rarely	Commonly
Fistulae present	Rarely	Commonly
Fissures present	Rarely	Commonly
Granulomas present	No	Yes
Cancer risk	Significantly raised	Slightly raised
Malabsorption	Rarely	Commonly

E

One method is to reduce the hernia, placing a finger over the deep inguinal ring (1.3 cm above the mid-inguinal point) and asking the patient to cough. Pressure over the deep inguinal ring controls the indirect but not the direct inguinal hernia. At operation, the hernial sac of the indirect inguinal hernia passes lateral to the inferior epigastric artery, whereas it passes medial to the artery for the direct inguinal hernia.

11.43

A

The appendix is a blind-ending tube that opens into the posteromedial wall of the caecum about 2 cm below the ileocaecal valve. The three taeniae of the caecum merge into a complete longitudinal muscle layer for the appendix.

B

On the surface of the abdomen, the appendix lies at McBurney's point. This is one-third of the way up the line joining the right anterior superior iliac spine to the umbilicus.

C

Before the sixth week, the developing alimentary canal is a simple tube lying in front of the aorta. By the sixth week, the liver has enlarged and the gut has lengthened to such an extent that there is insufficient space in the abdominal cavity. A loop of the gut therefore herniates into the umbilical cord until the 10th week, when the abdominal walls have grown in size. As the herniated loop of gut returns to the abdomen, there is a clockwise rotation (from the point of view of the fetus). The caecum is part of the midgut which returns to the abdomen last, and settles in the right iliac fossa.

D

The child has central dull umbilical pain initially. This is visceral pain and the site of the pain reflects the fact that the appendix develops from the midgut, which is a midline structure. At the later stage, the child develops sharp right iliac fossa pain due to irritation of the local peritoneum.

E

Although appendicitis is a common disorder, the aetiology is still ill understood. Factors thought to be responsible include hard pellets of faeces arising from dehydration and compaction (faecoliths), lymphoid hyperplasia (in childhood viral infections, known as mesenteric adenitis), and infections such as that caused by *Yersinia*. Rare causes include carcinoid tumour, tuberculosis and Crohn's disease.

The liver and biliary system

12.1 The liver:
   A Is attached to the abdominal wall via the falciform ligament
   B Is attached to the diaphragm via the falciform ligament
   C Is easier to palpate in a clinical examination during expiration than inspiration
   D Is covered with peritoneum for over 75% of its surface
   E Lies more interiorly in the supine than in the erect position

12.2 Extensive communications between the left and the right lobes of the liver exist between their:
   A Arterial blood supply
   B Venous drainage
   C Biliary drainage
   D Portal venous supply
   E Nerve supply

12.3 The portal venous system:
   A Provides a little less than 50% of the blood supply to the liver
   B Carries blood from the gastrointestinal tract to the liver
   C Carries blood from the spleen to the liver
   D Has a mean pressure of about 70 mmHg
   E Contains valves

12.4 Sites of communication between the portal and the systemic venous systems include the:
   A Gastro-oesophageal region
   B Ileal region
   C Caecal region
   D Anorectal region
   E Periumbilical region

12.5 Clinical portal hypertension may directly cause:
   A Haemorrhoids
   B An enlarged spleen
   C Oesophageal varices
   D Dilating tortuous veins radiating from the umbilicus
   E Elevated blood pressure

12.6 Functions of the liver include:
   A Synthesis of albumin
   B Synthesis of amino acids
   C Secretion of bile
   D Production of corticosteroids
   E Storage of glycogen

12.7 The following statements about a liver lobule are true:

   A Blood flow is outward from the central vein
   B Bile flows inwards towards the central vein
   C The tissues nearest the central vein are most vulnerable to anoxic injury
   D Each hepatocyte is adjacent to several bile canaliculi
   E Branches of the hepatic artery run in the centre of the lobule close to the central vein

12.8 The following substances are produced by the healthy liver:
   A Aspartate aminotransferase (AST)
   B Alkaline phosphatase
   C γ-Glutamyltransferase (γ-GT)
   D β-Human chorionic gonadotrophin (β-hCG)
   E α-Fetoprotein (AFP)

12.9 The following biochemical abnormalities are caused by primary liver failure:
   A Reduced albumin
   B Prolonged prothrombin time
   C Increased AST
   D Reduced γ-GT
   E Greatly elevated alkaline phosphatase

12.10 Causes for acute liver cell injury include:
   A Hepatitis A infection
   B Hepatitis C infection
   C α1-Antitrypsin deficiency
   D Primary biliary cirrhosis
   E Paracetamol

12.11 Liver diseases which may be caused by alcohol include:
   A Acute hepatitis
   B Chronic hepatitis
   C Fatty change
   D Micronodular cirrhosis
   E Liver cysts

12.12 Probable mechanisms for alcohol to cause liver disease include:
   A Accumulation of glycogen in liver cells
   B Accumulation of fats in liver cells
   C Toxicity of alcohol to liver cells
   D Deposition of elastin in liver cells
   E Stimulation of collagen synthesis in liver cells

12.13 Cirrhosis of the liver:
   A Often affects only one of the four lobes
   B May recover completely with time
   C Is usually caused by necrosis of individual liver cells (apoptosis)

D Is characterised by fibrosis
E Is characterised by nodular regeneration

12.14 Causes of cirrhosis include:
A Wilson's disease
B Hepatitis B infection
C Hepatitis A infection
D Haemochromatosis
E Primary biliary cirrhosis

12.15 Cirrhosis of the liver may lead to:
A Liver failure
B Liver cell carcinoma
C Gallstones
D Cardiac failure
E Portal hypertension

12.16 Liver cell carcinoma:
A Is commoner in Europe than South East Asia
B Is more commonly preceded by micronodular than macronodular cirrhosis
C Characteristically produces AFP
D Is often multifocal
E Is predisposed to by aflatotoxins

12.17 Significant constituents of bile include:
A Bilirubin
B Cholic acid
C Alkaline phosphatase
D Acid phosphatase
E Cholesterol

12.18 Substances whose absorption or excretion is severely reduced in the presence of obstruction in the bile ducts include:
A Carbohydrates
B Fats
C Proteins
D Bilirubin
E Vitamin K

12.19 The following statements about bile salts are true:
A They are mainly synthesised by the bile ducts
B They are discharged into the distal part of the stomach

C A little less than 30% are reabsorbed in the small intestine
D About 50% are reabsorbed in the large intestine
E The reabsorbed bile salts are transported back to the liver via the portal vein

12.20 Unconjugated bilirubin:
A Is formed by the breakdown of haemoglobin in the blood
B Is mostly bound to albumin in the circulation
C Is conjugated to glucuronic acid in the blood
D Cannot be absorbed in the intestine
E Can be excreted in the urine

12.21 Conjugated hyperbilirubinaemia may result from:
A Increased breakdown of red blood cells
B Reduced concentration of albumin
C Reduced entry of bilirubin into liver cells
D Intrahepatic bile duct obstruction
E Extrahepatic bile duct obstruction

12.22 Extrahepatic bile duct obstruction is associated with:
A Increased urinary urobilinogen concentration
B Pale stools
C Pruritus
D A markedly raised serum alkaline phosphatase level
E A low haemoglobin level

12.23 Significant functions of the gallbladder include:
A Secretion of cholesterol
B Formation of bile pigments
C Storage of bile between periods of digestion
D Concentration of bile
E Secretion of digestive enzymes

12.24 Cholecystokinin (CCK):
A Is secreted by the gallbladder
B Produces contraction of the gallbladder
C Increases the secretion of digestive enzyme from the pancreas
D Stimulates the secretion of secretin from the small intestine
E Is secreted in response to an increasing concentration of free bilirubin in the blood

12 **A**

SYSTEM-BASED MEDICAL SCIENCES

The liver and biliary system

12.1 A B D
The liver is the largest abdominal organ, and accounts for about 2% of the body weight in adults. The superior and anterior surfaces in contact with the diaphragm and the anterior abdominal wall respectively, and the falciform ligament attaches the liver to both these structures. As the diaphragm moves downwards with inspiration, the liver moves with it. Hence it is easier to palpate the liver during inspiration in a clinical examination. The liver also occupies a more inferior position in the erect than in the supine position due to gravity. As the liver develops between two layers of ventral mesentery embryologically, the surface of the liver is covered almost completely with peritoneum. The only exception is the bare area on its posterior surface.

12.2 –
The left and the right lobes of the liver are separated by the gallbladder fossa and the fossa for the inferior vena cava, and they function independently of each other. They receive their own arterial and portal venous blood supplies, and have their own venous and biliary drainage. The caudate lobe and most of the quadrate lobe of the liver function as the left lobe of the liver. The liver is innervated by the sympathetic and parasympathetic nervous systems via the hepatic plexus. However, there is no extensive communication between the nerve supplies to the right and the left lobes.

12.3 B C
The portal venous system carries blood from the gut, the spleen, the gallbladder and the pancreas to the liver. It provides about 70% of the blood supply to the liver, the other 30% being provided by the hepatic artery. Whilst the hepatic arterial pressure is about 90 mmHg, the portal venous pressure is only about 10 mmHg. The low portal venous pressure allows blood to flow from the mesenteric veins to the liver. In the presence of obstruction in the liver (e.g. due to cirrhosis), the portal venous pressure rises. As there are no valves in the portal veins, the blood flow can be reversed and portal venous blood can be returned to the inferior vena cava via the systemic-portal collateral circulation.

12.4 A D E
There are four main areas of portal – systemic anastomosis: in the gastrointestinal region, in the anorectal region, in the para-umbilical region and in the retroperitoneal region mainly between the splenic and the left renal veins. This is important clinically, as in the presence of portal hypertension dilated tortuous veins develop in these regions to cause haemorrhoids, oesophageal varices, caput medusae (veins radiating from the umbilicus) and enlarged spleen.

12.5 A B C D
See question 12.4 above. Ascites may also develop in portal hypertension. An increase in portal venous pressure (portal hypertension) does not affect the arterial blood pressure.

12.6 A C E
The liver performs many essential functions. The main functions are the formation and secretion of bile; inactivation of toxins and hormones; synthesis of important proteins (e.g. albumin, acute-phase proteins, some of the clotting factors, hormone-binding proteins); and the metabolism of carbohydrate, fats and proteins. The liver is the main storage site for glycogen. It breaks down amino acids to form urea (deamination).

12.7 C D
The liver is organised into lobules. In the centre is the central vein, which drains blood from branches of the portal vein and hepatic artery at the periphery. Hence blood flows inwards through the sinusoids towards the central vein. The central veins of the lobules then form the hepatic veins, which drain into the inferior vena cava. The blood in the sinusoids closest to the central vein is least oxygenated, and hence the tissues around the central vein are most prone to anoxic injury (e.g. in cardiac failure). Each liver cell is adjacent to several bile canaliculi, and the bile drains towards branches of the bile ducts in the portal space at the periphery of the lobule. Branches of the hepatic artery, portal vein and bile ducts run close together in the portal space.

Another way to describe the organisation of the liver is that it is divided into acini, with the portal space at the centre and the central veins in the periphery.

12.8 A C
AST, alanine aminotransferase (ALT) and γ-GT are produced by the healthy liver, and they are useful in diagnosing diseases of the liver cells. In the past, γ-GT was used clinically as a marker of excessive alcohol intake, although a raised level is not specific to liver injury by alcohol. Alkaline phosphatase is produced in the biliary system, and an elevated level indicates biliary obstruction. AFP is produced by primary liver cell tumour.

12.9 A B C
See question 12.8 above. As the liver is the prime producer of both albumin and the vitamin K-dependent clotting factors, a low albumin and a prolonged prothrombin time may occur in liver failure. A greatly elevated level of alkaline phosphatase occurs in biliary obstruction.

12.10 A B E
Causes of acute liver cell injury include viral infections (e.g. hepatitis viruses, alcohol), drugs (e.g. paracetamol) and

toxins. Primary biliary cirrhosis and α_1-antitrypsin deficiency usually cause chronic injury and cirrhosis.

12.11 A B C D
Alcohol causes a spectrum of liver diseases. Fatty change is a benign abnormality, and is characterised by fat globules within the cytoplasm of the liver cells. It may proceed to acute hepatitis with acute inflammation. Mallory's hyaline (intracytoplasmic aggregates of filaments in liver cells) is a characteristic histological feature. Alcohol may also cause chronic hepatitis and cirrhosis. Alcohol is the commonest cause of micronodular cirrhosis (i.e. with nodules less than 3 mm diameter).

12.12 B C E
The probable mechanisms for alcohol liver disease are diversion of cellular energy from fat metabolism (hence causing an accumulation of fats in liver cells), direct toxicity of alcohol to liver cells, and stimulation of collagen synthesis (hence causing fibrosis).

12.13 D E
Liver cells can usually regenerate in response to injury. However, if there are repeated injuries which affect the architecture of the liver, repair may not restore the architecture. In cirrhosis, there is diffuse irreversible disturbance of the liver architecture. Fibrosis and nodular regeneration are characteristic. In nodular regeneration, the organisation of the lobules is lost. Cirrhosis is more likely following bridging necrosis, with areas of necrosis in the lobules extending from the central area to the portal spaces.

12.14 A B D E
Hepatitis B, hepatitis C and alcohol are the common causes of cirrhosis. Other causes include haemochromatosis (associated with excess iron deposition), Wilson's disease (a genetic disease associated with abnormal copper deposition), primary biliary cirrhosis (an autoimmune disease) and α_1-antitripsin deficiency.

12.15 A B E
Cirrhosis of the liver may cause liver failure if a critical proportion of functioning liver cells are lost. Cirrhosis may cause portal hypertension by an increase in the vascular resistance at the sinusoids. Cirrhosis due to any aetiology predisposes to liver cell carcinoma.

12.16 C D E
All cases of cirrhosis predispose to liver cell carcinoma, but the risk is especially high for macronodular cirrhosis (i.e. nodules more than 3 mm in diameter). As nodules in cirrhosis are multifocal, liver cell carcinoma which occurs in cirrhotic livers also tends to be multifocal. Hepatitis B

infection is an important predisposing factor on its own, and may partly explain the higher prevalence in some parts of the world such as South East Asia. Aflatoxin (a toxin produced by the fungus *Aspergillus flavus*) may also cause liver cell carcinoma. Liver cell carcinoma characteristically produces AFP, which is clinically used as a diagnostic marker.

12.17 A B C E
Water constitutes over 95% of bile in the bile ducts. Bile salts, bile pigments, cholesterol and lecithin are important constituents. Bile salts are either sodium or potassium salts of bile acids, of which cholic acid and chenodeoxycholic acid are the most important. Bile pigments are mainly bilirubin and biliverdin, and account for the brown colour of the bile. The relative proportions of bile salt, cholesterol and lecithin determine the solubility of cholesterol, and are important in the formation of gallstones. Alkaline phosphatase is also present, and accounts for the greatly elevated level of the enzyme in obstructive jaundice compared with jaundice due to liver disease. Acid phosphatase is mainly secreted by the prostate gland.

12.18 B D E
The function of bile salts is to prepare for the digestion and absorption of fats. Bile salts reduce surface tension, and are important for the emulsification of fat before it is digested and absorbed in the small intestine. Also, bile salts have both a hydrophilic and a hydrophobic end. Hence bile salts tend to form cylindrical discs (micelles) and tend to keep fats in solution. In the absence of bile salts, the absorption of fat and fat-soluble vitamins (e.g. vitamins A, D, E and K) is severely reduced. Bile pigments consist mostly of biliverdin and bilirubin, and the biliary system is essential for their excretion.

12.19 E
Bile salts are synthesised in the liver. The bile enters the gallbladder, where the bile salts are concentrated by the reabsorption of water, and the bile passes through the cystic and the common bile ducts. The common bile duct joins the pancreatic duct and enters the second part of the duodenum. About 95% of the bile salts are reabsorbed in the small intestine, and re-enter the liver via the portal vein. This enterohepatic circulation is important. For example, fat malabsorption may result from the presence of severe small intestinal disease due to reduced absorption of bile salts, and the inability of the liver to keep up with its synthesis.

12.20 A B E
Most of the bilirubin is formed by the breakdown of haemoglobin. The unconjugated bilirubin is mostly bound

12 **A**

SYSTEM-BASED MEDICAL SCIENCES

The liver and biliary system

to albumin, and only a small proportion is free. Free bilirubin enters the liver cells and becomes conjugated to glucuronic acid. The reaction is catalysed by the enzyme glucuronyl transferase. The conjugated bilirubin is then secreted into the bile. Unlike unconjugated bilirubin, conjugated bilirubin cannot be absorbed in the intestine. Hence it is excreted by the gut, and accounts for the characteristic colour of the stool.

12.21 D E

Bilirubin is conjugated in the liver cells. Hence increased breakdown of red blood cells (i.e. haemolysis) and reduced entry of bilirubin into liver cell, or defective conjugation (e.g. due to glucoronyl transferase deficiency), result in unconjugated hyperbilirubinaemia. However, intrahepatic or extrahepatic bile duct obstruction results in conjugated hyperbilirubinaemia.

12.22 B C D

Extrahepatic bile duct obstruction results in conjugated hyperbilirubinaemia. Characteristic symptoms include jaundice, dark urine (due to conjugated bilirubin in the urine), pale stools (due to lack of bile pigments reaching the large intestine) and pruritus (due to increased bile salts in the blood). Increased urinary urobilinogen is due to unconjugated hyperbilirubinaemia.

12.23 C D

The gallbladder is not essential, as most subjects with their gallbladders removed surgically enjoy good health. The main functions of the gallbladder are to concentrate the bile and store the bile between periods of digestion.

12.24 B C D

In the past, it was thought that one hormone (cholecystokinin) stimulates the contraction of the gallbladder and another (pancreozymin) stimulates the production of enzyme-rich pancreatic secretion. They have been found to be the same hormone, and is now called cholecystokinin–pancreozymin (CCK-PZ). The hormone exists in several forms, and is secreted in both the small and large intestines. Its secretion is stimulated by the contact of digestive products with the intestinal mucosa, and especially the presence of fatty acids in the duodenum. Hence digestion is facilitated by the release of bile from the gallbladder and digestive enzymes from the pancreas. Furthermore, CCK-PZ stimulates the secretion of secretin from the small intestine. This increases the secretion of bicarbonate into the pancreatic juice.

The endocrine system ⓲

13.1 Physiological functions regulated by the hypothalamus include:
  A Temperature
  B Vomiting
  C 'Fight, fright and flight' defensive response
  D Blood pressure control
  E Sleep – wake cycle

13.2 Leptin:
  A Is a protein
  B Acts on the hypothalamus
  C Is found at a higher concentration in men than women
  D Is found at a higher concentration in obese than non-obese subjects
  E Increases food intake

13.3 The level of thirst is significantly increased by a reduction of:
  A Plasma osmolality
  B Plasma angiotensin II level
  C Plasma renin level
  D Extracellular volume
  E Intracellular volume

13.4 Physiological mechanisms for increasing the body temperature include:
  A Erection of hairs in the skin
  B Sweating
  C Shivering
  D Cutaneous vasoconstriction
  E Increased secretion of adrenaline (epinephrine)

13.5 Hormones secreted by the hypothalamus into the portal hypophyseal vessel include:
  A Vasopressin (ADH)
  B Thyrotrophin-releasing hormone (TRH)
  C Prolactin-prohibiting hormone
  D Adrenocorticotrophic hormone (ACTH)
  E Oxytocin

13.6 Vasopressin:
  A Is a nonapeptide (consists of nine amino acids)
  B Is secreted in the anterior pituitary gland
  C Is secreted directly by nerve cells
  D Has a half-life of about 24 h
  E Causes sodium retention

13.7 Factors which decrease the secretion of vasopressin include:
  A Consumption of alcohol
  B Haemorrhage
  C Oral consumption of water

  D Raised plasma osmolality
  E Erect posture

13.8 In nephrogenic diabetes insipidus:
  A The plasma vasopressin level is low
  B The subject often drinks a large quantity of water (polydipsia)
  C Urine output is low
  D The urine osmolality is high
  E Synthetic vasopressin may alleviate the symptoms

13.9 The following statements about inappropriate ADH secretion are true:
  A Bronchial carcinoma is a recognised cause
  B It often occurs following an operation
  C The plasma sodium concentration is often abnormally high
  D The extracellular volume increases
  E Demeclocycline is a recognised treatment

13.10 Direct actions of oxytocin include:
  A An increase in the volume of milk produced by the breast
  B Facilitation of the ejection of milk from the ducts of the breast
  C Contraction of the perineal muscle during labour
  D Contraction of the smooth muscle of the uterus
  E Contraction of the smooth muscle of the bladder

13.11 The following statements about the pituitary gland are true:
  A It lies inferior to the optic chiasma
  B It lies in the ethmoidal bones
  C It is supplied by branches of the internal carotid artery
  D The posterior pituitary develops from an evagination from the roof of the pharynx embryologically
  E The anterior pituitary develops from an evagination of the floor of the third ventricle embryologically

13.12 The following statements about thyroid hormones are true:
  A The thyroid gland produces more triiodothyronine (T_3) than levothyroxine (thyroxine) (T_4)
  B T_3 is more active than T_4
  C Reverse T_3 (RT_3) is more active than T_3
  D About 20% of T_4 in the plasma is bound to protein
  E T_4 can be converted into T_3 in the liver

175

13 **Q**

The endocrine system

13.13 Thyroid hormones:
  A Bind to receptors in the cytoplasm
  B Inhibit membrane-bound Na^+,K^+-ATPase activity
  C Alter the rate of protein synthesis by binding to the ribosomes
  D Increase the rate of mobilisation of fatty acids
  E Decrease the overall rate of oxygen consumption

13.14 Physiological effects of thyroid hormones include an increased rate of:
  A Carbohydrate absorption
  B Protein synthesis
  C Muscle breakdown
  D Glucagon synthesis
  E Fatty tissue synthesis

13.15 The following statements about the relationship between thyroid hormones and catecholamines are true:
  A Thyroid hormones increase the concentration of plasma catecholamines
  B Thyroid hormones are competitive inhibitors of plasma catecholamines
  C Thyroid hormones increase the number of β-adrenergic receptors
  D Thyroid hormones increase the affinity of catecholamines to β-adrenergic receptors
  E The effect of thyroid hormones may be partially reduced by propranolol

13.16 The following statements about the control of thyroid hormone secretion are true:
  A Increased free T_4 increases the rate of TRH secretion
  B Increased free T_4 decreases the rate of thyroid-stimulating hormone (TSH) secretion
  C Increased free T_3 decreases the rate of TSH synthesis
  D Increased catecholamines decrease the rate of TSH synthesis
  E Increased thyroxine-binding globulin (TBG) increases the rate of TSH secretion

13.17 Recognised clinical features of hyperthyroidism include:
  A Tremor
  B Weight gain
  C Hypothermia
  D Sweating
  E Increased heart rate

13.18 Recognised biochemical abnormalities of hypothyroidism due to thyroid disease include:
  A A raised free T_4 level
  B A raised plasma TSH level
  C A poor TSH response to a test dose of TRH
  D A raised plasma thyroxine-binding globulin
  E A low total plasma T_3 level

13.19 Carbimazole:
  A Is an antagonist of T_4 at the thyroid hormone receptor
  B Increases thyroid hormone synthesis
  C Exerts its maximal clinical effect within 24 h of administration
  D Usually results in reduction in the size of the goitre
  E May cause acute reduction in neutrophil count

13.20 Graves' disease:
  A Is the commonest cause of hyperthyroidism
  B Is usually associated with diffuse goitre
  C Is associated with autoantibodies to thyroglobulin
  D May be associated with exophthalmos
  E Occurs more frequently in men than women

13.21 Long-acting thyroid stimulator (LATS):
  A Is an autoantibody to thyroid epithelial cells
  B Is an IgM
  C Is associated with accumulation of mucopolysaccharides in the dermis of the shins (pretibial myxoedema)
  D Inhibits the formation of thyroid hormones
  E Is characteristically associated with Hashimoto's disease

13.22 The following statements about thyroid carcinomas are true:
  A They are commoner than benign thyroid tumours
  B Papillary carcinoma is commoner than other types of thyroid carcinomas
  C Anaplastic carcinoma has a worse prognosis than follicular carcinoma
  D Follicular carcinoma often metastasises to bone
  E Medullary carcinoma often secretes calcitonin

13.23 The following statements about the thyroid gland are true:
  A It is surrounded by a sheath derived from the pretracheal fascia
  B The isthmus lies anterior to the second to fourth rings of the trachea
  C It is developed from the endoderm embryologically
  D Embryological incomplete descent may result in lingual thyroid

E The recurrent laryngeal nerves lie posteromedial to the lobes

13.24 The following statements about calcium metabolism are true:
A Just less than half of the body calcium is in the skeleton
B Just over half of the calcium excretion takes place in the kidneys
C The amount of calcium bound to protein varies with the plasma protein concentration
D Calcium can be actively transported from the gut lumen into the capillaries
E There is usually no exchange of calcium between bones and extracellular fluid in healthy individuals

13.25 Total body calcium is generally higher in:
A Teenagers than childhood
B Those aged 50 than those aged 30
C The elderly than those aged 50
D Women than men of the same age
E Post-menopausal women than pre-menopausal women

13.26 Effects of vitamin D include increased:
A Active transport of calcium from the intestinal lumen to the capillaries
B Calcium reabsorption from the kidneys
C Calcium secretion in the kidneys
D Stimulation of osteoclasts in bone
E Stimulation of osteoblasts in bone

13.27 The following statements about the various forms of vitamin D are true:
A The normal diet contains colecalciferol (vitamin D_3)
B The synthesis of colecalciferol (vitamin D_3) from 7-dehydrocolecolesterol requires sunlight
C The conversion of 25-hydroxycolecalciferol to 1, 25-dihydroxycolecalciferol takes place in the kidneys
D The conversion of 25-hydroxycolecalciferol to 24, 25-dihydroxycolecalciferol takes place in the liver
E 24, 25-Dihydroxycolecalciferol is more active than 1, 25-dihydroxycolecalciferol

13.28 The following are important mechanisms for the regulation of the plasma level of the active form of vitamin D:
A High plasma calcium stimulates the formation of 25-hydroxycolecalciferol
B High plasma calcium stimulates the formation of 1, 25-dihydroxycolecalciferol

C High plasma phosphate stimulates the formation of 1, 25-dihydroxycolecalciferol
D High parathyroid hormone stimulates the formation of 1, 25-dihydroxycolecalciferol
E High parathyroid hormone stimulates the formation of 24, 25-dihydroxycolecalciferol

13.29 The following statements about the parathyroid glands are true:
A There are normally six parathyroid glands
B The superior parathyroid glands normally lie on the anterior surface of the thyroid gland
C The superior parathyroid glands normally lie outside the fascial sheath of the thyroid gland
D The inferior parathyroid glands are occasionally found within thymic tissue in the superior mediastinum
E They secrete calcitonin

13.30 Parathyroid hormone:
A Is a tripeptide
B Is secreted by the superior, but not the inferior, parathyroid glands
C Increases bone formation
D Increases plasma phosphate
E Indirectly increases calcium absorption from the intestine

13.31 Abnormal findings in pseudohypoparathyroidism include low:
A Plasma calcium
B Plasma phosphate
C Plasma parathyroid hormone
D Urinary phosphate excretion
E Plasma protein

13.32 Calcitonin:
A Increases plasma calcium
B Inhibits bone resorption
C Increases urinary calcium excretion
D Increases absorption of calcium from the gut
E Is a recognised treatment for Paget's disease

13.33 Clinical features of hypercalcaemia include:
A Tetany
B Convulsions
C Muscle weakness
D Polyuria
E Tiredness

13.34 Recognised causes of hypercalcaemia include:
A Bone metastases
B Ectopic PTH secretion from squamous bronchial carcinoma

13 **Q**

SYSTEM-BASED MEDICAL SCIENCES

The endocrine system

C Chronic renal failure
D Vitamin D deficiency
E Sarcoidosis

13.35 Secondary hyperparathyroidism:
A Is usually caused by a parathyroid adenoma
B Is associated with a high plasma calcium level
C May be due to renal failure
D May progress to tertiary hyperparathyroidism
E Is best treated by parathyroidectomy

13.36 Recognised temporary treatment for hypercalcaemia due to primary hyperparathroidism include:
A Adrenocortical steroid
B Intravenous saline and furosemide (frusemide)
C Thiazide diuretics
D Dialysis
E Calcitonin

13.37 Bisphosphonates may be used to treat:
A Osteoporosis
B Osteomalacia
C Hypercalcaemia
D Osteoarthritis
E Paget's disease

13.38 Hormones normally secreted by the islets of Langerhans in the pancreas include:
A Insulin
B Gastrin
C Glucagon
D Somatostatin
E Cholecystokinin–pancreozymin

13.39 The following statements about insulin are true:
A It consists of four amino acid chains
B Disulphide bridges link separate amino acid chains
C There are major differences in the structure between pig and human insulin
D Humans receiving beef insulin often develop antibodies against it
E Human insulin may be manufactured by recombinant DNA technique

13.40 Physiological effects of insulin include decreased:
A Transport of glucose into cells
B Transport of amino acids into cells
C Plasma potassium level
D Protein synthesis
E Glycogen synthesis

13.41 Insulin receptors:
A Are not found outside the pancreas

B Each consist of two α-and two β-glycoprotein subunits
C Are usually in the nuclei
D Decrease in number with increasing plasma insulin level
E Increase in number in obesity

13.42 The results of a standard glucose tolerance test depend significantly on:
A The rate of intestinal absorption of glucose
B The rate of entry of glucose into cells
C The uptake of glucose by the brain
D The rate of glycogen synthesis by the liver
E The rate of glucose uptake by red blood cells

13.43 Recognised effects of a high plasma glucose level include:
A Presence of glucose in the urine
B Dehydration
C Thirst
D Polyuria
E Reduction in HbA_{1c} level

13.44 Metabolic changes associated with diabetes mellitus include:
A Intracellular hyperglycaemia
B Glycogen depletion
C Increased formation of ketone bodies
D Greatly positive nitrogen balance
E Excess acetyl-CoA formation

13.45 In diabetic ketoacidosis:
A There is an accumulation of ketone bodies in the plasma
B There is an accumulation of total body sodium
C The total body potassium is depleted
D The plasma potassium is usually low
E The respiratory rate may be abnormally fast

13.46 Sulphonylureas:
A Increase insulin synthesis in the islet cells
B Are indicated for patients with total deficiency of insulin
C May cause hyperglycaemia in normal subjects
D Frequently cause weight loss
E Usually become more effective after regular usage for a few years

13.47 Biguanides:
A Include glibenclamide
B Are mainly used to treat insulin-dependent diabetes mellitus
C Reduce the production of glucose in the liver

178

    D May cause lactic acidosis
    E Are not suitable for obese patients

13.48 Compared to type II diabetes, type I diabetes (i.e. juvenile-onset, insulin-dependent diabetes)
    A Is more likely to present with ketoacidosis
    B Is associated with higher insulin secretion
    C Has a higher monozygotic twin concordance
    D Is more likely to be autoimmune in aetiology
    E Is more likely to be triggered by viral infection

13.49 The following diseases are commoner in patients with diabetes mellitus:
    A Myocardial infarction
    B Cerebrovascular disease
    C Peripheral vascular disease
    D Retinopathy
    E Nephropathy

13.50 Glucagon:
    A Increases the breakdown of glycogen
    B Increases the plasma glucose level
    C Is broken down in the liver
    D May act via cAMP as a second messenger
    E Stimulates the secretion of insulin

13.51 The following increase the secretion of glucagon:
    A High plasma glucose
    B High plasma insulin
    C Exercise
    D Sympathetic nervous stimulation
    E High plasma amino acids

13.52 Symptoms of hypoglycaemia may include:
    A Palpitations
    B Sweating
    C Confusion
    D Convulsions
    E Drowsiness

13.53 The following hormones increase as a compensatory response to hypoglycaemia:
    A Growth hormone
    B Adrenaline (epinephrine)
    C Aldosterone
    D Cortisol
    E Glucagon

13.54 Physiological effects of growth hormone include:
    A Linear elongation of long bones after the epiphyses have fused
    B An increase in the breakdown of proteins
    C A reduction of the breakdown of glycogen in the liver

    D Reduction in insulin secretion
    E An increase in the plasma free fatty acid

13.55 Somatomedins:
    A Are growth factors
    B Are secreted by the liver
    C Are secreted in response to growth hormone
    D Can stimulate both skeletal and cartilage growth
    E Are increased in untreated diabetes mellitus

13.56 The following hormones and the sites of secretion are correctly matched:
    A Mineralocorticoid – zona fasciculata of adrenal cortex
    B Sex hormones – zona glomerulosa of adrenal cortex
    C Dopamine – adrenal medulla
    D Adrenaline (epinephrine) – adrenal medulla
    E Glucocorticoids – zona reticularis of adrenal cortex

13.57 Compared to adrenaline (epinephrine), noradrenaline (norepinephrine) produces a significantly higher:
    A Peripheral resistance in the circulation
    B Heart rate
    C Diastolic blood pressure
    D Pulse pressure
    E Level of fear and anxiety

13.58 The following statements about the synthesis of glucocorticosteroids are true:
    A Cholesterol acts as the precursor
    B Mitochondrial enzymes are essential
    C Intracellular cyclic AMP acts as a second messenger
    D It is initiated by ACTH binding to a nuclear receptor
    E Some of the metabolic pathways are common to those for mineralocorticoid synthesis

13.59 Recognised pharmacological uses of systemic adrenal steroids include:
    A Collagen disorders (e.g. systemic lupus erythematosus)
    B Anaphylactic shock
    C Rejection of transplanted kidneys
    D Severe asthmatic attack
    E Idiopathic thrombocytopenia purpura

13.60 Recognised side effects of long-term administration of steroids include:
    A Postural hypotension
    B Osteomalacia

13 **Q**

The endocrine system

C Depression

D Peptic ulceration

E Increased susceptibility to infection

13.61 Conditions which are associated with a low plasma ACTH but a high plasma cortisol level include:

A Addison's disease

B Psychologically stressful situations

C Panhypopituitarism

D Primary adrenal tumour

E Ectopic ACTH-secreting bronchial carcinoma

13.62 A 29-year-old woman complained of tremor, sweatiness and weight loss. The doctor found a fast heart rate. A thyroid gland disorder was suspected, and thyroid function tests were performed. The blood test results were as follows:

• free levothyroxine (thyroxine): 80 pmol/l (reference 9–22 pmol/l)

• TSH: <0.1 miu/l (reference 0.5–5.7 miu/l).

A Where does the thyroid gland originate embryologically? Where is the normal adult thyroid gland in relation to the cricoid bone? Explain this from an embryological viewpoint.

B Name three hormones secreted by the thyroid gland. Which is the most active?

C Is the patient's thyroid gland overactive or underactive?

D Is the primary site of the lesion in the hypothalamus, pituitary gland or thyroid gland? Explain.

E How does the thyroid disease cause a fast heart rate? Suggest a drug (or a class of drug) which may be useful to reduce the heart rate in this patient quickly.

F How would the basal metabolic rate of the patient compare with normal individuals?

G Name one pathological cause for the condition of the thyroid.

13.63 The results of a patient's thyroid function tests are as follows:

• plasma T_3: 0.4 nmol/l (reference 1.2–3.0 nmol/l)

• plasma T_4: 25 nmol/l (reference 70–140 nmol/l)

• plasma TSH: 0.3 miu/l (reference 0.5–5.7 miu/l).

A Is the patient hypothyroid, hyperthyroid or euthyroid? Explain.

B What is the likely cause for the patient's condition? Explain.

C What test would you do to confirm your answer in (B)? Explain the rationale for this test.

13.64 A child from Central Europe develops a goitre. After investigations, he was diagnosed to have a goitre secondary to iodine deficiency.

A Explain how iodine deficiency can cause a goitre.

B What abnormalities (if any) would you expect to find in the levothyroxine (thyroxine) and TSH levels of this child?

13.65 A young adult had symptoms of polyuria (passing excessive quantities of urine), excessive thirst and failure to gain weight for some months and was admitted as an emergency, extremely unwell, dehydrated and acidotic. Ketones were detected in the urine.

A List the physiological functions of insulin in the following.

i Carbohydrate metabolism.

ii Fat metabolism.

iii Protein metabolism.

B Explain at the cellular level how insulin exerts the effects outlined in (A).

C Explain the mechanisms responsible for the following clinical features.

i Passing excessive quantities of urine.

ii Excessive thirst.

iii Failure to gain weight.

iv Acidosis and ketones in the urine.

D Which hormones tend to (1) raise and (2) lower the blood glucose level?

13.66 A 60-year-old man was diagnosed with diabetes mellitus and was initially treated with tolbutamide and metformin. As the diabetes remained uncontrolled, human insulin was prescribed. The general practitioner was called out as an emergency because the patient became unconscious. The doctor administered an injection of glucagon and the patient recovered consciousness.

A Briefly explain how tolbutamide and metformin might have helped to control diabetes mellitus.

B What was the reason for the patient's unconsciousness?

C What is the mechanism of action of glucagon?

13.67 A 50-year-old patient who had suffered from insulin-dependent diabetes since childhood was admitted with a myocardial infarct. Testing the level of control of his diabetes, his blood HbA_{1c} level was found to be 9.8% (reference 2.3–6.5%). On further examination and investigation, he was also found to have renal failure due to glomerulonephritis, impaired sensation in the lower limbs, ischaemic legs and haemorrhages in the retina.

A How is HbA$_{1C}$ produced in the body? Why might it indicate the level of control of diabetes?

B Interpret this patient's HbA$_{1C}$ results.

C Explain the mechanisms that may account for this patient's complications.

13.68 A patient was investigated for diabetes mellitus after his urine was found to contain glucose. The fasting blood glucose was 7.2 mmol/l (reference: diabetes excluded if <6 mmol/l, confirmed if >7.8 mmol/l). To investigate further, a glucose tolerance test was carried out. After fasting overnight, the patient was given 75 g of glucose with 300 ml of water to drink. The plasma glucose levels before and 2 h after the glucose was given were 7.2 mmol/l and 13.0 mmol/l, respectively (reference: 2 h after glucose given <11.1 mmol/l).

A Explain the advantage of fasting blood glucose level over random blood glucose level in the diagnosis of diabetes mellitus.

B Explain the underlying rationale for the glucose tolerance test. Why might it be a better test for diabetes mellitus than the fasting glucose level?

C Interpret the results in this patient.

13.69 The following are known causes of rickets and a low serum calcium level in children: dietary deficiency of vitamin D, lack of sunlight, intestinal malabsorption, liver disease and renal disease.

A List the various mechanisms by which a deficiency in vitamin D may result in a low serum calcium level.

B What is rickets? What is the corresponding condition in adults?

C What would you expect the serum phosphate level in children with rickets to be compared with normal children?

D Draw a simple diagram illustrating the biochemical pathway for the synthesis of the active form of vitamin D, and indicate why rickets may result from the causes listed above.

13.70 A 60-year-old patient complained of abdominal pain and constant tiredness. The following biochemical results were available:

- plasma calcium (total): 3.65 mmol/l (reference 2.12–2.65 mmol/l)
- plasma phosphate: 0.5 mmol/l (reference 0.8–1.45 mmol/l)
- plasma albumin: 40 g/l (reference 30–50 g/l)
- plasma urea: 6.0 mmol/l (reference 2.5–6.7 mmol/l)
- parathyroid hormone: 14.2 pmol/l (reference 0.8–8.5 pmol/l).

The patient was treated with intravenous rehydration, furosemide (frusemide) and pamidronate (bisphosphonates).

A What is the most likely diagnosis in this patient?

B What are the effects of parathyroid hormone on the serum calcium and phosphate levels? What are the mechanisms responsible?

C Explain how the secretion of parathyroid hormone is normally regulated?

D Why might the following drugs be effective in lowering plasma calcium levels?
  i Furosemide (frusemide).
  ii Pamidronate.

E Could thiazides be used for this condition? Explain.

13.71 A 65-year-old patient complained of excessive thirst. The following biochemical results were obtained:

- plasma calcium (total): 3.15 mmol/l (reference 2.12–2.65 mmol/l)
- plasma phosphate: 1.50 mmol/l (reference 0.8–1.45 mmol/l)
- plasma albumin: 41 g/l (reference 30–50 g/l)
- plasma urea: 5.1 mmol/l (reference 2.5–6.7 mmol/l)
- parathyroid hormone: 6.1 pmol/l (reference 0.8–8.5 pmol/l)
- parathyroid hormone-related protein (PTHrP): abnormally high.

A What is the most likely diagnosis in this patient? Explain.

B What abnormalities (if any) would you expect for the serum alkaline phosphatase and urinary phosphate levels in this patient?

C What is the mechanism responsible for the elevated serum calcium level?

13.72 A 50-year-old woman presented with buffalo hump, striae and myopathy, all suggestive of Cushing's syndrome. The following results were obtained:

- 24 h urinary free cortisol: 600 nmol/24 h (reference <280 nmol/24 h)
- simultaneous cortisol and ACTH levels (in the morning):
  cortisol: 1602 nmol/L (reference 450–700 nmol/l)
  ACTH: 302 ng/L (reference <80 ng/l).

A What are the features of Cushing's syndrome caused by?

B Draw a diagram to illustrate how the serum cortisol and ACTH levels are normally regulated.

C List the three main causes of Cushing's syndrome.

D Which is the most likely cause in this patient? Explain.

The endocrine system

E What other investigation can be performed to distinguish between these various causes? What would you expect to find for this patient?

F What abnormalities (if any) in the serum sodium and potassium levels would you expect to find in this patient? Explain.

13.73 A 22-year-old woman presented with secondary amenorrhoea (loss of menstrual periods). The following result was available:

• Plasma prolactin: 2040 iu/l (reference for women <600 iu/l)

After further investigations, bromocriptine was prescribed.

A What are the physiological functions of prolactin in women?

B Where is prolactin normally secreted?

C How is plasma prolactin level normally regulated?

D What is the likely cause for the endocrine abnormality in this patient?

E Explain the mechanism by which bromocriptine might reduce the plasma prolactin level.

13.74 A 40-year-old man presented with gradual onset of features suggesting acromegaly (large tongue, increased shoe size, coarse facial features). The following results were obtained:

• growth hormone level: 35 miu/L (reference <20 miu/l)

• serum IGF-1 (insulin-like growth factor 1): highly elevated.

After further tests, the patient was prescribed octreotide.

A Where is growth hormone usually secreted?

B What are the possible mechanisms by which growth hormone produces growth?

C What do these results suggest?

D What is acromegaly?

E Give one advantage of measurement of serum IGF-1 level over that of growth hormone level in the screening for acromegaly.

F What is the definitive test in the diagnosis of acromegaly?

G Describe the feedback control for the secretion of growth hormone.

H Explain the mechanism of action by which octreotide may reduce serum growth hormone level.

13.75 A patient presented with a raised blood pressure and a low serum potassium level. Investigations revealed:

• serum aldosterone: 1050 pmol/l (reference 100–500 pmol/L)

• serum renin (recumbent): 1.0 pmol/mL (reference 1.1–2.7 pmol/mL).

After further investigations, spironolactone was prescribed while treatment options were considered.

A Draw a diagram to illustrate the renin–angiotensin–aldosterone system.

B Explain why this patient has raised blood pressure and a reduced serum potassium level.

C What is the likely cause for the raised aldosterone level? Explain.

D How might spironolactone be beneficial in this patient?

The endocrine system

13.1 A C E
The hypothalamus plays an extremely important role for both endocrine control and the regulation of many autonomic functions. It exerts its endocrine control mainly via its neural connections with the posterior pituitary gland and its hormonal connections with the anterior pituitary gland. The hypothalamus also regulates several important physiological body functions. They include control of temperature, appetite, thirst, sexual behaviour and the defensive reactions. There is good evidence that the suprachiasmatic nuclei of the hypothalamus receive input from the eyes via the retinohypothalamic fibres, and control many circadian rhythms including body temperature rhythms and sleep–wake cycles. Vomiting, cough and blood pressure control are mediated by centres in the medulla oblongata.

13.2 A B D
Leptin is a protein containing 167 amino acids, and has only been recently isolated. It acts on the hypothalamus to decrease food intake and increase energy consumption. Leptin level can be measured by radioimmunoassay. Leptin levels appear to correlate directly with the proportion of body fat. Hence obese subjects have a higher concentration than non-obese subjects, and women have a higher concentration than men. It appears that leptin is important in controlling the body's store of fat by providing feedback to the hypothalamus on the total body fat store.

13.3 D
The level of thirst is usually controlled by two factors: plasma osmolality and the extracellular volume. An increase in plasma osmolality (e.g. in dehydration due to water loss, infusion of hypertonic solution) stimulates the osmoreceptors in the anterior hypothalamus, which results in an increased level of thirst. A reduction in extracellular volume (e.g. in haemorrhage) stimulates the baroreceptors, which causes an increase in the plasma level of renin and angiotensin II. This leads to an increased level of thirst.

13.4 A C D E
Body temperature may be increased either by producing more heat or reducing heat loss. Mechanisms for producing more heat include voluntary muscle contraction and shivering. Secretion of adrenaline (epinephrine) or noradrenaline (norepinephrine) will increase heat production in the short term, and thyroid hormone may increase heat production in the longer term. Mechanisms for minimising heat loss include constriction of the blood vessels in the skin and erection of hairs in the skin.

13.5 B C
The hypothalamus controls the release of anterior pituitary hormones by secreting releasing and inhibiting hormones into the portal hypophyseal vessel, but the secretion of posterior pituitary hormones is controlled by direct neural connection between the supraoptic and paraventricular nuclei of the hypothalamus and the posterior pituitary gland. Hormones secreted by the posterior pituitary gland include vasopressin (antidiuretic hormone) and oxytocin. Most of the anterior pituitary hormones are mainly controlled by releasing hormones, apart from prolactin, which is mainly controlled by prolactin-inhibiting hormone. The releasing hormones secreted by the hypothalamus into the portal hypophyseal vessel include corticotrophin-releasing hormone (CRH), TRH, luteinising hormone-releasing hormone (LHRH) and growth hormone-releasing hormone (GRH). There are only two types of inhibiting hormones: prolactin-inhibiting hormone (PIH) and growth hormone–inhibiting hormone (GHIH). ACTH is secreted by the anterior pituitary gland and its release is controlled by CRH.

13.6 A C
Vasopressin is secreted in the posterior pituitary gland by nerve cells and released directly into the circulation. Like oxytocin, it consists of nine amino acids (i.e. a nonapeptide). It has a short half-life (less than half an hour), and hence the plasma osmolality can be sensitively controlled. Its main effect is to decrease the urinary excretion of water.

13.7 A C
Factors controlling the secretion of vasopressin are similar to those controlling thirst: plasma osmolality and extracellular volume. Hence an increase of the osmotic pressure in the plasma results in stimulus of the osmoreceptors and release of vasopressin. Reduced extracellular volume is detected by the baroreceptors, which mediates the release of vasopressin. The occurs partly due to the release of angiotensin II. Standing slightly reduces the stimulation of the baroreceptors, and hence increases the secretion of vasopressin slightly. Alcohol reduces the secretion of vasopressin. This explains why diuresis occurs after alcohol consumption.

13.8 B
In diabetes insipidus, urinary excretion of water is increased due to reduced reabsorption in the collecting ducts. Hence the urinary volume increases, the urinary osmolality decreases and the plasma osmolality increases. This stimulates thirst, and the subject often drinks a large quantity of water (polydipsia). In most cases, the cause is reduced or absent secretion of vasopressin. In nephrogenic

SYSTEM-BASED MEDICAL SCIENCES

13

The endocrine system

diabetes insipidus, the plasma concentration of vasopressin is normal, but the kidneys fail to respond to the hormone due to a congenital defect of their receptors. Hence treatment with synthetic vasopressin does not usually alleviate the symptoms.

13.9   A B D E
The syndrome of inappropriate ADH secretion is said to occur if the secretion of vasopressin is high in spite of a low osmolality. This may occur because factors other than osmolality facilitate the secretion of vasopressin. An example is in the post-operative period when pain and reduced extracellular volume maintain a high level of vasopressin secretion. It may also occur as a result of autonomous secretion of vasopressin by bronchial carcinoma. There are also other causes such as head injury and cerebral tumour. The high level of vasopressin reduces the urinary excretion of water. Hence the extracellular volume and plasma sodium increase due to dilution effect. Demeclocycline (a tetracycline) has been found to reduce the response of the kidneys to vasopressin, and is often useful in treating the condition.

13.10   B D
The main sites of action for oxytocin are the breast and the uterus. Prolactin increases the volume of milk produced by the breast, whilst oxytocin facilitates the ejection of milk available in the breast. Oxytocin causes contraction of the uterine muscle, and the uterine muscle becomes more sensitive to oxytocin during pregnancy. Hence synthetic oxytocin is often used to accelerate labour, and also in the treatment of postpartum haemorrhage in conjunction with ergometrine.

13.11   A C
The pituitary gland is connected to the inferior surface of the brain via the infundibulum, and is well protected in the sella turcica of the sphenoid bone. It lies inferior to the optic chiasma. Hence a large pituitary tumour may involve the optic chiasma and give rise to characteristic visual field defects (bitemporal hemianopia). As a structure of the brain, it is supplied by branches of the internal carotid artery. Embryologically, the anterior and intermediate lobes of the pituitary gland develop from an evagination from the roof of the pharynx (Raphke's pouch), whilst the posterior lobe develops from an evagination of the floor of the third ventricle. Hence only the posterior pituitary belongs to the brain embryologically. This explains why posterior pituitary hormones are secreted directly from neurones with cell nuclei in the hypothalamus, whilst the anterior pituitary hormones are secreted in response to tropic hormones from the hypothalamus in the portal hypophyseal circulation.

13.12   B E
The main hormones secreted by the thyroid gland are T_4, T_3 and RT_3. T_4 constitutes over 90% of the hormones secreted, whilst T_3 accounts for less than 4% and RT_3 accounts for less than 2%. However, T_3 is more active than T_4, whilst RT_3 is inactive. Most of the plasma T_3 is produced by peripheral conversion from T_4 in tissues such as the liver and the kidneys. About 99.8% of plasma T_4 is bound to proteins. Hence the total plasma thyroid hormone may not reflect the true thyroid status of the subject. Measurement of free thyroid hormones or an indirect measure of their free concentration is important.

13.13   D
Thyroid hormones act by entering the cell and binding to receptors in the nucleus; the resulting hormone–receptor complex then binds to the DNA. This affects the rate of protein synthesis. In general, thyroid hormones increase the overall metabolic rate and rate of oxygen consumption. This is partly achieved by an increases in Na^+,K^+-ATPase activity. The rate of absorption of carbohydrates and mobilisation of fatty acids are increased.

13.14   A C
In general, thyroid hormones increase the rate of catabolism and decrease the rate of anabolism. Hence carbohydrates are absorbed and utilised at a high rate. The rate of fatty acid and protein breakdown is increased, but their rate of synthesis is reduced.

13.15   C D E
The actions of thyroid hormones and catecholamines are very similar and are closely interrelated. They both increase the metabolic rate. This is because thyroid hormones (T_3 and T_4) increase both the numbers of β-adrenergic receptors and the affinity of catecholamines to the receptors. Hence the tissue becomes more sensitive to catecholamines. This is important clinically. Thyroid hormones cause increased heart rate, sweating and tremor mainly through this effect, and this effect can be reduced by β-adrenergic antagonists. Hence it is essential to administer propranolol or other β-adrenergic antagonists in the immediate treatment of severe hyperthyroidism to protect against cardiotoxicity.

13.16   B C
The secretion of thyroid hormones is mostly regulated by the negative feedback control exerted by free T_3 and T_4 on both the hypothalamus and the pituitary gland. The main control mechanism is that an increase in either free T_3 or T_4 inhibits the secretion of TRH from the hypothalamus, which results in a reduction in both the synthesis and secretion of TSH from the pituitary gland. However, an

SELF-ASSESSMENT IN INTEGRATED MEDICAL SCIENCES

The endocrine system

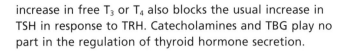

increase in free T_3 or T_4 also blocks the usual increase in TSH in response to TRH. Catecholamines and TBG play no part in the regulation of thyroid hormone secretion.

13.17   A D E
Many of the clinical features of hyperthyroidism can be deduced from the known effects of thyroid hormones. Increased sensitivity of the β-adrenergic receptors to catecholamines gives rise to increased heart rate, tremor, mental agitation and sweating. Weight loss and heat intolerance result from increased metabolic rate. Diarrhoea, palpitations, muscle weakness and increased tendon reflex are other features of hyperthyroidism.

13.18   B E
Hypothyroidism is most commonly due to primary disease of the thyroid, especially Hashimoto's disease (an autoimmune disorder). However, hypothyroidism may also be secondary to pituitary or hypothalamic failure. The biochemical abnormalities differ depending on the site of the disease. In primary hypothyroidism, all total and free thyroid hormones are low. This causes an increase in the secretion of TRH from the hypothalamus and TSH from the pituitary gland via its feedback loop. The TSH response to TRH is exaggerated. The concentration of plasma-binding proteins is not affected.

13.19   B E
Carbimazole belongs to a class of drugs known as thionamides. Its antithyroid action is due to a reduction in the synthesis of thyroid hormone both by inhibiting the incorporation of iodine and the conversion of T_3 and T_4 to iodotyrosines. The drug produces no significant clinical effects until the existing stores are exhausted, which may take up to three months. A decrease in T_4 results in increased synthesis and secretion of TSH from the pituitary gland, which may cause thyroid gland enlargement. Carbimazole and other thionamides rarely cause an acute aplastic anaemia or reduced granulocyte count, which may be fatal. Therefore it is essential to check the white cell count should a patient on carbimazole develop symptoms suggestive of an infection such as sore throat.

13.20   A B D
Grave's disease is the commonest cause of hyperthyroidism. It is a thyroid-specific autoimmune disease, and is usually associated with the production of long-acting thyroid stimulator (LATS). Autoantibodies to thyroglobulin are associated with Hashimoto's disease. Like most autoimmune disorders, it occurs more commonly in women than men. It causes a diffuse enlargement and increased vascularity of the thyroid gland. Clinically, the increased vascularity may be detected by a bruit over the gland. LATS mimics TSH by stimulating thyroid to secrete thyroid hormones. It also causes exophthalmos (accumulation of fat in orbital tissues), pretibial myxoedema and clubbing of the fingers (accumulation of mucopolysaccharides in the dermis).

13.21   A C
LATS is an autoantibody to thyroid epithelial cells and is characteristically associated with Grave's disease. It is an IgG, and hence may cross the placenta and give rise to symptoms of hyperthyroidism in the infant. It stimulates the thyroid gland to increase the formation of thyroid hormones. It is also associated with infiltration of the orbital tissues by fat (which results in exophthalmos) and accumulation of mucopolysaccharides in the dermis (which results in pretibial myxoedema and clubbing).

13.22   B C D E
Most thyroid tumours are benign, and thyroid carcinomas are quite rare. Amongst the thyroid carcinomas, about 60% are papillary carcinomas. They usually occur in young adults, and have the best prognosis. Follicular carcinoma constitutes about a quarter of all thyroid carcinomas. They occur in young adults and middle-aged people. They often spread via the bloodstream to the bones or lungs. However, they respond well to radioactive iodine. Anaplastic carcinomas constitutes only about 10–15% of all thyroid carcinomas. They usually occur in the elderly, and have the worst prognosis. Medullary carcinomas are derived from the C-cells and commonly secrete calcitonin. They are often associated with other endocrine neoplasia such as phaeochromocytoma.

13.23   A B C D E
The thyroid gland consists of two lobes connected by a narrow isthmus. It is surround by a sheath derived from the pretracheal fascia, which also adheres to the larynx. This explains why the thyroid gland moves with the larynx on swallowing. This phenomenon is valuable in deciding whether a neck swelling originates from the thyroid clinically. The thyroid gland develops from an endodermal outgrowth from the floor of the pharynx. The site of origin is on the tongue, the foramen caecum. Normally, the thyroid descends to its normal adult position. Incomplete descent may result in thyroid tissue being found at any point between the base of the tongue and the trachea. The isthmus lies anterior to the second and fourth rings of the trachea; the lobes of the thyroid gland lie lateral to the trachea. Hence clinical enlargement of the thyroid gland may compress the thyroid gland and cause airway obstruction. The recurrent laryngeal nerves lie posteromedial to the lobes in the groove between the trachea and the oesophagus, and may be liable to damage in a thyroidectomy operation.

185

13 **A**

SYSTEM-BASED MEDICAL SCIENCES

The endocrine system

13.24   C D
About 99% of the total body calcium is in the skeleton. Normally, about 90% of all calcium excreted appears in the faeces, and only 10% appears in the urine. This loss of calcium is replaced by net absorption of calcium from the diet. Calcium can be reabsorbed by either active transport or passive diffusion. There is usually a continuous exchange of calcium between the bones and extracellular fluid, although there might be little or no net transfer of calcium between two body compartments in healthy individuals. About half of the total plasma calcium is bound to proteins. This proportion increases with increasing plasma protein concentration and decreasing plasma pH.

13.25   A
Total body calcium is an index of bone mass. In osteoporosis, there is a net excess of bone resorption over bone formation, and people with osteoporosis are liable to develop fractures, especially of the femur. Normally, the bone mass increases in childhood during growth until early adulthood. Thereafter, the bone mass gradually declines. Men generally have higher bone mass than women. In women, the loss of bone mass accelerates after the menopause. Hence fracture of the femur is commoner in the elderly and in women especially after the menopause.

13.26   A B D E
Vitamin D increases the plasma calcium by its effect on the intestines, the kidneys and bone. It increases the absorption of calcium by stimulating the active transport of calcium from the intestinal lumen. The urinary excretion of calcium is reduced by increasing calcium reabsorption in the kidneys. It stimulates the maturation of both osteoblasts (which mobilise calcium from bone) and osteoclasts (which form bone utilising plasma calcium). However, the net effect is mobilisation of calcium from bone.

13.27   A B C
There are two sources of vitamin D_3: dietary and conversion from 7-dehydrocolecholesterol. Sunlight is required for the latter. Vitamin D_3 is converted to 25-hydroxycolecalciferol in the liver. It is then converted in the proximal tubules of the kidneys either to the active form, 1,25-dihydroxycolecalciferol, or to the relatively inactive form, 24,25-dihydroxycolecalciferol. The quantity of 24,25-dihydroxycolecalciferol is tightly controlled by the plasma calcium and phosphate level.

13.28   D
The most active form of vitamin D is 1,25-dihydroxycolecalciferol. It is tightly regulated, and is synthesised by conversion in the renal tubules from 25-hydroxycolecalciferol. The level of 25-hydroxycolecalciferol itself is not tightly regulated. When the synthesis of the 1,25-dihydroxycolecalciferol is increased, the synthesis of the inactive 24,25-dihydroxycolecalciferol is decreased, and vice versa. When the plasma calcium is high, the secretion of parathyroid hormone is decreased. This decreases the synthesis of 1,25-dihydroxycolecalciferol in the kidneys. A high plasma level of phosphate directly inhibits the synthesis of 1,25-dihydroxycolecalciferol in the kidneys.

13.29   D
There are normally two superior and two inferior parathyroid glands. They normally lie posterior to and within the fascial sheath of the thyroid gland. Hence the parathyroid glands can be accidentally removed in thyroidectomy. The superior glands are usually in their normal position. However, the inferior glands are sometimes found more caudal to their normal position, and are occasionally found amongst the thymic tissue in the superior mediastinum. This is because the inferior parathyroid glands and the thymus are closely related in their development, as they are both derived from the third pharyngeal pouch. During thyroidectomy, it is important for the surgeons to locate the parathyroid glands. The parathyroid glands only secrete parathyroid hormones. Calcitonin is secreted by the C-cells of the thyroid gland.

13.30   E
Parathyroid hormone (PTH) is a peptide with 84 amino acids. It is secreted by all four parathyroid glands. It increases plasma calcium and decreases plasma phosphate levels via its direct actions on bones and kidneys, and its indirect action on the intestines. It has an overall effect of mobilising calcium from the bones. PTH decreases the reabsorption of phosphates and increases the reabsorption of calcium from the kidneys. Hence the urinary excretion of phosphate is increased but the urinary excretion of calcium is decreased. PTH does not act directly on the intestine, but it increases the synthesis of 1,25-dihydroxycolecalciferol. This causes an increase in calcium absorption from the intestine.

13.31   A D
In hypoparathyroidism, the level of PTH is low. This leads to a low plasma calcium level, reduced urinary phosphate excretion and a high plasma phosphate level. In pseudohypoparathyroidism, the PTH receptors in the tissues fail to respond to the hormone. Hence, although the parathyroid hormone level is normal or increased, all other biochemical features are similar to hypoparathyroidism. Plasma protein level is not affected.

13.32   B C E
Calcitonin is secreted by the C-cells (parafollicular cells) of the thyroid gland. It acts mainly on the bones and the kidneys to lower the plasma calcium and phosphate levels. It inhibits the osteoclasts and hence inhibits bone resorption. As the disorganised new bone formation in Paget's disease is due to an increased osteoclastic activity, calcitonin is useful in the treatment of Paget's disease. Calcitonin also increases the urinary excretion of calcium, but it has no direct action on the intestine.

13.33   C D E
Calcium is essential for neuromuscular transmission. A low plasma calcium level has an excitatory effect on muscle and nerve cells. Hence hypocalcaemia may give rise to a 'pins and needles sensation', tetany or convulsions. Hypercalcaemia is associated with tiredness, muscle weakness, thirst or polyuria, and constipation.

13.34   A B E
Hypercalcaemia may be caused by primary or secondary bone diseases, excessive PTH secretion, excessive vitamin D or increased sensitivity of receptors to vitamin D. Bone metastases and multiple myeloma are important causes of hypercalcaemia. Excessive PTH may be due to primary or tertiary hyperparathyroidism or ectopic PTH secretion from malignancies. Increased sensitivity of tissues to vitamin D occurs in sarcoidosis.

13.35   C D
Primary hyperparathyroidism is usually caused by parathyroid hyperplasia or a parathyroid adenoma. The plasma calcium level is high, and the plasma PTH level is inappropriately high for the level of plasma calcium. Parathyroidectomy may be required. Secondary hyperparathyroidism is due to a physiological response to a low plasma calcium level caused by a disease outside the parathyroid gland. The parathyroid gland attempts to compensate for the low calcium level by producing more PTH. Renal failure is a common cause. Treatment of the underlying disease is essential. The parathyroid gland in chronic secondary hyperparathyroidsm may become autonomous. This is tertiary hyperparathyroidism, when the plasma calcium level is high.

13.36   B D E
Medical treatment for hypercalcaemia is only a temporary measure to allow more time for the underlying cause to be treated. The first line of treatment is to rehydrate with intravenous saline in order to increase the urinary excretion of calcium. This can be augmented with a loop diuretic such as furosemide (frusemide). However, thiazide diuretics must not be used as it increases renal reabsorption of calcium. Calcitonin reduces plasma calcium by inhibiting bone resorption and increasing urinary calcium excretion. Bisphosphonates may also be used, although they are more useful in hypercalcaemia due to malignancy. Adrenocortical steroid acts by reducing intestinal absorption of calcium, and is useful in hypercalcaemia due to vitamin D intoxication or sarcoidosis with associated hypersensitivity to vitamin D. However, adrenocortical steroid is not useful in hyperparathyroidism. Dialysis may be required for severe cases or in the presence of renal failure.

13.37   A C E
Bisphosphonates reduce the reabsorption of bone by adsorbing onto bone crystals and by inhibiting osteoclast activity. Hence they have been used to treat Paget's disease (which is characterised by increased bone resorption and formation), osteoporosis (with abnormal reduction in the bone mass) and hypercalcaemia due to neoplasia. Osteomalacia is caused by vitamin D deficiency, and the treatment is vitamin D.

13.38   A C D
The islets of Langerhans of the pancreas secrete at least four hormones. Insulin and glucagon are important for regulating the metabolism of carbohydrates, fats and proteins. Somatostatin is important for regulating islet cell secretion. The fourth hormone, pancreatic polypeptide, is primarily concerned with gastrointestinal function. Gastrin is secreted by G-cells in the stomach. Cholecystokinin–pancreozymin is secreted in the upper small intestine, and mediates the contraction of the gallbladder and enzymatic secretion of the pancreas.

13.39   B D E
Insulin consists of two amino acid chains linked by disulphide bridges. There are only minor variations in amino acid sequences amongst species. For example, pig insulin only differs from human insulin by one amino acid, and beef insulin by three amino acids. Hence pig and beef insulin are active when given to diabetic humans. However, humans almost invariably develop antibodies to beef insulin after a few months of treatment, although the antigenicity of pig insulin is lower. This reduces the effectiveness of the treatment. Fortunately, this problem can now be avoided as human insulin can be manufactured by recombinant DNA technique.

13.40   C
The overall net effect of insulin is to increase storage of carbohydrates, protein and fat. Hence the transport of glucose and amino acids into cells is increased. The transport of potassium into cells is also increased, and insulin and glucose together are sometimes used to treat hyperkalaemia. Protein synthesis is increased, and protein

13 The endocrine system

degradation is reduced. The synthesis of both glycogen and fat is increased.

13.41 B D
Insulin receptors are found in a large variety of cells, and are found on the cell membranes. Each receptor consists of two α- and two β-glycoprotein subunits, but these are synthesised by a single mRNA. When insulin binds to its receptors, they aggregate and are endocytosed into the cytoplasm, where they exert their effects of increasing transport of glucose, amino acids into cells, as well as their effects on other mediators. The insulin–receptor complexes are eventually destroyed in lysosomes. The number and affinity of insulin receptors are closely regulated. Hence the number of receptors decreases with increasing plasma insulin level, and the affinity of receptors increases with decreasing plasma insulin level. The number of receptors decreases in obesity. This is partly explained by a higher plasma insulin level.

13.42 B D
Glucose tolerance refers to the rate of decline of the plasma glucose level to normal after an oral glucose meal. In the glucose tolerance test, a standard glucose load is given orally, and the rate of decline of the plasma glucose level is monitored. The result depends mainly on the rate of entry of glucose into the cells (peripheral utilisation) and the rate of glycogen synthesis by the liver. The rate of glucose absorption is not an important factor. The rates of glucose uptake by the brain and red blood cells do not usually vary much with plasma glucose level.

13.43 A B C D
Some of the clinical features of diabetes result directly from the high plasma glucose level. When the renal threshold for glucose is exceeded, glucose may appear in the urine, and may be detected with a dipstick. High plasma glucose increases the plasma osmolality. This leads to the stimulation of thirst as well as osmotic diuresis. If the plasma level is elevated over a period of time, small amounts of haemoglobin A may be glycosylated to form HbA_{1c}. This is used clinically to monitor diabetic patients in clinical practice, as elevated levels of HbA_{1c} may indicate poor control of diabetes over the previous six weeks.

13.44 B C E
Deficiency of insulin in diabetes mellitus leads to decreased entry of glucose into cells. Hence there is intracellular glucose deficiency. Glycogen synthesis is reduced, and glycogen breakdown increases. Breakdown of adipose tissue and fats leads to an accumulation of acetyl-CoA. Entry to the citric acid cycle is decreased due to a deficiency of enzyme converting acetyl-CoA to malonyl-CoA. Hence, the excess acetyl-CoA is converted to ketone bodies, which also appear in the urine. The ketone bodies can be detected in diabetic patients clinically. Deficiency of insulin also leads to decreased entry of amino acids into cells. These amino acids may be used to synthesis glucose in the liver. Hence there is a net breakdown of protein, and there is an overall negative nitrogen balance.

13.45 A C E
In diabetic ketoacidosis, the accumulation of ketone bodies causes excessive hydrogen ions to be released in the plasma. The low plasma pH stimulates the respiratory centre, and results in abnormally deep and fast breathing. Urinary loss of sodium and potassium is excessive partly due to the polyuria associated with increased plasma osmolality. Hence the total body sodium and potassium are depleted. However, the plasma potassium is usually normal. This is partly because the extracellular volume is diminished, and partly because the low insulin level and high plasma H^+ favour potassium to stay in the extracellular fluid rather than in cells.

13.46 –
Sulphonylureas include drugs such as tolbutamide and chlorpropamide. They lower the blood glucose mainly by releasing stored insulin from the islet cells. However, they do not increase insulin synthesis. Hence they should not be used in patients with total deficiency of insulin (e.g. type I diabetes). Sulphonylureas also seem to increase the sensitivity of tissues to insulin. They cause hypoglycaemia in the same way in normal subjects. Sulphonylureas frequently cause weight gain. As diabetes is usually associated with progressive loss of β-cell function, the effectiveness of sulphonylureas usually decreases with time.

13.47 C D
Metformin is the commonest biguanide used in clinical practice. It reduces plasma glucose by decreasing the production of glucose in the liver and enhancing peripheral utilisation of glucose. It does not increase the formation of insulin, and hence is unsuitable for insulin-dependent diabetes mellitus. As it has an anorexic effect and may reduce weight in obese patients, its main use is for obese patients with non-insulin-dependent diabetes mellitus. It may be used in combination with sulphonylureas. It usually does not cause hypoglycaemia on its own. However, it may occasionally cause lactic acidosis, especially if there are other underlying diseases such as septicaemia, liver or renal failure.

13.48 A D E
Type I diabetes is due to impaired β-cell function and inadequate insulin secretion. Subjects often present in

childhood with diabetic ketoacidosis, and usually require long-term insulin treatment. There are several hypotheses regarding its aetiology. Subjects often have circulating antibodies to different islet cells, and the disease is thought to be autoimmune. Subjects with certain HLA types (e.g. HLA-DR4) are more likely to develop the disease. The autoimmune disease is thought to be triggered by certain viruses such as Coxsackie B viruses. The monozygotic twin concordance rate is 40%. By contrast, type II diabetes secretes a normal amount of insulin, but there is a reduction in the number of insulin receptors. The disease usually develops in middle age, and ketoacidosis is uncommon. Genetic factors play an extremely important part, as the monozygotic concordance is almost 100%. There is no evidence that it is an autoimmune disease.

13.49 A B C D E
Diabetes mellitus affects both large and small blood vessels. Hence patients with diabetes often develop atherosclerosis at an earlier age, and hence are more at risk of myocardial infarction, cerebrovascular disease and peripheral vascular diseases. It also affects small blood vessels of the kidneys and the retina. Hence subjects may develop nephropathy and retinopathy.

13.50 A B C D E
Glucagon is a polypeptide with 29 amino acids. In the liver, glucagon mediates its effect by increasing cAMP. Glucagon increases the breakdown of glycogen in the liver, which also increases the plasma glucose level. It also increases the conversion of amino acids in the liver to glucose, and increases ketone body formation and the breakdown of fats. Physiologically, it is important that the available glucose is taken up and used by the cells. This is achieved as glucagon is a potent stimulator of insulin secretion, and insulin increases the uptake of glucose by the cells. Glucagon is broken down in the liver. Hence, in patients with liver diseases, the amount of glucagon reaching the circulation may be increased.

13.51 C D E
The secretion of glucagon is mainly stimulated by a reduced plasma glucose level. This provides a feedback mechanism to control the plasma glucose level. Although a high plasma insulin level would result in a reduced plasma glucose level, insulin increases the secretion of GABA from A-cells, which in turn inhibits glucagon secretion. Stimulation of the β-adrenergic receptors results in increased secretion of glucagon. This is important in the 'fight, fright, flight' response of the sympathetic nervous system. Exercise increases the secretion of glucagon at least partly via stimulating the sympathetic nervous system. A high level of plasma amino acids increases the

secretion of glucagon, as glucagon is necessary for the conversion of amino acids into glucose.

13.52 A B C D E
When the plasma glucose decreases, the first symptoms to appear are due to increased sympathetic discharge. Hence sweating, palpitations and nervousness occur. As glucose is the only source of fuel for the neural tissues, neurological symptoms appear if the plasma glucose decreases further. Lethargy, coma, convulsions and permanent brain damage may occur depending on the level of hypoglycaemia.

13.53 A B D E
Whilst insulin is the only hormone which lowers the plasma glucose level, there are at least four hormones which increase the plasma glucose level: glucagon, adrenaline (epinephrine), growth hormone and cortisol. All four hormones increase the breakdown of glycogen in the liver. Growth hormone and cortisol increase peripheral utilisation of glucose.

13.54 E
The physiological effects of growth hormone include the growth of long bones before the epiphyses have fused, and metabolic effects on carbohydrates, fat and protein metabolism. Linear growth of the long bones is no longer possible after the epiphyses have fused. Hence excessive growth hormone may cause bone and soft tissue deformities as in acromegaly. Growth hormone increases the breakdown of glycogen in the liver, and hence increases the plasma glucose level. Although growth hormone enhances the response of the tissues to insulin, it has no effect on the plasma insulin level. Growth hormone breaks down fat and increases the plasma fatty acid level, which can be used by tissues as an alternative source of energy.

13.55 A B C D
Somatomedins are polypeptide growth factors which are secreted by the liver and other tissue in response to growth hormone. One of the factors (IGF-1) can stimulate both skeletal and cartilage growth. It is not clear exactly what role somatomedins play in mediating the actions of growth hormone. Somatomedins are decreased in untreated diabetes mellitus, which partly accounts for the increased breakdown of protein.

13.56 C D E
The adrenal medulla secretes catecholamines (adrenaline (epinephrine), noradrenaline (norepinephrine) and dopamine). The adrenal cortex consists of an outer layer (zona glomerulosa), a middle layer (zona fasciculata) and an inner layer (zona reticularis). The zona glomerulosa secretes mineralocorticoid. Sex hormones are secreted by

13 The endocrine system

both the zona fasciculata and zona reticularis. Glucocorticoids are secreted by all three layers.

13.57 A D

Both adrenaline (epinephrine) and noradrenaline (norepinephrine) are produced by the adrenal medulla and the sympathetic nervous system. Whilst the physiological effects of adrenaline and noradrenaline are very similar, there are some minor differences. Both adrenaline and noradrenaline act on the β_1 receptors to increase the force and rate of cardiac contractions. However, noradrenaline produces vasoconstriction in most organs (via α_1 receptors) whilst adrenaline dilates the blood vessels in skeletal muscles and the liver (via β_2 receptors). Hence, whilst the peripheral resistance increases with noradrenaline, it may decrease with adrenaline. Whilst noradrenaline produces an increase of both systolic and diastolic blood pressure, adrenaline tends to produce an increase in systolic blood pressure but decreases the diastolic pressure, hence widening the pulse pressure. Adrenaline tends to produce a higher level of fear and anxiety. It has been found that the ratio of noradrenaline to adrenaline is increased in certain situations (e.g. hypoxia). The significance of this is still not properly understood.

13.58 A B C E

In the synthesis of glucocorticoids, ACTH acts on receptors on the plasma membrane of a cortisol-secreting cells in the zona fasciculata or zona reticularis of the adrenal cortex. This leads to activation of membrane adenyl cyclase, and an increase in intracellular cAMP. The cAMP activates protein kinase, which converts cholesterol esters to cholesterol. Cholesterol is the precursor of all steroids. The cholesterol is transported into mitochondria by a carrier protein. The enzymes responsible for the synthesis of various glucocorticoids and mineralocorticoids are the mitochondrial cytochrome P_{450}s. The products are shuttled between the mitochondria and the smooth endoplasmic reticulum, before the final products are released outside the cell. Mineralocorticoids (e.g. aldosterone) are synthesised by enzymatic conversion of corticosterone.

13.59 A B C D E

Systemic adrenal steroids are used in a wide variety of conditions for their anti-inflammatory and immunosuppressive actions. These include collagen disorders and other autoimmune disorders such as idiopathic thrombocytopenia purpura, anaphylactic shock, organ rejection, severe asthma attack, severe dermatitis, active chronic hepatitis, sarcoidosis and rheumatic fever. Adrenal steroids are occasionally used to replace physiological deficiencies as in Addison's disease.

13.60 C D E

Long-term administration of steroids may induce features of Cushing's syndrome. These include characteristic deposition of fat in the body and face (moon face), striae, hypertension, acne and hirsuitism, and osteoporosis of bone with associated fractures. Other recognised side effects include peptic ulceration, mental symptoms (e.g. depression or psychosis), and increased susceptibility to infection.

13.61 D

Cortisol is normally secreted in the adrenal cortex in response to ACTH. Hence psychologically stressful situations and ectopic ACTH-secreting tumours are associated with raised ACTH and cortisol levels. On the other hand, panhypopituitarism is associated with reduced ACTH and cortisol levels. In Addison's disease, the secretion of cortisol by the adrenal cortex is reduced. This stimulates ACTH secretion. Hence the cortisol level is low but the ACTH level is high. In primary adrenal tumour, the cortisol level may be high. Plasma ACTH level is low due to feedback inhibition from the raised plasma cortisol level.

13.62

A
The thyroid gland develops from an endodermal outgrowth from the floor of the pharynx. The site of origin is on the tongue, the foramen caecum. Normally, the thyroid descends to its normal adult position, which is below the cricoid bone.

B
Levo thyroxine (thyroxine) (T_4), tri-iodothyronine (T_3) and reverse tri-iodothyronine (RT_3). T_3 is the most active.

C
Overactive.

D
In the thyroid gland. This would explain a low TSH level due to feedback inhibition by the increased T_4 level. In hyperthyroidism caused by pituitary or hypothalamic lesions, the TSH level is abnormally high.

E
The excess thyroid hormones cause an increase in the number and affinity of β-adrenergic receptors in the heart. Hence, the sensitivity of the heart to circulating catecholamines is increased.
  A β-receptor antagonist (e.g. propranolol) may reduce the patient's heart rate quickly.

F
Increased.

G

Autoimmune thyroid disease (Graves' disease). (Other possible answers: solitary toxic adenoma, toxic multinodular goitre, thyroiditis.)

13.63

A

The patient is hypothyroid because both the plasma T_3 and T_4 levels are abnormally low.

B

As the plasma TSH level is also low, the likely cause is secondary hypothyroidism due to pituitary failure to secrete TSH. The plasma TSH level is normally grossly elevated in primary hypothyroidism.

C

A TRH stimulation test is necessary to confirm this diagnosis. Baseline levels of T_4 and TSH are first taken; 200 g TRH is given intravenously; TSH levels are measured 20 and 60 min after TRH is administered and levels of less than 3.9 and 3.0 miu/l, respectively, indicate some degree of pituitary deficiency in TSH secretion.

13.64

A

Iodine is a raw material essential for the synthesis of all thyroid hormones: deficiency of dietary iodine results in inadequate secretion of these hormones. TSH secretion from the anterior pituitary increases as its secretion is normally suppressed by a negative feedback mechanism by T_4. The increased TSH level causes the thyroid gland to hypertrophy, giving rise to a large goitre.

B

The T_4 level would be low and the TSH level would be high.

13.65

A

i • Facilitating entry of glucose into the peripheral tissues.
  • Releasing glucose into the circulation from the liver (hepatic glucogenesis).
ii • Increasing fatty synthesis in adipose tissue.
  • Increasing lipid synthesis and decreasing production of ketone bodies in the liver.
  • increasing uptake of ketone in muscle.
iii • Increasing protein synthesis in the liver.
  • Increasing amino acid uptake and protein synthesis in muscle.
  • Reducing catabolism of amino acids to carbon dioxide and water.

B

The insulin receptors are found on cell membranes and consist of two α and two β glycoprotein subunits. Insulin acts by first binding to these receptors and triggering the tyrosine kinase activity of the β subunits. This produces autophosphorylation, which in turn triggers a variety of responses, including phosphorylation of some cytoplasmic proteins, dephosphorylation of other cytoplasmic proteins, glucose transport, activation of other effector systems and secondary mediators, and events in the nucleus such as DNA synthesis and gene transcription.

C

i The presence of large amounts of glucose in the renal tubules exerts considerable osmotic effects, which tend to hold water in the renal tubules. Hence, osmotic diuresis occurs.
ii Excessive loss of water through osmotic diuresis and the high plasma level of glucose result in dehydration and an increase in osmolality, both of which induce thirst.
iii The lack of insulin results in a reduction in protein synthesis and an increased catabolism of amino acids to carbon dioxide and water. Hence, the child fails to gain weight.
iv Increased breakdown of fat into fatty acids and acetyl-CoA results in increased production of ketone bodies (including acetoacetate and β-hydroxybutyrate). When the capacity to buffer these acids is exceeded, metabolic acidosis results and ketones appear in the urine.

D

Glucocorticoids, growth hormone, somatostatin, glucagon and catecholamines may all raise the blood glucose level. Insulin is the only hormone that lowers blood glucose level, which is why the effects of the inadequate insulin cannot be compensated for in diabetes mellitus.

13.66

A

Tolbutamide is a sulphonyurea. It reduces plasma glucose concentration by stimulating the B-cells of the islets in the pancreas to secrete insulin. Metformin is a biguanide. It acts mainly by increasing glucose uptake in skeletal muscle. It also inhibits glucose output from the liver and glucose absorption from the intestines.

B

The reason for the patient's unconsciousness is likely to be hypoglycaemia (low blood glucose) induced by the oral hypoglycaemic drugs. This is confirmed by the effectiveness of glucagon in the patient's treatment.

13 **A** SYSTEM-BASED MEDICAL SCIENCES

The endocrine system

C

Glucagon acts on specific membrane receptors via G protein to activate adenylate cyclase. Glucagon's action is similar to that of adrenaline (epinephrine) mediated via β-adrenoceptors. Its main actions are to stimulate glycogen breakdown and gluconeogenesis and to inhibit glycogen synthesis and glucose oxidation.

13.67
A

HbA_{1C} is formed by non-enzymatic glycosylation of haemoglobin A. Hence, each molecule has a glucose attached to the terminal valine in each chain. The rate of HbA_{1C} formation increases with the length of time the plasma glucose level is elevated. Hence, HbA_{1C} levels in diabetic patients reflect the level of control of their diabetes in the recent 8 weeks (half-life of red blood cells).

B

The HbA_{1C} level of this patient is above the normal reference range. This may suggest that his diabetes has been relatively poorly controlled within the past 8 weeks.

C

The mechanisms responsible for the complications are:
- Myocardial infarct and ischaemic legs: accelerated atheroma formation in the large blood vessels
- Renal damage and retinopathy: damage to the endothelial cells and basal lamina of small blood vessels
- Impaired sensation in the legs: disease of the small blood vessels of the nerves supplying the legs.

13.68
A

The blood glucose level increases after ingestion of food, and the rate and extent of this increase depend on numerous factors; it is therefore difficult to interpret a random blood glucose level.

B

The glucose tolerance test assesses the rate of entry of glucose into cells (i.e. peripheral utilisation). A standard load of glucose is given orally and the rate of disappearance of the glucose reflects entry into cells, especially skeletal and cardiac cells. Since insulin facilitates the entry of glucose into cells, the peripheral utilisation is impaired in diabetes mellitus. The glucose tolerance test might be a better test then fasting glucose level in patients with partial lack of insulin because the fasting glucose may be normal in spite of impaired glucose uptake into cells.

C

For this patient, the fasting glucose was borderline but the glucose tolerance test shows that the patient has reduced rate of uptake of glucose into cells. He can thus be diagnosed as suffering from diabetes (according to WHO guidelines).

13.69
A

A deficiency of vitamin D may result in a decreased serum calcium level because 1,25-dihydroxycholecalciferol normally:
- facilitates calcium reabsorption in the kidneys
- increases calcium (and phosphate) absorption from the intestines (probably by increasing the number of Ca^{2+},H^+-ATPase)
- mobilises calcium (and phosphate) from the bones by increasing the activity of osteoclasts.

B

Rickets is a condition in children in which there is inadequate mineralisation (due to lack of calcium) of the organic bone matrix. The disease is characterised by bone deformities. The corresponding condition in adults is osteomalacia.

C

The phosphate level in children with rickets is usually low.

D

See Fig 13.1. Rickets may result from:
- Dietary deficiency and intestinal malabsorption: synthesis depends on a constant supply of cholecalciferol or 7-dehydrocholesterol
- lack of sunlight: ultraviolet light is required to convert 7-dehydrocholesterol to previtamin D_3
- liver disease: the conversion of vitamin D3 to 25-hydroxycholecalciferol takes place in the liver
- renal disease: the conversion of 25-hydroxycholecalciferol to either 24,25-dihydroxycholecalciferol or 1,25-Dihydroxycholecalciferol takes place in the kidneys.

13.70
A

The most likely diagnosis is primary hyperparathyroidism. The high level of parathyroid hormone points to hyperparathyroidism. The high plasma calcium level and low plasma phosphate level suggests primary hyperparathyroidism. Primary hyperparathyroidism is a condition with excessive secretion of parathyroid hormone (PTH) by an adenoma or hyperplasia of the parathyroid gland. (*Note* The calcium level is abnormally low in

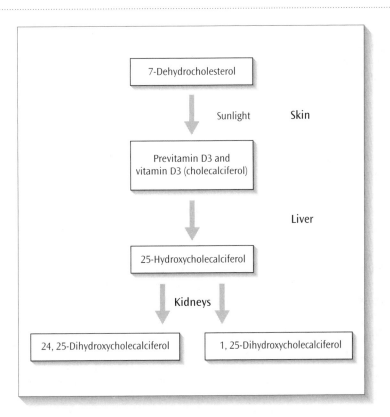

Fig. 13.1 Synthesis of vitamin D.

secondary hyerparathyroidism. The increased PTH level in this condition reflects the physiological response of the parathyroid glands to a low calcium level.)

B
PTH results in a high serum calcium level and a low phosphate level because it:
- increases the reabsorption of calcium in the distal tubules and decreases the reabsorption of phosphates in the proximal tubules
- acts directly on bone to increase bone reabsorption
- increases the formation of 1,25-dihydroxycholecalciferol and hence increases calcium absorption from the intestine.

C
The main mechanisms for the regulation of PTH level:
- Serum ionised calcium acts directly on the calcium receptor on the parathyroid gland to reduce PTH secretion.
- 1,25-Dihydroxycholecalciferol acts directly on parathyroid glands to reduce PTH synthesis by decreasing prepro-PTH mRNA.
- Mg^{2+} level may decrease the secretion of PTH from the parathyroid gland.

D
i Furosemide (frusemide) is a loop diuretic and acts by increasing the renal excretion of calcium.
ii Pamidronate is one of the bisphosphonates. Bisphosphonates are analogues of pyrophosphates which normally inhibit mineralisation of bone. Hence, it reduces the turnover of bone by both inhibiting osteoclast and stimulating osteoblast activity.

E
Thiazides must not be used in hypercalcaemia because they tend to increase the renal reabsorption of calcium.

13.71
A
Thirst is likely to be due to hypercalcaemia. It is not due to hyperparathyroidism as the PTH level is normal. Abnormally high levels of PTH-related protein are usually the result of ectopic production from malignant tumours (such as breast, kidney and ovarian tumours).

B
The serum phosphate level is usually normal or raised due to mobilisation from bone. The alkaline phosphatase level is characteristically high.

193

C

The elevated calcium is likely to be due to the effects of parathyroid-related protein, which both increases osteoclast activity and the tubular reabsorption of urinary calcium.

13.72

A

The features of Cushing's syndrome are due to the effects of excessive circulating glucocorticoids.

B

See Fig. 13.2.

C

- Adrenal gland adenoma (or corticosteroid administration).
- Cushing's disease (i.e. excessive ACTH secretion from a pituitary tumour).
- Ectopic ACTH secretion (e.g. from small cell lung cancer or ACTH administration).

D

The patient had simultaneously raised cortisol and ACTH levels. Adrenal gland adenoma can be ruled out, as the ACTH level is usually undetectable in this condition due to cortisol suppression. In Cushing's disease, although the ACTH level is high, it seldom exceeds 250 ng/l. The most likely diagnosis is ectopic ACTH secretion.

E

To differentiate between Cushing's disease and ectopic ACTH secretion, dexamethasone suppression test is necessary. Dexamethasone is given every 6 h for 2 days. The serum cortisol and the 24 h urinary cortisol during the second day are measured. One would expect no suppression of cortisol by dexamethasone in ectopic ACTH secretion, but partial suppression in Cushing's disease.

F

Glucocorticoids have mild mineralocorticoid activity. Hence, the potassium level is likely to be low and the sodium level is likely to be high.

13.73

A

- Milk secretion after parturition (in the presence of oestrogen and progesterone priming).
- Prevention of ovulation in lactating women (hence reducing the likelihood of women conceiving while lactating).

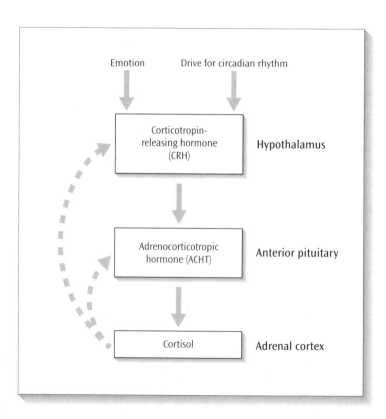

Fig. 13.2 Control of the secretion of cortisol.

B
In the anterior pituitary gland.

C
The secretion of prolactin is normally tonically inhibited by dopamine secreted by the hypothalamus. It can be affected by factors (e.g. stress, circadian rhythm, etc.) acting on the hypothalamus. Prolactin facilitates the secretion of dopamine in the hypothalamus, thus creating a negative feedback system.

D
Given that the prolactin level is grossly elevated, the diagnosis is likely to be due to a chromophobe pituitary adenoma.

E
Bromocriptine is a dopamine-receptor agonist. It stimulates the dopamine receptor in the hypothalamus, which in turn inhibits the secretion of prolactin.

13.74
A
Growth hormone is secreted from the anterior pituitary gland.

B
It is not entirely clear how growth hormone produces growth. Possible mechanisms include:
- direct action on tissues such as cartilage
- action via somatomedins

- action on cartilage to convert stem cells into cells that respond to IGF-1 and then locally produce IGF-1 to make cartilage grow.

C
Random growth hormone was elevated; however, this is not diagnostic of acromegaly as growth hormone level varies with the time of the day and other factors. Serum IGF-1 level is highly elevated.

D
Acromegaly is a condition due to excessive secretion of growth hormone, usually from a pituitary tumour.

E
This is a better test than random growth hormone as it provides a measure of growth hormone secretion over the past 24 h.

F
The oral glucose tolerance test. After oral glucose is given, blood is taken for growth hormone, glucose and insulin at 0, 30, 60, 90, 120 and 150 min. Glucose usually suppresses the secretion of growth hormone. Acromegaly can be diagnosed if the growth hormone level does not fall below 2 miu/l.

G
See Fig. 13.3. The secretion of growth hormone from the anterior pituitary gland is stimulated by growth releasing

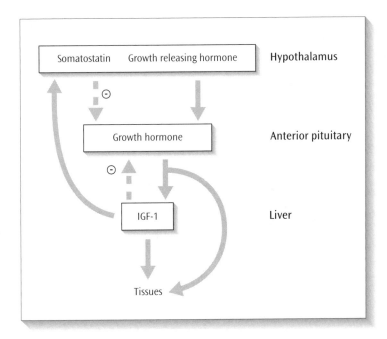

Fig. 13.3 Feedback control for the secretion of growth hormone.

The endocrine system

hormone and inhibited by somatostatin secreted by the hypothalamus. Growth hormone increases circulating insulin growth factor 1 (IGF-1), which provides two negative feedback mechanisms. First, it inhibits the secretion of growth hormone from the anterior pituitary. Second, it stimulates the secretion of somatostatin from the hypothalamus.

H
Octreotide is a long-acting analogue of somatostatin. It acts by directly inhibiting the secretion of growth hormone from the anterior pituitary gland.

13.75
A
See Fig. 13.4.

B
This patient has a high blood pressure and a low serum K⁺ level due to the effects of a high serum aldosterone level.

C
The serum renin concentration is at the lower end of normal in spite of a high aldosterone level. Hence, the high aldosterone level is not driven by excessive renin. The likely cause is primary hyperaldosteronism (e.g. due to adrenocortical adenoma, adrenocortical hyperplasia or adrenal carcinoma).

D
Spironolactone is an antagonist of aldosterone and acts by competing for intracellular aldosterone receptors in the cells of the distal tubule.

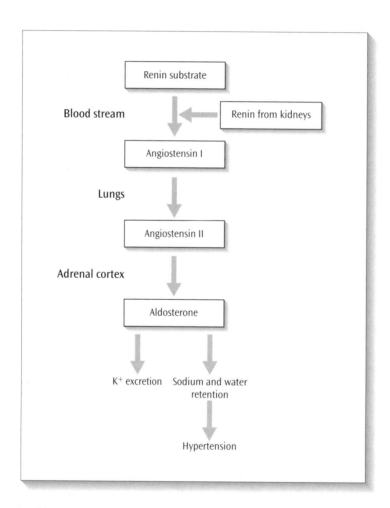

Fig. 13.4   The renin–angiotensin–aldosterone system.

The reuctive system

14.1 People with the following sex chromosomal constitutions usually have testes:

A XX
B XXY
C XO
D XYY
E XXX

14.2 People with the following sex chromosomal constitutions have significantly abnormal gonadal function:

A XO
B XX
C XY
D XXY
E XYY

14.3 The following statements about the genetic control of the embryological development of the gonads are true:

A A sex-determining region on the X chromosomes (SRX) directs the primordial germ cells to develop into ovaries
B A sex-determining region on the Y chromosome (SRY) directs the primordial germ cells to develop into testes
C The structural genes for developing the gonads are located in the sex chromosomes
D XXY individuals may have both testes and ovaries
E Testosterone is essential for the development of testes

14.4 The following structures develop from the embryological Wolffian (mesonephric) system:

A Testes
B The penis
C Ovaries
D Epididymis
E Oviducts

14.5 Structures developed from the Mullerian (paramesonephric) ducts are usually absent in the following individuals:

A Normal people with XY sex chromosomes
B Normal people with XX sex chromosomes
C Complete testicular feminisation syndrome with XY sex chromosomes
D Adrenogenital syndrome (XX individuals with excessive secretion of androgens)
E Turner's syndrome with sex chromosomes XO

14.6 Individuals with complete testicular feminisation syndrome and reared unambiguously as girls from birth usually have female:

A Genetic sex
B External genitalia
C Internal genitalia
D Gender identity
E Gender role

14.7 Prior to any medical treatment, a male to female transsexual almost always has male:

A Genetic sex
B External genitalia
C Internal genitalia
D Gender identity
E Sexual preference

14.8 Compared to puberty in girls, boys have:

A An earlier growth spurt
B A higher growth velocity
C More conspicuous voice changes
D A higher increase in the proportion of body fat
E A higher increase in skeletal mass

14.9 According to the hypothalamic maturation hypothesis for the initiation of puberty:

A The key mechanism is a change in the pituitary sensitivity to gonadotrophin-releasing hormone (GnRH)
B The key mechanism is the secretion of GnRH in a pulsatile manner
C Hypothalamic maturation is not possible in people without functioning gonads
D Gonads of young children cannot be made to respond to hypothalamic signals
E The gonadostat hypothesis is impossible

14.10 The following statements about puberty in developed countries are true:

A There has been a secular trend towards earlier puberty for girls
B There has been a secular trend towards later puberty in boys
C Girls with a body weight below 45 kg are unlikely to have menstruation
D Reduction in exposure to sunlight is associated with earlier puberty
E A low protein diet is associated with earlier puberty

14.11 Causes of delayed puberty in girls include:

A Anorexia nervosa
B Constitutional delay
C Anterior hypothalamic tumour
D Turner's syndrome
E Oestrogen-secreting ovarian tumour

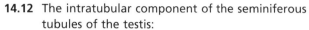

The reproductive system

14.12 The intratubular component of the seminiferous tubules of the testis:

A Is associated with the synthesis of spermatozoa

B Is associated with the synthesis of androgens

C Is associated with the synthesis of inhibin

D Is lined by Leydig cells

E Exchanges freely with the extratubular component

14.13 The following statements about the regulation of androgen and spermatozoa synthesis are true:

A Luteinising hormone (LH) is essential for the secretion of testosterone

B Follicule-stimulating hormone (FSH) is essential for the secretion of testosterone

C Oestrogen is essential for effective spermatogenesis

D FSH is essential for effective spermatogenesis

E Testosterone is essential for effective spermatogenesis

14.14 The following statements about ovarian germ cells in a human female are correct:

A The total number reaches a maximum at about 25 years of age

B The total number increases rapidly during puberty

C About 10% result in a functioning corpus luteum

D Selection for pre-antral follicular development is regulated by the pituitary gland

E The ovarian germ cells of a 10-year-old girl can undergo mitosis

14.15 The release of GnRH:

A Stimulates the secretion of FSH

B Stimulates the secretion of LH

C Is usually at a constant rate

D Is from the hypothalamus

E Is usually increased by a high progesterone concentration

14.16 The LH surge in the menstrual cycle:

A Is an example of a positive feedback system

B Is associated with reduced sensitivity of the anterior pituitary to GnRH

C Is associated with increased secretion of GnRH

D Is necessary for ovulation to occur

E Is induced by a progesterone surge

14.17 In females, inhibin:

A Is secreted by the corpus luteum

B Acts to reduce the plasma FSH level

C Acts to reduce the plasma LH level

D Is important in the positive feedback regulation of gonadotrophins

E Acts in a similar way to activin

14.18 The following hormones are generally significantly higher in the luteal than in the early follicular phase in the menstrual cycle:

A Oestrogen

B Progesterone

C FSH

D LH

E Inhibin

14.19 During the late luteal phase of the menstrual cycle:

A The number of progesterone receptors in the uterus increases

B The basal body temperature is higher than in the follicular phase

C The cervix produces thick mucus

D Sperm penetration into cervical mucus is enhanced

E Stromal proliferation occurs in the uterus

14.20 Most combined oral contraceptives ('the pill') consist of:

A Androgen

B Oestrogen

C Progestagen

D Corticosteroids

E Prostaglandins

14.21 Mechanisms of action of combined oral contraceptives include:

A Production of anti-sperm antibodies

B Prevention of fertilisation

C Facilitation of implanted zygote to abort

D Spermicidal activity

E Inhibition of ovulation

14.22 Advantages of combined oral contraceptives over progestagen-only contraceptive ('mini-pills') include reduced likelihood of:

A Contraceptive failure

B Deep-vein thrombosis

C Inhibition of lactation during pregnancy

D Irregular bleeding

E Contraceptive failure if the administration of a pill is inadvertently delayed

14.23 Inhibition of ovulation is a significant mechanism of action for the following contraceptives:

A Progestagen-only pills

B Intramuscular progesterone

C Intrauterine contraceptive device

D Subcutaneous progestagen implant (e.g. Norplant)

E Female surgical sterilisation procedure

14.24 Significant predisposing factors for endometrial carcinoma include:

A Oestrogen replacement therapy after menopause
B Late menarche
C Obesity
D Premature menopause
E Multiple sexual partners

14.25 Primary ovarian tumours:
A May be familial
B Are often associated with an increased plasma CA125 level
C Cause more deaths than endometrial carcinoma
D Are almost always malignant
E May produce oestrogen

14.26 Significant predisposing factors for carcinoma of the cervix include:
A Cigarette smoking
B Frequent sexual intercourse
C Multiple sexual partners
D Human papillomavirus infection
E Late menopause

14.27 The following statements about the female breast are correct:
A Accessory nipples are usually found in the midline
B The lobes secrete milk independent of one another
C The epithelial cells do not produce secretions
D The myoepithelial cells contain contractile proteins
E Each lobe is drained by one lactiferous duct

14.28 The female breasts:
A Require progesterone for their development
B Require oestrogens for their development
C Enlarge rapidly during puberty
D Enlarge rapidly during pregnancy
E Undergo cyclical changes in the absence of pregnancy

14.29 The following substances increase the secretion of prolactin:
A Dopamine
B Bromocriptine
C Phenothiazines (e.g. chlorpromazine)
D Vasoactive intestinal polypeptide (VIP)
E Digoxin

14.30 The following are associated with unusually high plasma prolactin levels in women:
A Breast-feeding
B Pregnancy
C Recent university entry
D Hyperthyroidism
E Pituitary tumour

14.31 An abnormally high plasma level of prolactin in women may cause:
A Impaired fertility
B Loss of menstruation
C Headache
D Loss of libido
E Abnormal milk secretion

14.32 Significant factors for maintaining milk production during breast-feeding include:
A A high oestrogen level
B A high progesterone level
C Suckling
D A high prolactin level
E A high corticosteroid level

14.33 Pharmacological actions of cyproterone acetate in men include:
A Competitive inhibition of peripheral testosterone receptors
B A reduction in sperm counts
C A reduction in sex drive
D Impotence
E Breast enlargement

14.34 Recognised indications for cyproterone acetate include:
A Male contraception
B Male hypersexuality
C Prostatic carcinoma
D Severe acne in women
E Failure to ovulate in women

14.35 After spermatogenesis, the sperms must pass through the following structures before ejaculation:
A Epididymis
B Vas deferens
C Prostatic duct
D Seminal vesicle
E Penile urethra

14.36 Events which normally occur during penile erection include:
A Inhibition of the parasympathetic nervous supply
B Inhibition of the sympathetic nervous supply
C An increase in the arterial smooth muscle tone
D An increase of blood flow into the corpora cavernosa
E An increase in the venous outflow from the corpora cavernosa

14.37 The following neurotransmitters play significant roles in initiating and sustaining penile erection:
A GABA

199

B Acetylcholine
C Gastrin
D Nitric oxide
E Vasoactive intestinal polypeptide (VIP)

14.38 Recognised local drug treatment for impotence include:
A α-Adrenergic antagonists (e.g. papaverine)
B β-Adrenergic antagonists (e.g. propranolol)
C Corticosteroids (e.g. prednisolone)
D Prostaglandin E_1 (e.g. alprostadil)
E Calcium antagonists (e.g. nifedipine)

14.39 Oral sildenafil (Viagra):
A Is effective in improving spermatogenesis
B Is effective in treating impotence
C Is an inhibitor of cGMP-specific phosphodiesterase
D Increase nitric oxide level in the corpora cavernosum
E Is particularly useful if there is a recent history of myocardial infarct

14.40 The following statements about fertilisation are correct:
A It takes place in the endometrium of the uterus
B Sperm capacitation occurs after the acrosome reaction
C The acrosome reaction occurs after fusion with the oocyte
D Down's syndrome may result if an oocyte is fertilised by two sperms
E The oocyte contains a haploid set of chromosomes before fertilisation

14.41 The following events between fertilisation and implantation and their outcomes are appropriately matched:
A Division of the conceptus into two distinct groups of cells – monozygotic twins
B Two oocytes are separately fertilised by two sperms in the same ovulatory cycle – dizygotic twins
C One oocyte is fertilised by two sperms in the same ovulatory cycle – monozygotic twins
D Two oocytes are fertilised by two sperms in different ovulatory cycles – polyploidy
E Two separately fertilised conceptuses sticking together to form a single conceptus – triploidy

14.42 Human chorionic gonadotrophin (hCG):
A Is secreted by the ovaries
B Binds to LH receptors
C Increases during the luteal phase of the menstrual cycle in the absence of pregnancy

D Consists of two α chains and two β chains
E May be used as a marker of pregnancy

14.43 The following hormones are secreted by the placenta during pregnancy:
A Oestrogen
B Progesterone
C Prolactin
D hCG
E Human placental lactogen

14.44 Amniotic fluid:
A Has a total volume of about 2 litres at 20 weeks pregnancy
B Has a protein content higher than that of normal serum
C Is removed by the fetus from the amniotic cavity by swallowing
D Is partly produced by the fetus micturating into the amniotic cavity
E Contains fetal epithelial cells

14.45 The following abnormalities of amniotic fluid and their possible fetal causes are correctly matched:
A Low amniotic fluid volume (in late pregnancy) – oesophageal atresia
B Excessive amniotic fluid (in late pregnancy) – renal agenesis
C Low α-fetoprotein (AFP) level (in early pregnancy) – spina bifida
D High bilibrubin level (in late pregnancy) – rhesus incompatibility
E Low sphingomyelin: lecithin ratio – immature fetal lungs

14.46 The following diseases may be diagnosed antenatally by amniocentesis or chorionic villous biopsy:
A Duchenne muscular dystrophy
B Cystic fibrosis
C Down's syndrome
D Haemophilia
E Turner's syndrome

14.47 Significant mechanisms protecting the fetus against rejection by the mother's immune system include:
A General immunosuppression by fetal corticosteroids
B Inert properties of the chorionic trophoblast
C Induced tolerance of the mother's immune system
D Barriers to maternal–fetal transmission of antibodies or immune cells
E Binding of fetal antigens to hostile maternal antibodies or immune cells

TAble 14.1

	Turner's syndrome	Klinefelter's syndrome	Testicular feminisation syndrome	Adrenogenital syndrome in females	True hermaphroditism
Basic defect					
Sex chromosomes					
Presence of testes					
Presence of ovaries					
Presence of male internal genitalia					
Presence of female internal genitalia					
External genitalia					
Likely gender assignment					

14.48 Endocrine changes just before parturition include an increase of:
   A Oestrogen to progesterone ratio
   B Prostaglandin locally in the uterus
   C Inhibin
   D Oxytocin
   E Relaxin

14.49 The following statements about uterine muscle contraction at parturition are true:
   A The muscle cells act as a syncytium
   B Prostaglandin increase contractility by direct action on prostaglandin receptors
   C Oxytocin increases contractility by lowering the excitation threshold
   D Contraction is initiated by the release of intracellular calcium
   E Pacemakers are usually located near the cervix

14.50 The following measures are effective in initiating labour:
   A Prostaglandin vaginal pessary
   B Intravenous salbutamol
   C Intravenous syntocinon (analogue of oxytocin)
   D Artificial rupture of membrane
   E Intravenous corticosteroids

14.51 **A** In human embryological development, describe how the following features are determined.
       i   Genetic sex.
       ii Presence of testes.

   iii Presence of ovaries.
   iv   Male internal genitalia.
   v   Female internal genitalia.
   vi   Male external genitalia.
   vii Female external genitalia.
   viii Likely gender assignment.

   B From your answers above, complete Table 14.1.

14.52 For a male-to-female transsexual before medical treatment, give the status of the following:
   • genetic sex
   • gonads
   • internal genitalia
   • external genitalia
   • sex reared as in childhood
   • gender identity
   • sexual preference.

14.53 In a mixed class of 10-year-olds in 1993, the average heights of boys and girls were similar. In 1995, girls were on average significantly taller than boys. In 1999 when they were taking the GCSE examinations, boys were on average much taller than girls.
   A Explain these observations.
   B List other changes associated with this rapid increase in height for (1) boys and (2) girls.
   C Describe the endocrine mechanism that initiates this process. What are the associated endocrine changes for (1) boys and (2) girls?

The reproductive system

D How has the age at which children undergo this process altered over the last century? Give two hypotheses for this change over the last century.

14.54 A 20-year-old woman presented to her general practitioner with a history of never having had a period, although she had normal breast development.
  A Would you regard this as abnormal?
  B Where might the lesion be and what might be the underlying cause?

14.55 A 55-year-old woman complained of hut flushes. The following endocrine results were obtained:
  • follicle-stimulating hormone: 80 iu/l (reference 2–8 iu/l)
  • luteinizing hormone: 60 iu/l (reference 3–16 iu/l).
  A What is the most likely diagnosis?
  B What are her symptoms due to?
  C Explain the FSH and LH results.
  D What would you expect the 17 β-estradiol level to be if it were measured?
  E What is the treatment for this condition?

14.56 A couple were investigated for infertility. The following report shows part of the results of the semen analysis:
  • volume: 3.2 ml (reference >2.75 ml)
  • sperm count: 80×10^6 sperm/ml (reference $>40 \times 10^6$ sperm/ml)
  • % motile: 10% (reference >40%)
  • % normal form: 80% (reference >40%)
  A Briefly trace the development of the sperm from the primary spermatocyte stage to the final stage ready for fertilisation. What hormones are particularly important for the their maturation and motility?
  B What effects (if any) does temperature have on the results of semen analysis? Explain.
  C What abnormalities are revealed in this semen analysis? Are these abnormalities sufficient to account for the couple's infertility?

14.57 A 34-year-old man presented with impotence. After appropriate history, examination and investigations, the doctor discussed a range of possible treatments with him.
  A Describe the normal process of penile erection.
  B What are the roles of various neurotransmitters in erection?
  C What are the mechanisms of action of the following treatments?

  i Local papaverine.
  ii Local alprostadil (prostaglandin E).
  iii Oral sildenafil (Viagra).

14.58 **A** List the physiological functions of androgens in men in adulthood.
  B i Where are androgens secreted?
     ii What are the active forms of androgens?
     iii Explain at a cellular level how they exert their effects?
  C Give an example of an antiandrogen drug. What might it be used for clinically?

14.59 A 22-year-old woman presented with infertility and it is important to monitor whether ovulation has occurred during her menstrual cycle.
  A Describe the development of the ovarian follicle before ovulation.
  B What is ovulation? When does it usually occur in the menstrual cycle?
  C Assuming that ovulation occurs, compare features 4 days before and 4 days after ovulation by completing Table 14.2.
  D Explain the mechanisms for the changes in the uterus and the cervix after ovulation.
  E Explain the mechanisms for the LH surge at the time of ovulation.
  F List all clinical indicators for ovulation, including the history, hormonal and other investigations.
  G Why don't the changes outlined in (C) occur in the absence of ovulation?

14.60 **A** Outline the steps from the release of the sperm in the vagina to the implantation of the blastocytes.
  B Explain what events would lead to pregnancy with the following.
     i Monozygotic twins.
     ii Dizygotic twins.

14.61 A woman was seen for infertility. After investigations, the gynaecologist prescribed clomifene.
  A What does the gynaecologist consider the most likely reason for her infertility?
  B What is the mechanism of action of clomifene?

14.62 A woman sought contraceptive advice from her general practitioner. The options of a combined oral contraceptive and progesterone-only pills were discussed.
  A What are the mechanisms of action for both types of contraceptive?

Table 14.2

	4 days before ovulation	4 days after ovulation
General		
Basal body temperature		
Uterus		
Phase		
Thickness of endometrium		
Uterine glands		
Cervix		
Thickness of mucus		
Cellularity of mucus		
Breasts		
Lobules and alveoli		
Symptoms		
Endocrine		
Progesterone		
17 β-estradiol		
LH		
FSH		

B List the advantages and disadvantages of combined oral contraceptives over progesterone-only pills?

14.63 A A 39-week pregnant mother was admitted in early labour.
   i What changes in the cervix and uterus are necessary before the baby is born?
   ii Describe the mechanisms which ensure that the contractions of the uterus increase progressively until the baby is born.

B Another mother was 41 weeks into her pregnancy, but there were no signs of labour. The obstetrician admitted the mother, administered a vaginal prostaglandin pessary, set up an oxytocin (Syntocinon) infusion, and ruptured the membranes with a sterile instrument. Explain how these interventions may help the mother to go into labour.

C A 32-week pregnant woman was admitted with uterine contractions. What pharmacological interventions can be used to prolong the pregnancy?

The reproductive system

14.1 B D

The key determinant to whether a person develops testes is the presence of the 'sex-determining region' on the Y chromosome. A person with a Y chromosome has the potential to develop testes, whilst the female gonads (the ovaries) develop in the absence of a Y chromosome. The Y chromosome contains a regulatory gene which controls the expression of other structural genes for developing the testes. The sex chromosomal constitution for normal males and normal females is XY and XX respectively. Turner's syndrome has XO constitution, and 'super females' have XXX constitution. They develop ovaries, although the ovaries of Turner's syndrome often under-develop and fail prematurely. XYY and XXY are the sex chromosomal constitution for 'super males' and Kleinefelter's syndrome respectively. They both develop testes. However, in Klinefelter's syndrome, the germ cells die when they enter meiosis, and the person may become infertile.

14.2 A D

See question 14.1 above. A Y chromosome is necessary for the initial formation of testes, and ovaries develop in the absence of a Y chromosome. However, the subsequent abnormal testicular development in Klinefelter's syndrome demonstrates that normal testicular development cannot take place with more than one X chromosome. Similarly, the abnormal ovarian development in Turner's syndrome demonstrates that the presence of more than one X chromosome is necessary for the subsequent normal ovarian development.

14.3 B

See also question 14.1. Whilst the formation of testes is dependent on the sex-determining region on the Y chromosome (SRY), the formation of ovaries is by default. The sex-determining region on the Y chromosome is located at the end of the short arm of the Y chromosome, and regulates the activities of many structural genes on various other chromosomes which are required to make the tests. Whilst the testes make testosterone, the development of testes is not dependent on testosterone.

14.4 D

The embryological gonads and external genitalia are capable of differentiating into either male or female structures. However, the embryological internal genitalia of males and females have different origins: the male internal genitalia develop from the embryological Wolffian (mesonephric) ducts to form the epididymis, vas deferens and seminal vesicles, whilst the female internal genitalia develop from the embryological Mullerian (paramesonephric) ducts to form the oviducts, the uterus and the cervix.

14.5 A C

The development of the Wolffian (male) and Mullerian (female) ducts is controlled by different hormones, and is not necessarily related to the genetic sex. The Wolffian ducts persist only in the presence of testosterone secreted by the testes, otherwise they will disappear. On the other hand, the Mullerian ducts will disappear only in the presence of Mullerian inhibiting hormone (MIH) secreted by the testes, otherwise they will persist. Hence, the structures developed from the Wolffian ducts (epididymis, vas deferens, seminal vesicles) are only found in males, and those from the Mullerian ducts (oviducts, uterus, cervix) are only found in females. In testicular feminisation syndrome, the genetic sex is male, and the secretion of androgens is normal. The peripheral tissues are insensitive to androgens, and hence the Wolffian ducts disappear. However, MIH is secreted and causes the Mullerian system to disappear as well. Hence individuals with testicular feminisation syndrome have no internal genitalia structures. Individuals with adrenogenital syndrome have female genetic sex and secrete androgens. However, they do not secrete MIH. Hence they develop the structures derived from both Mullerian and Wolffian ducts. People with Turner's syndrome secrete neither androgens nor MIH, and they develop normal Mullerian duct structures.

14.6 B D E

Individuals with complete testicular feminisation syndrome have XY sex chromosomes and therefore have male genetic sex. The tissues are insensitive to androgens, and hence they have female external genitalia. They have neither female nor male internal genitalia (see question 14.5 above). Gender identity is the self-awareness and personal experience of one's identity as male or female. This depends mainly on the sex assignment at birth and subsequent rearing. Hence individuals with complete testicular feminisation syndromes and reared as girls usually have a female gender identity. Gender role is defined by the way the individuals relate to others about their gender identity.

14.7 A B C

A male to female transsexual is an XY individual with testes and male external genitalia, and yet feels psychologically that he is a female. Hence their genetic sex is male, they have male internal and external genitalia, but they have female gender identity. Prior to medical treatment, their sexual preference may be either male or female.

14.8 B C E

Although many physiological and behavioural changes during puberty are similar in boys and girls, there are a few differences. Puberty in boys is initiated by androgens, but oestrogen is essential for puberty in girls. Whilst the onset of menarche (first menstrual bleeding) in girls is quite definitive, the first ejaculation in boys is less so. The growth spurt in boys is later than in girls, although the average peak height velocity is higher in boys than girls. This partly explains why, although girls are usually taller than boys between the ages of 11 and 14, men are taller than women. The changes in body shape are considerable during puberty. There is a much higher increase in the proportion of body fat in girls than boys, but boys achieve a higher increase in skeletal mass.

14.9 B
There are two main hypotheses for the mechanism for the initiation of puberty: the gonadostat hypothesis and the hypothalamic maturation hypothesis. According to the gonadostat hypothesis, maturation of the feedback system of the hypothalmic–pituitary–gonadal axis is important. Hence changes in the responsiveness of the hypothalamus to oestrogen or testosterone levels and the pituitary of GnRH are important. According to the hypothalamic maturation hypothesis, the maturation of the hypothalamus is the key element, and is independent of the pituitary–gonadal axis. The hypothalamus releases GnRH in a pulsatile manner. According to this hypothesis, hypothalamic maturation may occur in individuals without functioning gonads (e.g. Turner's syndrome), and gonads of young children can be made to respond to pulsatile release of GnRH. Experimental and clinical evidence supports the hypothalamic maturation hypothesis. However, the two hypotheses are not mutually exclusive.

14.10 A C
There has been a secular trend towards earlier puberty in the developed countries amongst both boys and girls. There are many hypothesis for this observation. Firstly, longer days created by artificial light are associated with earlier puberty in some animals. However, this is unlikely to be important in humans. Secondly, improved nutrition may be important. Body weight has been shown to correlate closely with the onset of puberty. Girls under about 47kg and boys under about 55kg are unlikely to undergo puberty. However, the precise mechanism for triggering pulsatile secretion of GnRH in the hypothalamus is still unknown.

14.11 A B C D
Delayed puberty in girls is said to occur if menstruation has not occurred by 16 years of age. The commonest cause is constitutional delayed puberty with no organic pathology, and there is often a family history. It appears that the hypothalamic maturation is programmed to be delayed. Pathological causes include pathology in the

hypothalamus, pituitary and the ovaries. Girls with anorexia nervosa may fail to reach the critical body weight necessary to trigger hypothalamic maturation. Tumours in the anterior hypothalamus cause delayed puberty, whilst tumours in the posterior hypothalamus cause precocious puberty. Prolactin-secreting pituitary tumours or craniopharyngioma (tumour of Rathke's pouch) are associated with delayed puberty, whilst gonadotrophin-secreting pituitary tumours are associated with precocious puberty. Premature ovarian failure (e.g. Turner's syndrome) is associated with delayed puberty due to lack of oestrogen. On the other hand, oestrogen-secreting ovarian tumour causes precocious puberty.

14.12 A
Two intratubular and extratubular components of the seminiferous tubules of the testis are completely separate. Spermatozoa are synthesised in the intratubular compartment in association with Sertoli cells, whilst hormones (androgens, inhibin, oestrogens) are secreted in the Leydig cells within the extratubular compartment. The two compartments are separated by junctional barriers between adjacent Sertoli cells, and form the blood–testis barrier. As the body's immune system will produce antibodies against spermatozoal antigens which may lead to subfertility, this barrier is important in preventing spermatozoa from leaking into the lymphatic or venous system.

14.13 A D E
The secretion of testosterone by Leydig cells is stimulated by LH secreted by the anterior pituitary gland, and is facilitated by both inhibin and prolactin. Effective spermatogenesis depends on the actions of both testosterone and FSH.

14.14 –
Unlike spermatogenesis, mitosis of ovarian germ cells cease at the time of birth, and meiosis is initiated. Hence a human female has all the egg cells she will ever have (about 7 million) within her ovaries at birth. Thereafter, the total number declines until menopause. About 15–20 follicles are recruited for early antral follicle development in each cycle, and only one becomes the dominant follicle. Hence the proportion of ovarian germ cells which results in a functioning corpus luteum is very small (less than 1%). The mechanisms for selection of cells for pre-antral follicular development are not subject to regulation by factors outside the ovaries, although the exact mechanism is still unclear.

14.15 A B D
GnRH is secreted by the hypothalamus. It is secreted in pulses, and stimulates the secretion of both FSH and LH.

14 **A**

SYSTEM-BASED MEDICAL SCIENCES

The reproductive system

Hence the gonadotrophins are also secreted in a pulsatile manner. Both the secretion of GnRH and the response of the pituitary gland to GnRH are important mechanisms for the control of the menstrual cycle in the female. In general, oestrogen usually reduces the pulse amplitude of GnRH secretion at relatively low secretion, and progesterone reduces the pulse frequency of GnRH secretion. This usually acts as a negative feedback system. However, in the luteal phase, a very high level of oestrogen may increase GnRH (and hence LHRH) secretion by a positive feedback system.

14.16   A C D
The LH surge marks the end of the follicular phase of the menstrual cycle, and is essential for the luteal phase and ovulation to take place. The LH surge is an example of a positive feedback system, and is triggered by an oestrogen surge at the end of the follicular phase. This positive feedback system is brought about by a combination of increased pulse amplitude of the GnRH secretion, and increased sensitivity of the anterior pituitary to the released GnRH.

14.17   A B
In the female, inhibin is secreted by the granulosa cells in the late follicular phase and by the corpus luteum. Hence, the plasma level of inhibin starts to increase in late follicular phase, and is highest in the early luteal phase. It acts to reduce plasma FSH level by reducing the anterior pituitary response to GnRH. It has no effect on LH level. It is thought to be important in the negative feedback regulation of gonadotrophins. Activin is another cytokine with an opposite mode of action to inhibin. It generally increases FSH level, but its physiological role is still unclear.

14.18   A B E
In the luteal phase, the corpus luteum secretes large quantities of progesterone, as well as oestrogen and inhibin. Inhibin acts to reduce the FSH level. Oestrogen and progesterone act to suppress the gonadotrophin levels. The presence of progesterone also prevents positive feedback regulation leading to LH surge.

14.19   A B C E
In the early luteal phase of the menstrual cycle, oestrogen induces the synthesis of progesterone receptors in the uterus. This, together with the increasing concentration of progesterone, stimulates secretions from the endometrium (lining of the uterus), stromal proliferation, as well as enlargement of the uterine muscle cells (myometrium). These changes prepare for the implantation of the embryo should fertilisation occur. In the cervix, progesterone changes the nature and amount of glycoproteins produced in the cervical epithelium, and produces a small volume of thick mucus which can only be stretched a short distance before snapping (a low spinnbarkeit). This mucus is relatively impenetrable to sperms. The body temperature also increases slightly under the influence of progesterone. This increase in body temperature and changes in cervical mucus allow women to detect ovulation and work out the 'safe period' using the 'natural' contraceptive method.

14.20   B C
Most combined oral contraceptives consist of an oestrogen and a progestagen. Most combined oral contraceptives contain low-dose oestrogen (20–35 μg), and contraceptives containing 50 μg oestrogen are now seldomly used.

14.21   B E
Combined oral contraceptives act mainly by inhibiting ovulation. This is achieved by oestrogen acting on the hypothalamus to prevent release of GnRH. However, progesterone in the combined oral contraceptives also makes cervical mucus more viscous and hence spermatozoa are less likely to reach the egg cell. Whilst combined oral contraceptives might inhibit the implantation of the zygote into the endometrium, they do not cause an implanted zygote to abort.

14.22   A D E
Combined oral contraceptives have a lower failure rate, and are less susceptible to contraceptive failure due to inadvertent delay or omission of a pill. Whereas an alternative contraceptive method must be used if a mini-pill is delayed for more than 3 h, the combined oral contraceptives are still effective even if an oral pill is delayed for up to 12 h. Furthermore, as the combined oral contraceptives are taken 21 days out of 28, women on combined oral contraceptives experience regular withdrawal bleeding, whereas women on progestagen-only pill may experience either absent, irregular or excessive vaginal bleeding. However, as the oral combined contraceptives contain oestrogen, there is a small increased risk of arterial or venous thromboembolism. As oestrogen inhibits lactation, it is not suitable whilst breast-feeding.

14.23   A B D
Although the key mechanism of action for the progestagen-only contraception method may be to render the cervical mucus inhospitable to sperms, it also inhibits ovulation. This applies whether the progestagens are taken orally, intramuscularly or subcutaneously. Intrauterine contraceptive devices act mainly by preventing implantation of the zygote in the endometrium. In female sterilisation, the oviducts (Fallopian tubes) are blocked by surgical clips. This prevents fertilisation from taking place.

14.24   A C
Endometrial carcinomas are mostly adenocarcinomas. The main risk factor is oestrogen stimulation unopposed by progesterone. Hence hormone replacement therapy with oestrogen (without progesterone) and polycystic ovarian syndrome are significant risk factors. They also occur more commonly in obese women, probably reflecting their higher oestrogen level. Multiple sexual partners are a significant risk factor for cervical but not endometrial carcinoma.

14.25   A B C E
There are many types of primary ovarian tumours, and they may arise from epithelial cells, germs cells or the sex cord stroma. They may be benign or malignant. Some ovarian carcinomas are familial, and a few ovarian cancer genes have recently been identified. As ovarian carcinomas often present late, they cause more deaths than any other gynaecological cancers. The protein CA125 has been found to be raised in cases of ovarian cancer, and it is now widely used as a tumour marker both to aid diagnosis and to monitor therapy.

14.26   A B C D
Squamous carcinoma is the commonest cervical carcinoma. It is likely to be caused by a sexually transmitted agent, such as human papillomaviruses and perhaps herpes simplex virus type 2. In general, increased sexual exposure (e.g. early age of sexual intercourse, frequent sexual intercourse and multiple sexual partners) is a predisposing factor. Cigarette smoking is an independent risk factor. Squamous cervical carcinoma is not hormone-dependent.

14.27   B D E
The female breasts consist of about 15–20 lobes. The lobes are separated from each other by fat and connective tissue. Milk is secreted by acini in each lobule. The acini are lined by epithelial cells which secrete milk. The myoepithelial cells surround the epithelial cells. They contain contractile proteins which contract in response to oxytocin and help to expel any milk synthesised into the ducts. The intralobular ducts drain into extralobular ducts, and they finally drain into the lactiferous ducts and sinuses. Each lobe is drained by one lactiferous duct. Accessory nipples are developmental abnormalities, and they are almost always found along the embryological 'milk line' between the axilla and the groin.

14.28   A B C D E
The hormonal regulation for breast development is complex and still not fully understood. However, it is clear that oestrogen and progesterone are essential. Other hormones which may be important include prolactin, growth hormone, glucocorticoids and insulin. The female breasts grow rapidly during puberty and in pregnancy. This involves both ductular and glandular proliferation, as well as deposition of adipose and connective tissue. The female breasts vary slightly in size and consistency due to variations in oestrogen and progesterone levels throughout the menstrual cycle. After menopause, the ductules and glandular structure involute. In the elderly, the breasts consist of mainly adipose tissue.

14.29   C D E
In diseases associated with a disconnection in the vascular links between the hypothalamus and the anterior pituitary gland, the secretion of prolactin is greatly increased whilst that of other hormones is reduced. Hence the secretion of prolactin from the anterior pituitary is mostly controlled via inhibitory factors from the hypothalamus. Dopamine is the main prolactin inhibitory factor, but GABA (γ-aminobutyric acid) and GnRH may also inhibit the release of prolactin. Bromocriptine is a dopamine agonist, and therefore inhibits the secretion of prolactin. Phenothiazines are dopamine antagonists and hence they increase prolactin secretion. It has been found recently that prolactin-releasing factors also exist. The main prolactin-releasing factor is VIP, but thyrotrophin-releasing hormone (TRH) and oestrogens also stimulate prolactin secretion. Digoxin increases prolactin secretion and may cause breast enlargement in men.

14.30   A B C E
Plasma prolactin levels are usually higher during sleep and decrease when awake. They are also abnormally high in the presence of psychological stress. As the main function of prolactin is to initiate and maintain milk secretion, the plasma level is physiologically high during pregnancy and breast-feeding. An elevated TRH level (e.g. in primary hypothyroidism) may increase prolactin secretion. Greatly elevated levels of prolactin may be due to a prolactin-secreting pituitary microadenoma.

14.31   A B D E
Hyperprolactinaemia is commoner in women than in men. In men a high prolactin level may cause impaired fertility and loss of libido. In women it may cause loss of libido, loss of menstruation, impaired fertility and abnormal milk secretion. Headache may be a symptom of a pituitary tumour, but not hyperprolactinaemia itself.

14.32   C D
Whilst oestrogen and progesterone are important in promoting ductal and lobular growth of the breasts during pregnancy, they inhibit milk secretion. Suckling is important in inducing prolactin release during breast-feeding and hence maintains milk production. Conditioned reflex (e.g. to a baby's cry) may increase the secretion of

SYSTEM-BASED MEDICAL SCIENCES

14 **The reproductive system**

oxytocin and induce the expulsion of milk into the ducts. However, it does not increase milk production on its own.

14.33   A B C D
Cyproterone acetate is a competitive inhibitor of testosterone receptors in the peripheral tissues. Hence cyproterone acetate would reduce spermatogenesis, sex drive and the ability to sustain erection in men. It does not have an oestrogenic effect, and does not cause breast enlargement.

14.34   B C D
As cyproterone acetate is anti-androgenic, it may be used for management of male hypersexuality. However, it is particularly important to obtain informed consent. Cyproterone acetate is used in prostatic carcinoma as the disease is often androgen-dependent. The anti-androgenic effect of cyproterone may also be useful in treating severe acne or polycystic ovarian syndrome in women. Cyproterone acetate has no effect on ovulation.

14.35   A B E
After spermatogenesis, the spermatozoa are carried through vasa efferentia, and via the epididymis into the vas deferens and the posterior urethra. Semen is formed by a mixture of the spermatozoa with secretions from the prostate and the seminal vesicles.

14.36   B D
Erection is caused by increased blood flow to the corpora cavernosa. This causes venous compression and reduced venous outflow, and hence erection occurs. The initial increase in blood flow is initiated by a reduction in the arterial smooth muscle tone, which is controlled by the opposing effects of sympathetic and parasympathetic nervous supplies. Stimulation of the parasympathetic nervous system stimulates the α-adrenergic receptors, and causes a reduction in the arterial smooth muscle tone and hence penile erection, whilst stimulation of the sympathetic nervous system causes an increase in the arterial smooth muscle tone and hence penile flaccidity.

14.37   B D E
Stimulation of the sympathetic nervous system causes penile flaccidity. Stimulation of the parasympathetic nervous system causes penile erection, and the neurotransmitters implicated are acetylcholine, VIP and nitric oxide. The levels of these neurotransmitters are raised during erection.

14.38   A D
α-Adrenergic antagonists (e.g. papaverine) injected into the corpora cavernosa may be effective in treating impotence as it blocks the sympathetic tone which tends to increase the tone of the arterial smooth muscle. β-Adrenergic antagonists have no effect. Prostaglandin E$_1$ (e.g. alprostadil) is a vasodilator and may increase arterial inflow if injected into the corpora cavernosa. Corticosteroids and calcium antagonists have no effect on penile erection.

14.39   B C D
Sildenafil (Viagra) was licensed for the treatment of male impotence in Britain in 1998. It is a potent inhibitor of cGMP phosphodiesterase type 5, the specific isoenzyme found in corpora cavernosa. Hence sildenafil increases cGMP, which in turns increase nitric oxide and decreases the tone of arterial smooth muscle. Its possible cardiovascular side effects have been well publicised, and the drug should not be given to anyone with a history of myocardial infarct within the last six months.

14.40   –
Fertilisation takes place in the Fallopian tube (oviduct). Before the sperm can fuse with the oocyte, it must undergo the acrosome reaction. Before the acrosomal reaction can occur, it must be prepared by the process of sperm capacitation, during which the surface components of the spermatozoa undergo changes. In this acrosome reaction, the acrosomal membrane of the sperm fuses with the overlying plasma membrane, and the contents of the acrosomal vesicle are discharged. This is associated with a large increase in intracellular calcium and cAMP, and the exposed plasma membrane in the equatorial and post-acrosomal membrane is now capable of fusion with the occyte. If the oocyte is fertilised by two sperms, the zygote contains three sets of chromosomes and triploidy results. The resulting triploidy is termed androgenetic triploidy. Before fusion of the gametes, the oocyte is in its second meiotic division, and still contains two sets of chromosomes. It must complete the second meiotic division and get rid of one set of chromosomes via the second polar body. Otherwise, gynogenetic triploidy occurs.

14.41   A B
Normally, the zona keeps the cells of the conceptus together after fertilisation but before implantation. Monozygotic twins result from the division of the conceptus shortly after fertilisation into two distinct groups of cells. The twins are genetically identical. Dizygotic twins result if two oocytes are separately fertilised in the same ovulatory cycle. Their genetic similarities are the same as those between other siblings. Androgenetic triploidy results if one oocyte is fertilised by two sperms in the same ovulatory cycle. Two oocytes fertilised in different ovulatory cycles result in normal siblings. Two separately fertilised conceptuses sticking

together to form a single conceptus result in a chimaeric conceptus. The resulting fetus has two genetically different sets of cells.

14.42   B D E
hCG is structurally similar to LH, and consists of two α chains and two β chains. It signals the presence of the conceptus to the mother so that the uterus can be maintained in the luteal phase. It is initially secreted by the cytotrophoblast, and later by the syncytiotrophoblast of the implanting blastocyte from a few days after implantation. Urinary test for the β unit of hCG is widely used for the diagnosis of pregnancy.

14.43   A B D E
The placenta produces several hormones during pregnancy. hCG is important from two to seven weeks of pregnancy. Oestrogen and progesterone are important in maintaining the uterus in the luteal phase thereafter. Human placental lactogen and a placental variant of human growth hormone is produced after the first trimester, but their functions are not entirely clear. In the past, the maternal serum level of some of these hormones has been used as indicators of placental function, and 16α-hydroxylated steroids have been used as indicators of fetal well-being. However, these biochemical markers are now seldom used as ultrasound and Doppler findings have been found to be more reliable.

14.44   C D E
The volume of amniotic fluid produced in pregnancy increases until about 34 weeks. The average amniotic fluid volume at 20 weeks is about 500 ml. Apart from a much lower protein content, the composition of the amniotic fluid is broadly similar to that of normal serum. Before about 20 weeks into pregnancy, the amniotic fluid exchanges freely with the extracellular fluid of the fetus via its lungs, gut and skin. In later stages of pregnancy, micturition of the fetus contributes significantly to amniotic fluid volume. Hence renal agenesis of the fetus (Potter's syndrome) is associated with a low volume of amniotic fluid (oligohydramnios). The fetus swallowing contributes significantly to the removal of amniotic fluid in late pregnancy. Hence an excess of amniotic fluid (polyhydramnios) occurs in mechanical gastrointestinal obstruction (e.g. oesophageal atresia). Skin epithelial cells of the fetus can be found in the amniotic fluid. Hence chromosomal and genetic diseases may be diagnosed by sampling the amniotic fluid (amniocentesis) in early pregnancy.

14.45   D E
As the amniotic fluid exchanges freely with the extracellular fluid of the fetus, abnormalities in the fetus may cause abnormalities in the amniotic fluid. Abnormally low or abnormally high amniotic fluid volume may be due to renal agenesis or oesophageal atresia respectively (see question 14.44 above). A high AFP level in the amniotic fluid may indicate open neural tube defect in the fetus. The maternal serum AFP level may also be raised, although the result is not as reliable as the amniotic fluid level. Maternal AFP level and ultrasound are used as initial screening tests. A high unconjugated bilirubin level in the amniotic fluid in late pregnancy is likely to be due to haemolytic diseases in the fetus. This is usually due to rhesus incompatibility, although the disease is now rare due to the use of anti-D in rhesus-negative mothers after delivery. Amniotic bilirubin level may be used to monitor the disease antenatally. The fetal lung secretes surfactant during late pregnancy, and a lack of surfactant may cause idiopathic respiratory distress syndrome in the newborn baby. A component of the surfactant may be detected in the amniotic fluid in late pregnancy. This is valuable in predicting whether the fetus would develop idiopathic respiratory distress syndrome if delivered prematurely. If the sphingomyelin: lecithin ratio is low (<2), intramuscular corticosteroid or ACTH may be given to the mother at least 48 h before delivery in order to stimulate the fetus lung to produce sufficient surfactant.

14.46   A B C D E
Fetal cells are obtained from both amniocentesis and chorionic villous biopsy. Hence the karyotype of the fetus can be examined for chromosomal abnormalities such as Down's syndrome and Turner's syndrome. Genetic diseases may be diagnosed using recombinant DNA techniques if the relevant gene probes are available. These are now available for cystic fibrosis, haemophilia, Duchenne muscular dystrophy and most haemoglobinopathies.

14.47   B D E
Fetal antigens are different from the maternal antigens. Hence the mother's immune system would reject the fetus if there are no protecting mechanisms. It has been shown that the mother is neither generally immunosuppressed nor tolerant to the fetal antigens during pregnancy. Hence a rhesus-negative mother would react against rhesus-positive antigen on the fetal red cell membrane. The major protecting mechanisms are that the chorionic trophoblast is inert and acts as an immunological filter; some maternal immune cells may not cross the placenta (although IgG does cross the human placenta); and that free fetal antigens may bind to and hence 'mop up' a small quantity of maternal antibodies or immune cells. The last mechanism fails in rhesus incompatibility because the antigen is only present in a small proportion of cells in the body (red blood cells).

The reproductive system

14.48   A B D E

To prepare for parturition, the cervix needs to be softened ('ripened'), and the uterus needs to be capable of contracting strongly and in a coordinated manner to expel the fetus. Prostaglandin both softens the cervix and increases the contractility of the uterus, and it is released locally from the cervix and uterus. Oxytocin also increases the contractility of the uterus. The release of both prostaglandin and oxytocin is facilitated by an increase in the oestrogen to progesterone ratio. Relaxin is also released in late pregnancy. It also softens the cervix. It might also soften the ligaments joining individual pelvic bones, and hence facilitate delivery.

14.49   A C D

The uterine muscle cells hypertrophy during pregnancy. They also act as a syncytium so that action potentials can spread via gap junctions. This allows effective and coordinated contraction of the uterus during parturition. The pacemakers are usually at the upper end of the uterus, so that contraction results in expulsion of the fetus. Uterine contraction is initiated by an increase of intracellular calcium. This is regulated by both prostaglandin and oxytocin. Prostaglandin increases the release of calcium from intracellular stores, whilst oxytocin lowers the excitation threshold of the muscle cells.

14.50   A C D

See question 14.49. Clinically, induction of labour may be achieved by artificial rupture of membranes, prostaglandin pessary and intravenous syntocinon. Artificial rupture of membranes causes an sudden release of prostaglandin from the cervix and uterus. Intravenous salbutamol (β-adrengergic agonist) tends to inhibit uterine contraction and prolong labour.

14.51

A

i *Genetic sex* is determined by the sex chromosomes. Normal males are XY and normal females are XX.

ii *Presence of testes* is determined by the sex-determining region of the Y chromosome (SRY). SRY is located near the tip of the short arm of the human Y chromosome. It initiates the transcription of a cascade of genes essential for testicular differentiation.

iii Ovaries develop in the absence of the Y chromosome.

iv Male internal genitalia (i.e. epididymis, vas deferens) develop from the Wolffian ducts. The Wolffian ducts persist only in the presence of testosterone secreted by the testes; otherwise, they will disappear.

v Female internal genitalia (Fallopian tubes and uterus) develop from the Mullerian duct system. The Mullerian ducts regress by apoptosis in the presence of Mullerian

inhibiting substance (MIS) secreted by Sertoli cells in the testes; otherwise, they persist.

vi Testosterone induces the formation of male external genitalia (i.e. the penis).

vii Female external genitalia develop in the absence of testosterone.

viii Gender assignment is usually determined by the appearance of the external genitalia.

B

See Table 14.3.

14.52

Male-to-female transsexuals have XY chromosome and testes, with normal male internal and external genitalia. They are reared as boys in childhood but psychologically feel that they are females (i.e. female gender identity). They may choose either males or females as sexual partners (i.e. either male or female sexual preference).

14.53

A

The onset of puberty is associated with growth spurts. In boys it occurs on average about 2 years later than in girls, which explains the common observation that, although men are in general taller than women in adulthood, girls are taller than boys between the ages of about 11 to 14.

B

Changes associated with puberty in boys include:
- deepening of voice
- development of beard, axillary and pubic hair
- enlargement of testes, increase in length and width of penis, pigmentation of scrotum
- becoming more aggressive; developing interest in opposite sex.

Changes associated with puberty for girls include:
- breast development (thelarche)
- development of axillary and pubic hair (pubarche)
- onset of menstruation (menarche).

C

According to the hypothalamic maturation hypothesis, the maturation of the hypothalamus is central to the initiation of puberty, independent of the pituitary–gonadal axis. The onset of puberty is initiated by pulsatile release of gonadotropin releasing hormone (GnRH). According to the gonadostat hypothesis, maturation of the feedback system of the hypothalamo–pituitary–gonadal axis is important. Puberty in boys is due mostly to androgens, particularly testosterone. In girls, oestrogen plays an important part.

Table 14.3

	Turner's syndrome	Klinefelter's syndrome	Testicular feminisation syndrome	Adrenogenital syndrome in females	True hermaphroditism
Basic defect	Lack of an X chromosome compared with normal females	An extra X chromosome in normal males	Peripheral tissues insensitive to androgen	Enzyme deficiency in steroid biosynthesis	Mosaicism of cells with XX and XY sex chromosomes
Sex chromosomes constitution	XO	XXY	XY	XX	XX/XY
Presence of testes	No	Yes	Yes (undescended)	No	Yes
Presence of ovaries	Streak or absent	No	No	Yes	Yes
Presence of male internal genitalia	No	Yes	No	No	Either, but often yes
Presence of female internal genitalia	Yes	No	No	Yes	Either, but often no
External genitalia	Female	Male	Female	May appear male	Either, but often male
Likely gender assignment	Female	Male	Female	Female (if detected and treated)	Either

D

Over the last century, the age of puberty has been gradually declining in developed countries, for both boys and girls. Two possible hypotheses are:
- Puberty does not occur until a critical weight is reached (about 47 kg for girls and 55 kg for boys). Children now achieve the critical weight earlier as a result of improved nutrition.
- Longer days achieved by artificial light (although this is unlikely to be important for humans).

14.54
A

Menarche (first menstrual period) is considered pathologically delayed if it has not occurred by the age of about 16. It is definitely abnormal if menstruation has not occurred by 20 years of age.

B

As she had normal breast development, testicular feminisation is excluded.
   The site of lesion may be in the:
- *hypothalamus* – e.g. due to anorexia nervosa, constitutional delay (usually with a family history)
- *pituitary* – e.g. due to prolactinoma

- *ovary* – e.g. streak ovaries in Turner's syndrome
- *uterus* – e.g. absent uterus, imperforate hymen

14.55
A

The endocrine results show very high levels of follicle-stimulating hormone (FSH) and luteinizing hormone (LH). As she was 55 years old and suffered from hot flushes, the diagnosis is almost certainly menopause. In menopause, the ovaries become unresponsive to gonadotrophins. This results in a decline of the number of primordial follicles in the ovaries.

B

Hot flushes are associated with declining oestrogen levels and can be prevented by oestrogen treatment; however, these symptoms seem to coincide with beginning of surges of LH release. The exact mechanism is not entirely clear.

C

Normally, the secretion of FSH and LH is subject to negative feedback control from circulating oestrogen levels. If the production of oestrogen is reduced, this negative feedback control is lost and the levels of both FSH and LH rise.

SYSTEM-BASED MEDICAL SCIENCES

The reproductive system

D

The 17 β-estradiol level would be very low.

E

Menopause is a physiological process. Its symptoms may be controlled by oestrogen replacement. Hormone replacement therapy may be given orally, as skin patches or as an implant. It is usually given together with progesterone to reduce the risk of uterine cancer, unless a total hysterectomy has been carried out.

14.56

A

1. *Primary spermatocytes* develop from the primitive germ cells in the seminiferous tubules from adolescence.
2. Meiosis of primary spermatocytes results in *secondary spermatocytes, spermatids* and sperm. (This process is dependent on the presence of *androgens*.)
3. Mature sperms are released from the Sertoli cells and appear in the lumen of the tubules.
4. Sperm acquire motility during passage through the epididymis.
5. Sperm motility is further improved by *relaxin* released from the prostate gland.
6. Sperm enter the vagina.
7. Sperm acquire the ability to produce fertilisation (better adherence to the ovum) in the time spent in the female reproductive tract (capacitation).

B

Exposure of the scrotum to periods of high temperature can considerably reduce the sperm count because spermatogenesis requires a temperature considerably lower than that of the interior of the body.

C

The main abnormality is the severe reduction of the percentage of motile sperm (to 10%), which is certainly sufficient to account for the couple's infertility.

14.57

A

Penile erection is initiated by penile arteriole dilatation. The erectile tissue of the penis is filled with blood. The veins are compressed and the outflow of blood from the penis is blocked. Hence, the penis becomes turgid.

B

The afferent nerves from the genitalia travel to the lumbar segments of the spinal cord. The efferent fibres are the parasympathetic fibres in the pelvic splanchnic nerves. These fibres contain acetylcholine and vasoactive intestinal peptide (VIP). Acetylcholine acts on the muscarinic

receptors to decrease the release of noradrenaline (norepinephrine). VIP produces vasodilatation. There are also nonadrenergic noncholinergic fibres which contain large quantities of nitric oxide (NO) synthase; it appears that NO is an important mediator of erection.

C

i Papaverine is a phosphodiesterase inhibitor and increases cellular cyclic AMP. It also blocks calcium channels. Its action is to relax vascular smooth muscle. Hence, direct injection of papaverine into the corpus cavernosum of the penis relaxes smooth muscle in the blood vessels and produces erection.
ii *Local alprostodil (prostaglandin E)* is a vasodilator and causes penile arteriole dilatation.
iii *Oral sildenafil* (Viagra) is a potent inhibitor of cGMP phophodiesterase type V; hence, sildenafil increases cGMP, which in turn increases NO levels and decreases arteriolar smooth muscle tone.

14.58

A

- Male sex drive.
- Libido.
- Spermatogenesis.
- Increase in muscle mass.
- Regulation of secretion of LH by negative feedback.

B

i Testosterone is synthesised from cholesterol in the Leydig cells and is also formed from androstenedione secreted by the adrenal cortex.
ii Testosterone and dihydrotestosterone (DHT). DHT is converted from testosterone in the peripheral cells by the enzyme 5α-reductase. Testosterone is particularly important for sex drive and libido and DHT is particularly important for the development of facial hair, acne and hairline recession.
iii Testosterone enters the cell and binds to intracellular receptors to form complexes, which then bind to DNA in the nucleus to facilitate the transcription of various genes to produce the desired effects.

C

An example of an antiandrogen drug is cyproterone. It has been proposed for use in the treatment of severe hypersexuality in male sexual offenders. It is also used to treat precocious puberty in males and severe masculinisation or acne in women.

14.59

A

1. At birth, there are numerous primordial follicles in the ovaries.

Table 14.4

	4 days before ovulation	4 days after ovulation
General		
Basal body temperature		Increases by about 0.5°C
Uterus		
Phase	Proliferative	Secretory
Thickness of endometrium	Rapidly increasing under the influence of oestrogen, moderately thick	Thick
Uterine glands	Lengthen, but are not convoluted and do not secrete	Convoluted and secrete clear fluid
Cervix		
Thickness of mucus	Thin, exhibit fern-like pattern	Thick
Cellularity of mucus	Not cellular	Highly cellular
Breasts		
Lobules and alveoli		Growth of lobules and alveoli
Symptoms	Nil	Breast swelling and tenderness
Endocrine		
Progesterone	Very low	High
17 β-estradiol	Moderate (but increase to a peak at ovulation)	High (reduced from peak at ovulation)
LH	Moderate (before surge at ovulation)	Moderate (after surge at ovulation)
FSH	Moderate (before surge at ovulation)	Moderate (after surge at ovulation)

2. At each ovarian cycle, several of these follicles enlarge, with a cavity around the ovum (antrum formation).
3. One of these follicles grows rapidly at the sixth day, and becomes the dominant follicle.
4. Other follicles regress by apoptosis.
5. Theca interna cells of the follicle secrete oestrogen.

B

Ovulation is the process by which the distended follicle ruptures and the ovum is extruded into the abdominal cavity. It usually occurs at about 14 days of the cycle.

C

See Table 14.4.

D

After ovulation, the luteal cells of the corpus luteum secrete progesterone and oestrogen. These hormones are responsible for the changes observed in the uterus and cervix.

E

The LH surge at the time of ovulation is due to a positive feedback effect of oestrogen on LH secretion. Normally, if oestrogen is moderately elevated, the secretion of LH is inhibited (negative feedback effect). However, if the elevation of oestrogen is pronounced and prolonged, a positive feedback effect occurs, which results in the LH surge.

F

Clinical indicators for ovulation are mainly concerned with the increase in progesterone level and include:
- increase in basal body temperature
- thinning and increased elasticity of cervical mucus
- raised serum progesterone level 7 days before menstruation
- sudden reduction in size of the dominant follicle, shown by ultrasound.

G

Changes observed in the uterus and cervix do not occur in the absence of ovulation because there is no corpus luteum to produce oestrogen and progesterone.

14.60

A

1. Sperm are attracted by the chemotactic factor released by the ovum.
2. Many sperm reach the ovum.
3. Sperm bind to a sperm receptor in the zona pellucida.
4. The acrosome of the sperm is broken down (acrosomal reaction) and several enzymes (including acrosin) are released.
5. Acrosin facilitates the penetration of the zona pellucida by the sperm.
6. Sperm and ovum are fused and the blastocyte is formed.
7. The blastocyte moves down the Fallopian tube to the uterus.
8. The blastocyte is implanted in the uterus.

The reproductive system

B

i   Monozygotic (identical) twins occur when one sperm fertilises the ovum, but the conceptus then divides into two distinct groups of cells. The twins are then genetically identical.

ii Dizygotic twins occur when two ova are fertilised within the same menstrual cycle. The genetic similarity of the twins is the same as that between any siblings.

14.61

A

Clomifene induces ovulation. The gynaecologist may consider the absence of ovulation as the most likely reason for the patient's infertility.

B

Clomifene is an anti-oestrogen drug. It inhibits oestrogen binding in the anterior pituitary gland to prevent the normal feedback inhibition of the release of GnRH and gonadotrophins. Hence, the release of GnRH, LH and FSH is increased, which results in ovulation.

14.62

A

Combined oral contraceptives consist of a combination of oestrogen and progesterone. They are taken cyclically for 21 days followed by 7 pill-free days. They act as follows:

*   Oestrogen inhibits the release of FSH and suppresses ovarian follicular development.
*   Progesterone inhibits the release of LH and prevents ovulation.
*   Both oestrogen and progesterone alter the endometrium, discouraging implantation.

Progesterone-only pills are taken daily without interruption. Progesterone acts as follows:

*   It alters cervical mucus to make sperms less likely to survive.
*   It hinders implantation through its effects on endometrium.

B

Advantages are:

*   much more effective (smaller failure rate)

*   less risk of irregular periods and bleeding between periods.

Disadvantages are:

*   minor side effects: weight gain, nausea
*   very small increased risk of thromboembolism
*   small increased risk of reversible hypertension
*   possibly very small increased risk of breast cancer.

14.63

A

i   The changes in the cervix and uterus required for parturition include:

*   softening and dilatation of the cervix
*   increased sensitivity of the uterine muscles to oxytocin.

ii For parturition to progress smoothly, contractions of the uterus must increase progressively until the baby is born. This is achieved by a positive feedback system. Uterine contraction causes increased dilatation and distension of the vagina. This stimulus causes an increased secretion of oxytocin, which causes further uterine contraction. The number of oxytocin receptors in the uterine muscles also increases.

B

*   *A prostaglandin vaginal pessary* (prostaglandin E and F) relaxes and softens the cervix. It also promotes a series of coordinated contractions of the body of the uterus.
*   Syntocinon is a synthetic oxytocin, to which the pregnant uterus is very sensitive. It causes regular coordinated contractions, which travel from the fundus to the cervix, as well as increasing the frequency of contractions.
*   *Artificial rupture of the membranes* releases prostaglandins locally and has the same effects as a prostaglandin vaginal pessary.

C

In the uterus, α-adrenergic agonists (e.g. noradrenaline (norepinephrine)) stimulate muscle contraction and β₂-adrenergic agonists (e.g. adrenaline (epinephrine), ritodrine) inhibit muscle contraction. Hence, ritodrine infusion may be used in an attempt to prolong the pregnancy.

The renal and urinary system

15.1 The urinary concentration is normally significantly higher than the plasma concentration for the following substances:
- **A** Glucose
- **B** Urea
- **C** Sodium ions
- **D** Creatinine
- **E** Albumin

15.2 The following substances are produced by the kidneys:
- **A** Renin
- **B** Aldosterone
- **C** Erythropoietin
- **D** 1,25-Dihydroxycholecalciferol
- **E** Angiotensin II

15.3 The following statements about the kidneys are true:
- **A** The left kidney lies slightly more inferior than the right kidney
- **B** They normally move downwards on inspiration
- **C** They lie in the peritoneal cavity
- **D** They mainly receive parasympathetic innervation
- **E** They are surrounded by fatty tissue

15.4 In contrast to cortical nephrons, juxtamedullary nephrons:
- **A** Are more abundant
- **B** Have longer loops of Henle
- **C** Have glomeruli on the outer portions of the renal cortex
- **D** Do not have vasa recta
- **E** Produce more concentrated urine

15.5 The following structures of juxtamedullary nephrons can be found in the renal medulla:
- **A** Renal glomeruli
- **B** Distal convoluted tubules
- **C** Thin descending limb of the loops of Henle
- **D** Vasa recta
- **E** Collecting ducts

15.6 The ureters:
- **A** Open into the anterior surface of the bladder
- **B** Have fibrous walls
- **C** Are partially innervated via the testicular plexus in the male
- **D** Are separated from the bladder by bicuspid ureteric sphincters
- **E** Run anterior to the parietal peritoneum

15.7 The following structures originate from the ureteric bud in their embryological development:
- **A** The renal pelvis
- **B** Glomeruli
- **C** Loops of Henle
- **D** Collecting ducts
- **E** The ureters

15.8 A horseshoe kidney:
- **A** Results from the degeneration of the ureteric bud
- **B** Results from a defect in the function of the proximal convoluted tubule
- **C** Occurs as a result of abnormal descent of the metanephric mesoderm in its development
- **D** Occurs in less than one out of a million people
- **E** Is associated with fusion of the upper poles of both kidneys

15.9 An inert substance X is not produced, stored or metabolised by the kidneys. It is freely filtered by the kidneys. It is actively secreted but not reabsorbed by the renal tubules. It does not affect renal blood flow. The urine flow is 10 ml/min, the urinary concentration of X is 20 mg/ml, and its plasma concentration is 0.2 mg/ml.
- **A** Substance X is ideal for measuring glomerular filtration rate (GFR)
- **B** Substance X is ideal for measuring effective renal plasma flow
- **C** The effective renal plasma flow is 1 litre/min
- **D** The GFR is less than 1 litre/min
- **E** The clearance of X is greater than the GFR

15.10 Which of the following increase renal blood flow?
- **A** Noradrenaline (norepinephrine)
- **B** Dopamine
- **C** Exercise
- **D** Renin
- **E** Changing from supine to erect position

15.11 The GFR:
- **A** Is higher in women than in men
- **B** Is higher in neonates than in adults after correction for surface area
- **C** Is higher in the elderly than in younger adults.
- **D** Is normally about 1.8 litres per day (1.25 ml/min) in adults
- **E** May be estimated by creatinine clearance in clinical practice

15.12 The following substances are correctly matched to the mechanism of reabsorption in the proximal renal tubules:
- **A** Mannitol – passive diffusion
- **B** Water – secondary active transport via carrier proteins

215

SYSTEM-BASED MEDICAL SCIENCES

The renal and urinary system

C Glucose – primary active transport
D Sodium ions – secondary active transport via carrier proteins
E Lactic acid – passive diffusion

15.13 Fluid at the following sites of the nephron is significantly hypertonic:
A The glomerulus
B Thin descending loop of Henle
C The top of the thick ascending loop of Henle
D Distal tubule
E Medullary portion of the collecting duct

15.14 In the absence of vasopressin (antidiuretic hormone):
A The collecting ducts are highly permeable to water
B Reabsorption of sodium ions in the proximal renal tubules is reduced
C The osmolality of the urine is abnormally low
D The osmolality of the plasma is abnormally low
E The urine volume is abnormally low

15.15 A reduction in the transport of sodium and chloride ions from the thick segment of the ascending loop of Henle:
A May result in increased urinary potassium excretion
B May result in diuresis
C May increase the osmolality in the medullary interstitium
D May be caused by furosemide (frusemide)
E May be caused by thiazides

15.16 Spironolactone:
A Is an aldosterone antagonist
B Decreases the sodium reabsorption in the distal tubule
C May cause hypokalaemia
D Is a more powerful diuretic than furosemide (frusemide)
E Antagonises the diuretic effect of furosemide (frusemide)

15.17 Osmotic diuresis occurs in:
A Mannitol infusion
B Diabetes insipidus
C Diabetes mellitus
D Compulsive water drinking
E Inappropriate ADH secretion

15.18 Recognised indications for furosemide (frusemide) include:
A Congestive heart failure
B Hypokalaemia (low potassium level)

C Hypercalcaemia (high calcium level)
D Hypertension
E Hyponatraemia (low sodium level)

15.19 Sodium excretion from the kidneys increases with:
A Shock
B Massive gastrointestinal haemorrhage
C A high-salt dietary intake
D An abnormally high plasma level of aldosterone
E Hypotension

15.20 The following changes occur in dehydration:
A Renal blood flow decreases
B GFR increases
C The medullary interstitial fluid becomes more hypertonic
D The urine becomes less concentrated
E Less vasopressin is secreted

15.21 The following statements about the transport of hydrogen ions from renal tubular cells into the tubular lumen are true:
A It occurs mainly in the loop of Henle
B Passive diffusion is an important mechanism
C Primary active transport is an important mechanism
D It is coupled with the entry of a sodium ion from the tubular lumen into the tubular cell
E It fails to occur if the pH of the urine is less than 3

15.22 Acetazolamide:
A Is an inhibitor of carbonic anhydrase
B Increases the production of aqueous humour
C Is an effective and commonly used diuretic
D Usually increases the plasma pH
E May be useful in preventing mountain sickness and facilitating acclimatisation at high altitude

15.23 The following buffer systems in the renal tubular lumen are important for effective excretion of hydrogen ions:
A Bicarbonate
B Sulphate
C Phosphate
D Ammonia
E Chloride

15.24 Alkalisation of urine:
A May be achieved by oral ammonium chloride
B Discourages the growth of *Escherichia coli* in urine
C Is useful in the treatment of amphetamine poisoning

D Is useful in the treatment of aspirin poisoning

E Is useful in the treatment of phenobarbitone poisoning

15.25 Recognised pharmacological effects of thiazide diuretics include:

A Increased plasma potassium

B Decreased plasma sodium

C Increased plasma magnesium

D Glucose intolerance

E Increased plasma uric acid

15.26 The following abnormalities frequently occur in renal failure:

A Anaemia

B Metabolic alkalosis

C High plasma urea

D Low plasma creatinine

E High plasma calcium

15.27 The presence of significant quantities of the following substances in urine is characteristic of glomerular damage:

A Urea

B Blood

C Protein

D Amino acids

E Glucose

15.28 Recognised causes of glomerular diseases include:

A Anti-glomerular basement membrane antibodies

B Diabetes mellitus

C Connective tissue disease

D Drugs

E Post-streptococcal infection

15.29 Recognised pathological features of obstructive nephropathy due to ureteric calculi include:

A Dilated renal pelvis

B Constricted renal calyces

C Atrophic renal tissues

D Hydronephrosis

E Dilated bladder

15.30 Pyelonephritis occurs more frequently:

A During pregnancy than at other times for women

B In the presence of vesico-ureteric reflux

C In the presence of urinary tract infection

D In the presence of septicaemia

E Following urethral catheterisation

15.31 Factors which favour the formation of stones in the urinary tract include:

A *Proteus* urinary tract infection

B Hypocalcaemia

C Excess excretion of calcium in urine

D High plasma uric acid level

E High blood cholesterol level

15.32 The following statements about renal cell carcinoma (hypernephroma) are true:

A It is the commonest malignant tumour in men

B It occurs less frequently than transitional cell tumour of the kidney

C Patients frequently present after metastasis has occurred

D It may be associated with polycythaemia (high red cell number)

E It is associated with exposure to aniline dye

15.33 The empty bladder:

A Lies entirely in the pelvis in adults

B Lies entirely in the pelvis in young children

C Can be palpated through the abdominal wall in adults

D Is approximately cuboid in shape

E Is joined at the middle portion of its anterior surface by the two ureters

15.34 The following groups of muscles usually contract during voluntary micturition:

A Perineal muscles

B External urethral sphincter

C Detrusor muscle

D Internal urethral sphincter

E Abdominal wall muscles

15.35 The following statements about neural control of the bladder are true:

A Micturition may occur as a spinal reflex action

B Micturition may be controlled via the higher cortical centre

C The parasympathetic nervous supply to the bladder is active during micturition

D Sympathetic stimulation is associated with contraction of the detrusor muscles

E Sympathetic stimulation is associated with contraction of the external urethral sphincter

15.36 The following groups of drugs are recognised treatment for incontinence of urine due to instability of the detrusor muscle:

A Noradrenaline (norepinephrine)

B Tricyclic antidepressants

C Antimuscarinic agents

D Cholinergic agents

E Inhibitors of serotonin reuptake

The renal and urinary system

15.37 Causes of muscular hypertrophy of the bladder include:
- **A** Renal cell carcinoma
- **B** Benign prostatic hypertrophy
- **C** Carcinoma of the prostate
- **D** Urethral stricture
- **E** Ureteric calculi

15.38 The following statements about bladder tumours are true:
- **A** Sarcomas are commoner than epithelial tumours
- **B** Squamous cell carcinoma is the commonest epithelial tumour
- **C** They are commonly of the papillary type
- **D** Hydronephrosis in one kidney is a recognised complication
- **E** They are more commonly solitary than multiple

15.39 Significant predisposing factors for transitional cell bladder tumours include:
- **A** Aniline dyes
- **B** Schistosomiasis
- **C** Diabetes mellitus
- **D** Smoking
- **E** Excessive alcohol intake

15.40 Acquired bladder diverticula:
- **A** Predispose to calculi formation
- **B** Predispose to urinary tract infection
- **C** Are usually solitary
- **D** Occur more frequently in women than in men
- **E** Are frequently associated with bladder muscle hypertrophy

15.41 The prostate gland:
- **A** Lies lateral to the rectum
- **B** Lies superior to the neck of the bladder
- **C** Can be palpated in a rectal examination
- **D** Surrounds the prostatic urethra
- **E** Produces an acidic secretion

15.42 Benign enlargement of the prostate gland:
- **A** Has a higher incidence in older men
- **B** Is associated with hypertrophy of glandular tissue
- **C** Is caused by a reduction in oestrogen level
- **D** Is associated with multiple circumscribed solid nodules
- **E** May cause trabeculation of the bladder

15.43 Symptoms of benign prostatic enlargement may be partially relieved by:
- **A** Loop diuretics
- **B** α_1-Adrenoceptor antagonist
- **C** β-Adrenoceptor antagonists
- **D** 5 α-Reductase inhibitors
- **E** Synthetic oestrogen

15.44 Clinical prostatic carcinoma:
- **A** Arises most commonly in the lateral lobes
- **B** Is mostly of the squamous cell type
- **C** Is often associated with an abnormal low serum acid phosphatase level
- **D** Is often associated with a raised serum prostatic specific antigen level
- **E** Seldom metastasise to bone

15.45 **A** Inulin is a substance that is freely filtered in the glomeruli and neither reabsorbed nor secreted in the renal tubules. In an experiment, a loading dose of inulin is given intravenously to a subject, followed by a sustained infusion to keep the arterial plasma level constant. At equilibrium, a urine specimen was collected for 3 h. A plasma sample was collected at 90 min. Exactly 1 litre of urine was collected and the urinary concentration of inulin was 10 mg/ml. The plasma concentration was 0.46 mg/ml.
  - i Calculate the renal clearance of inulin. Show your workings carefully.
  - ii Is your answer in (Ai) a good estimate of renal plasma flow or glomerular filtration rate? Explain. List any other assumptions about the property of inulin which are not stated in the question.

  B p-Aminohippuric acid (PAH) is a substance filtered by the glomeuli and secreted by the tubular cells with a high extraction ratio, so that the renal venous concentration is very low. In a similar experiment with PAH rather than inulin, 1 litre of urine was collected over 2 h, and the urinary concentration of PAH was 25 mg/ml. The plasma concentration was 0.35 mg/ml.
  - i Calculate the renal clearance of PAH. Show your workings carefully.
  - ii Is your answer in (Bi) a good estimate of renal blood flow or glomerular filtration rate? Explain. The renal venous concentration of PAH, although low, is not zero. What effect would it have on the estimate?

  C What is meant by filtration fraction? Calculate the filtration fraction from your previous answers.

  D What is the effect of a sudden decrease in blood pressure on renal blood flow and glomerular filtration rate? What is the effect on filtration fraction? Explain.

15.46 A sample of venous blood and urine was taken from a normal young adult, a diabetic young adult and a non-diabetic elderly person. The blood samples were tested for glucose levels and the urine samples were tested for glucose. The results were as follows:
- normal young adult: plasma glucose level 4 mmol/l; no glucose detected in urine
- diabetic young adult: plasma glucose level 16 mmol/l; glucose +++ detected in urine
- non-diabetic elderly person: plasma glucose level 4 mmol/l; glucose ++ detected in urine.

  A For the normal young adult, explain why glucose is present in the plasma and yet no glucose is detected in the urine. Explain in detail any transport mechanism involved and where it occurs in the kidney. Draw a diagram to illustrate the transport mechanisms involved.

  B Glucose appears in the urine of the diabetic young adult but not in the normal young adult. Explain this difference in terms of the transport mechanisms you outlined in (A).

  C Glucose also appears in the urine of the non-diabetic elderly person in spite of a normal plasma glucose level. Explain this observation in terms of the transport mechanisms you outlined.

  D Explain why diabetic patients with a high plasma glucose level often produce large volumes of urine in spite of dehydration.

15.47 A previously healthy subject becomes dehydrated through lack of fluid intake during a long trip. The plasma became hypertonic.

  A Describe the physiological mechanism that enables the subject to drink water to restore the plasma tonicity?

  B Complete Table 15.1 to show the permeability of the various segments of the nephrons to water, both in the presence and absence of vasopressin (ADH). (Use – to indicate non-permeability; and +, ++ and +++ to indicate minimal, moderate and high permeability, respectively.)

Table 15.1

Segment	ADH present	ADH absent
Loop of Henle		
Thin descending limb		
Thin ascending limb		
Thick ascending limb		
Distal convoluted tubule		
Collecting duct		
Cortical portion		
Medullary portion		

  C Using your answer to (B), explain how the kidneys prevent further loss of excess water in the subject.

  D What is free water clearance? Would you expect the 'free water clearance' for this subject to be positive or negative? Explain.

  E What criterion relating to the tonicity of the renal cortex or medulla must be satisfied for the mechanism in (C) to work?

  F Explain the roles of the following in fulfilling this criterion.
    i Countercurrent mechanism.
    ii Vasa recta.
    iii Urea.

  G Give the mechanism of action of the following diuretics:
    i Thiazide diuretics.
    ii Furosemide (frusemide).

15.48 **A** Draw a simple diagram of a renal proximal tubule cell and illustrate how the cell can excrete acid.

  B A patient with severe chronic obstructive airway disease had a high partial pressure of carbon dioxide.
    i What type of acidosis does the high partial pressure of carbon dioxide cause?
    ii Write down the Henderson–Hasselbalch equation and explain the effect of this high partial pressure of carbon dioxide on plasma pH.
    iii Using your diagram in (A), explain how the kidney compensates for this change in pH.

15.49 An adult patient usually took a high therapeutic dose of aspirin. One day, he took a toxic overdose and was admitted to hospital with a high temperature. His respiratory rate became abnormally low and he had severe acidosis.

  A Given that the patient normally takes a high therapeutic dose of aspirin, in what ways might the oxygen consumption and carbon dioxide production be abnormal? Explain.

  B What type of acid/base abnormality was the patient likely to have had before the overdose?

  C What role does the kidney play? Explain.

  D List the principal acid/base buffers in the blood. Are there any acid/base buffers in the interstitial fluid and inside cells?

  E How might aspirin cause the patient to have a high temperature on admission?

  F Give three possible reasons for the severe acidosis on admission.

  G How might the renal excretion of aspirin be increased in this patient? Explain.

The renal and urinary system

15.50 An adult patient presented with high blood pressure and blood and protein in the urine but without any symptoms of pain. After appropriate investigations, the cause was thought to be due to a primary glomerular disease.

   A What is meant by 'primary' and 'secondary' glomerular diseases? Give two examples of secondary glomerular diseases.

   B Describe how primary glomerular diseases might by classified according to the following.

     i Aetiology.

     ii Histology.

   C What does the glomerular capillary comprise and what are the functions of its components?

   D Explain why the patient had the following.

     i High blood pressure.

     ii Blood in the urine.

     iii Protein in the urine.

15.51 Compare and contrast renal cell tumours and bladder tumours by completing Table 15.2.

Table 15.2

	Renal cell tumour	Bladder tumour
Histological types		
Unifocal/multifocal		
Smoking as risk factor		
Chemicals as risk factors		
Other predisposing factors		
Association with hypercalcaemia		
Association with polycythaemia		

The renal and urinary system

15.1   B D
The kidneys filter a fluid (glomerular filtrate) which resembles plasma in composition. In the renal tubules, over 99% of water and about 99% of solutes are reabsorbed. The proportion of urea and creatinine reabsorbed is only about 53% and 8% respectively, and hence their concentrations in urine are higher than their plasma concentrations. Over 99% of sodium is reabsorbed, and its urinary concentration is normally less than its plasma concentration. Normally, almost 100% of the glucose is reabsorbed, and it is absent in the urine. The presence of glucose in urine may be caused by excessive blood glucose (e.g. in diabetes) or reduced reabsorption of glucose by the kidneys (e.g. renal glycosuria). Although albumin is a relatively small molecule (about 7 nm in diameter), it is negatively charged, and is repelled by the negative charges on the glomerular walls. Hence the urinary concentration of albumin in urine is normally very low.

15.2   A C D
Substances produced by the kidneys include renin, erythropoietin and vitamin D (1,25-dihydroxycholecalciferol). Erythropoietin stimulates red cell production, and is useful clinically for the treatment of anaemia in renal failure. 1,25-Dihydroxycholecalciferol is an active metabolite of vitamin D, and is converted from the less active metabolite 25-hydroxycholecalciferol in the proximal tubules of the kidneys. Renin is produced in the kidneys. Renin converts angiotensionogen into angiotensin I, which is in turn converted by angiotensin-converting enzyme into angiotensin II in the lungs. Aldosterone is produced by the adrenal cortex.

15.3   B E
The kidneys lie behind the peritoneum on the posterior abdominal wall under the costal margin. They are surrounded by fatty tissues (perirenal fat, renal fascia and pararenal fat) which support the kidneys and hold them in position. The right kidney lies lower than the left kidney due to the large size of the right lobe of the liver. Both kidneys move downward during inspiration when the diaphragm contracts. This movement may be detected clinically if the kidneys are abnormally large. The kidneys receive mainly sympathetic innervation via the renal sympathetic plexus. This innervation is important in the control of renin secretion and renal blood flow.

15.4   B C E
There are two types of nephrons. In humans, 85% of nephrons are of the juxtamedullary type and 15% are of the cortical type. The cortical nephrons have their glomeruli in the outer portions of the renal cortex, they have shorter loops of Henle, and consequently are less able to produce concentrated urine. By contrast, the juxtamedullary type have their glomeruli on the outer portions of the renal cortex, have longer loops of Henle, and can produce more concentrated urine. There are also more mitochondria as much energy is required to concentrate the urine in the loops of Henle. Vasa recta are vessels that form hairpin loops alongside the loops of Henle which the efferent arterioles of the juxtamedullary glomeruli drain into. Vasa recta are absent in cortical nephrons.

15.5   C D E
The glomerulus and proximal convoluted tubule can be found in the renal cortex. The loops of Henle lie in the outer and inner medulla. The ascending loops of Henle emerge in the cortex from the medulla and form the distal convoluted tubules. The distal tubules coalesce to form the collecting ducts, which then pass through both the renal cortex and medulla to empty into the pelvis of the kidney. Vasa recta are alongside the loops of Henle and are therefore in the renal medulla.

15.6   C
The ureters drain urine from the pelvis of the kidneys to the posterior surface of the urinary bladder. They are retroperitoneal and run immediately behind the parietal peritoneum. Urine is propelled by peristaltic contraction of the smooth muscle walls. Hence patients with ureteric stones may complain of colicky pain. The ureters pass obliquely through the bladder wall, which tends to keep the ureters closed except during peristaltic waves. This usually prevents reflux of urine up the ureters in adults and older children. However, there are no anatomical ureteric sphincters. Renal scarring may result in children under 5 years of age in the presence of both urinary tract infection and reflux of urine into the ureters. The ureters are innervated by renal, testicular (or ovarian in women) and hypogastric plexuses. The innervation from the testicular plexus explains why patients with ureteric colic may complain of referred testicular pain.

15.7   A D E
The kidneys develop from two different sources of embryological tissues: the metanephric mesoderm and the ureteric bud. The ureteric bud gives rise to the ureter, the renal pelvis, the major and minor calyces and the collecting ducts. The metanephric mesoderm gives rise to the glomeruli, the proximal convoluted tubule, the loop of Henle and the distal convoluted tubule. Hence early splitting of the ureteric bud may result in duplication of the ureter and renal pelvis.

15.8   –
The embryological kidneys usually ascend in the cranial direction during their development. If the two kidneys are

SYSTEM-BASED MEDICAL SCIENCES

The renal and urinary system

very close together during their ascent, the lower poles may fuse, and their ascent may be prevented by the root of the inferior mesenteric artery. This results in the formation of a horseshoe kidney. It is a relatively common congenital abnormality and can be found in about one in every 600 people.

15.9   B C D E

Substances for measuring effective renal plasma flow should have the following characteristics: freely filtered by the kidneys; not affecting the renal blood flow; and not stored, produced or metabolised by the kidneys. Substances actively secreted by the renal tubules would be more suitable, as the venous concentration can be ignored, being much smaller than the arterial concentration. The effective renal plasma flow can then be estimated by the clearance of the substance

$$clearance = \frac{\text{urinary concentration} \times \text{urine flow}}{\text{plasma concentration}}$$

Hence,

$$clearance\ of \times (ml/min) = \frac{20 \times 10}{0.2} = 1000\ ml/min = 1\ litre/min$$

Substances for measuring GFR must also be freely filtered by the kidneys, produce no effect on the renal blood flow, and not stored, produced or metabolised by the kidneys. However, there must be no net reabsorption or secretion by renal tubules. The GFR can be calculated by their clearance as above.

   For substances with no net tubular secretion or reabsorption, the clearance equals the GFR. For substances with a net tubular secretion, the clearance exceeds the GFR. For substances with net tubular reabsorption, the clearance is less than the GFR.

15.10   B

Renal blood flow is increased by vasodilatation of the renal afferent arterioles. Noradrenaline (norepinephrine) or stimulation of the sympathetic noradrenergic nerves to the kidneys causes marked vasoconstriction and reduced renal blood flow. This is mediated via the adrenergic receptors, and partially explains the reduction in renal blood flow observed clinically in shock. Renin is released on stimulation of the renal nerves or by direct action of noradrenaline (norepinephrine) on the juxtaglomerular cells. It causes renal vasoconstriction with reduction in renal blood flow and GFR. Dopamine causes renal vasodilatation and an increase in renal blood flow. During exercise, blood is directed away from the kidneys. Changing from supine to standing position also slightly reduces renal blood flow.

15.11   E

The GFR is generally proportional to the body surface area. However, even after correction for surface area, the GFR is higher in men than in women, in adults than in neonates, and in younger adults than in the elderly. This is important clinically in prescribing, as smaller doses should be prescribed for neonates and the elderly. The normal GFR for an average man is 125 ml/min (i.e. 180 litres per day). This is about 60 times the plasma volume. Although inulin clearance is ideal for estimating GFR, creatinine clearance is often sufficiently accurate to be used in clinical practice.

15.12   –

In the proximal renal tubules, sodium ions are reabsorbed by primary active transport with energy derived from Na^+, K^+-ATPase. Some substances such as glucose, amino acids, lactate, citrate, phosphate, hydrogen and chloride ions are reabsorbed using secondary active transport via carrier proteins. For example, glucose and sodium ions bind to the common carrier SGLT 2, and glucose molecules are carried from the renal tubules into the cells as sodium ions move down its electrical and chemical gradient. Water is reabsorbed mainly by passive diffusion down the osmotic gradient created by the reabsorption of sodium ions. Mannitol acts as an osmotic diuretic, as it is not reabsorbed in the proximal convoluted tubule. Hence the osmotic pressure in the proximal renal tubules is increased, and less water is reabsorbed.

15.13   B E

Fluid at the glomerulus and proximal renal tubule is essentially plasma, and is isotonic. As it enters the water-permeable thin descending loop of Henle, water is drawn into the hypertonic interstitium. Hence the fluid becomes hypertonic. At the thick ascending loop of Henle, active transport of sodium into the interstitial fluid takes place but it is impermeable to water. Hence the fluid becomes hypotonic at the top of the thick ascending loop of Henle and the distal tubule. Water moves into the hypertonic interstitial fluid of the medulla at the medullary portion of the collecting duct. Hence it becomes hypertonic.

15.14   C

Vasopressin is produced by the posterior pituitary gland. It acts by increasing the permeability of the collecting ducts to water. Hence, in the absence of vasopressin (as in diabetes insipidus), the collecting ducts are impermeable to water. Therefore less water is reabsorbed from the collecting ducts, the urine volume increases and the urine osmolality decreases. As a result of water loss, the plasma osmolality increases.

15.15   A B D

Loop diuretics such as furosemide (frusemide) and bumetanide inhibit the transport of sodium and chloride ions at the medullary (thick) ascending loop of Henle. As a result, the countercurrent multiplier mechanism cannot function, and the normal hyperosmolality in the medullary interstitium is lost. Hence less water is reabsorbed in the collecting ducts, which results in the production of a large volume of dilute urine. As more sodium ions reach the distal tubule, they exchange with potassium ions, which leads to increased urinary potassium loss and hypokalaemia. Thiazide diuretics act by inhibiting sodium reabsorption at the cortical (thin) segment of the ascending limb of Henle.

15.16   A B
Spironolactone is a competitive inhibitor of aldosterone. Aldosterone increases the sodium reabsorption in exchange for potassium. Hence spironolactone increases urinary potassium loss and may cause hyperkalaemia. Spironolactone is a much less powerful diuretic than furosemide (frusemide). However, it may act synergistically with a loop diuretic such as furosemide (frusemide), as they act on different sites.

15.17   A C
If large quantities of solutes are present in the proximal renal tubules which cannot be reabsorbed, then the osmotic pressure increases and the amount of water reabsorbed increases. This is known as osmotic diuresis. This may result from infusion of mannitol, sodium chloride or urea. Alternatively, the excessive solutes (e.g. glucose) may be produced in disease states (e.g. diabetes mellitus). In inappropriate ADH secretion, the urine volume is reduced. In diabetes insipidus, urine volume increases due to reduced reabsorption of water in the collecting ducts. The reabsorption of water in the proximal renal tubules is normal in compulsive water drinking.

15.18   A C D
Furosemide (frusemide) is an effective diuretic, and reduces the intravascular volume. Hence it is used in the treatment of congestive cardiac failure and pulmonary oedema. It increases the urinary loss of sodium, potassium and calcium by its action on the ascending loop of Henle, and is sometimes used in the emergency treatment of hypercalcaemia.

15.19   C
The extracellular fluid volume depends primarily on the amount of sodium in the body, which in turn depends on the sodium excretion from the kidneys. Hence sodium excretion is delicately controlled by several mechanisms. A reduction in extracellular volume (e.g. in hypotension, in shock and in massive gastrointestinal haemorrhage) results in a reduction of sodium excretion. A high-salt dietary intake results in increased sodium excretion. Aldosterone increases the tubular reabsorption of sodium.

15.20   A C
In dehydration, the kidneys attempt to compensate by increasing the urine concentration and decreasing the urine volume. This is achieved in two ways. Firstly, a reduction in renal blood flow leads to a decrease in the GFR. Hence less fluid is presented to the countercurrent mechanism, and the fluid flow rate in the loop of Henle decreases. The medullary interstitial fluid becomes more concentrated, and hence more water is reabsorbed from the collecting duct. Secondly, the secretion of ADH is increased due to an increase in plasma osmolality. This renders the collecting duct more permeable to water.

15.21   D E
Hydrogen ion is actively secreted into the renal tubular lumen mainly in the proximal and distal renal tubules. This occurs by secondary active transport. The Na^+, K^+-ATPase actively transports sodium from the renal tubule cell into the interstitial fluid. This lowers the concentration of sodium in the renal tubule cell, and sodium diffuses into the tubule cell passively from the tubular lumen in exchange for a hydrogen ion moving into the lumen. The source of hydrogen ions in the renal tubule cell is carbonic anhydrase, which catalyses the formation of H_2CO_3, which dissociates into hydrogen and bicarbonate ions. If the pH of the tubular fluid is less than 4.5, this transport mechanism fails. Hence the minimum possible urinary pH is 4.5.

15.22   A E
Acetazolamide is the most commonly used carbonic anhydrase inhibitor. Carbonic anhydrase is present in tissues secreting either acid or alkaline fluids, such as the gastric mucosa, renal tubule cells, the eye and the pancreas. It catalyses the formation of hydrogen and bicarbonate ions from water and carbon dioxide, which are essential in any acid or alkaline secretor processes. As acids are usually actively secreted in the renal tubular lumen, inhibition of carbonic anhydrase usually decreases urinary acid secretion and reduces the plasma pH. Acetazolamide is not commonly used as a diuretic. As the formation of aqueous humour depends on the availability of bicarbonate ions, acetazolamide reduces the formation of aqueous humour and is used clinically to lower the intraocular pressure in glaucoma. It is also occasionally used to facilitate acclimatisation at high altitude. Mountain sickness is caused by hypoxia, and the acidosis induced by acetazolamide may help to increase respiratory drive.

15.23   A C D
The secretion of acid into the tubular lumen cannot occur if the urinary pH is less than 4.5. However, excretion of acid may be increased if free hydrogen ions are removed

15 The renal and urinary system

from the urine in the tubular lumen by buffer systems. There are three main buffer systems: reaction with bicarbonate ions to form water and carbon dioxide; reaction with HPO_4^{2-} to form $H_2PO_4^-$, and reaction with ammonia to form ammonium ions.

15.24 B D E
Alkalisation of urine may be achieved either by sodium bicarbonate infusion or oral potassium citrate. Alkalisation of urine discourages bacterial growth in the urinary tract and reduces urinary tract inflammation, and is occassionally used to treat urinary tract infection in combination with antibiotics. Acidification of urine may be achieved by oral ammonium chloride. In poisoning by acidic drugs such as salicylate or phenobarbitone, alkalisation of urine increases the proportion of the ionised form of the drug in the tubular fluid which is lipid-insoluble and remains in the renal tubules. This increases its excretion in urine. Conversely, acidification of basic drugs such as amphetamine increases their urinary excretion.

15.25 B D E
Thiazide diuretics act by reducing sodium reabsorption at the cortical diluting segment between the ascending loop of Henle and the distal renal tubules. This leads to increased sodium excretion and a low plasma sodium level. The increased sodium at the distal renal tubule leads to increased Na^+–K^+ exchange at the distal tubule, and hence urinary potassium excretion is also increased. Potassium supplements may be required clinically. Both loop and thiazide diuretics may cause increased urinary excretion of magnesium, and may rarely cause cardiac arrhythmia. The urinary uric acid excretion is reduced for two reasons. Firstly, thiazide diuretics may compete for the transport of uric acid secretion into the renal tubules. Secondly, the volume depletion may lead to a reduction of GFR and an increased reabsorption of all solutes including uric acid. Both thiazides and loop diuretics may cause glucose intolerance due to prolonged hypokalaemia.

15.26 A C
In renal failure, the function of the kidneys is impaired, and the breakdown products of protein metabolism accumulate in the blood. Urea and creatinine are only two of many such substances. This clinical picture is known as uraemia, and symptoms may include anorexia, nausea, vomiting, lethargy, confusion and convulsions. As acid is normally actively excreted by the kidneys, abnormal accumulation of acid in the blood occurs in renal failure. Renal failure also results in failure to produce erythropoietin, which leads to anaemia. As the kidneys normally manufacture an active metabolite of vitamin D (1,25-dihydroxycholecalciferol), renal failure may be

associated with renal rickets and a low plasma calcium level.

15.27 B C
Normally, large particles such as proteins and red blood cells are filtered by the glomeruli. Hence the presence of large quantities of blood and protein in urine is characteristic of glomerular disease. Smaller molecules (e.g. glucose and amino acids) are reabsorbed in the proximal and distal renal tubules. Thus the urinary excretion of these substances is increased in tubular diseases. As hydrogen ions are normally secreted in the renal tubules from the tubular lumen, renal tubular diseases are often associated with an abnormally high urinary pH and metabolic acidosis. The presence of urea in urine is normal.

15.28 A B C D E
There are numerous causes of glomerular diseases. They may be divided into immunological and non-immunological causes. Immunological causes may be primary (e.g. anti-glomerular basement membrane antibodies in Goodpasture's disease) or secondary to non-glomerular antigens (e.g. post-streptococcal glomerulonephritis). Non-immunological causes are usually secondary to diseases outside the kidneys (e.g. infections, metabolic diseases, vasculitis, drugs). Metabolic diseases which cause glomerular damage include diabetes mellitus and amyloidosis. Vasculitis may be caused by polyarteritis nodosa, systemic lupus erythematosus, and Henoch–Schönlein purpura. Drugs which may cause glomerular damage include gold and penicillamine.

15.29 A C D
Obstructive nephropathy may be due to any cause of urinary tract obstruction, and includes uretero-pelvic stenosis, ureteric stones, carcinoma of the bladder, carcinoma of the prostate and benign prostatic hyperplasia. The clinical and pathological features depend on the level of obstruction. If the obstruction is at the level of the ureter, the back-pressure causes dilatation of the renal pelvis and calyceal system. The kidney may become dilated, and the renal tissue may undergo atrophy due to compression. This is hydronephrosis. The bladder would not be affected as it is below the level of obstruction.

15.30 A B C D E
Pyelonephritis is defined as infection of the kidney. The infecting organisms may originate either in the bloodstream (i.e. in septicaemia) or from retrograde spread from the lower urinary tract. Ascending infection from the lower urinary tract may occur if the urine is infected and there is reflux of urine into the kidney.

Urinary tract infection is commoner in women (due to short urethra), in pregnancy and following instrumentation of the urethra (e.g. urethral catheterisation). Reflux urine is more likely in patients with vesico-ureteric reflux, which may be due either to congenital abnormalities in children or to urinary tract obstruction in adults.

15.31 A C D

The commonest type of urinary calculi consists of calcium oxalate, followed by magensium ammonium phosphate and uric acid. The risk of calcium oxalate stones is increased in the presence of high urinary calcium, which may be due either to high serum calcium or idiopathic hypercalcuria (high urinary calcium with normal serum calcium). Magnesium ammonium phosphate calculi characteristically form large staghorn calculi. They are often associated with *Proteus* urinary tract infection, as *Proteus* breaks down urea to form ammonia. The formation of magnesium ammonium phosphate calculi is facilitated by alkaline urine. Gout is caused by an increased serum uric acid level, which also increases the risk of uric acid calculi formation.

15.32 C D

The commonest malignant tumours in men are bronchial carcinoma and colorectal carcinoma, and renal tumours are relatively uncommon. Amongst the primary malignant renal tumours, renal cell carcinoma is the commonest. Other less common histological types include Wilms' tumour (which occurs in children) and transitional cell tumour of the renal pelvis. Renal cell tumour has a small association with smoking, and occurs more frequently in a rare hereditary condition (Hippel–Lindau disease). Transitional cell tumours of the renal pelvis, like transitional cell tumours of the bladder, are associated with exposure to aniline dye and other chemical agents. Renal cell tumour may be associated with inappropriate erythropoietin secretion, which causes polycythaemia.

15.33 A

The empty bladder lies completely in the pelvis in adults, but rises to the hypogastric region of the abdominal cavity when it is filled with urine. Hence the empty bladder cannot be palpated through the anterior abdominal wall. However, in children under five years of age, the empty bladder lies partially in the abdominal cavity. The empty bladder is approximately pyramidal in shape, with its apex facing anteriorly and its base facing posteriorly. The ureters join the bladder obliquely at the superolateral angles of its posterior surface. This arrangement normally prevents the retrograde flow of urine from the bladder up the ureters.

15.34 C E

Micturition may be either a reflex action, a voluntary action, or a combination of both. Detrusor muscle forms the smooth muscular coat of the bladder, and is arranged in longitudinal, circular and spiral bundles. Its contraction helps to increase the pressure in the bladder during micturition. In voluntary micturition, the abdominal wall muscles also contract to increase the intra-abdominal pressure. The external urethral sphincter consists of skeletal (voluntary) muscles surrounding the membranous urethra. It is relaxed during micturition. It and the perineal muscles may be voluntarily contracted to postpone emptying of the bladder. The internal urethral sphincter consists of smooth muscles, and it plays no part in micturition.

15.35 A B C E

Micturition may occur as a spinal reflex action, as in a newborn baby. However, after about 18 months of age, it may be controlled and moderated by higher cortical centres. The bladder is supplied by both the sympathetic and parasympathetic nervous systems. Stimulation of the parasympathetic nerves causes contraction of the detrusor muscle and relaxation of the external urethral sphincter. This occurs during micturition. Conversely, stimulation of the sympathetic nerves causes relaxation of the detrusor muscle and contraction of the external urethral sphincter.

15.36 B C

Antimuscarinic agents (e.g. propantheline) relax the detrusor muscle, and may be useful in the treatment of incontinence due to detrusor instability. Tricyclic antidepressants (e.g. imipramine, amitriptyline) have antimuscarinic properties and may also be useful.

15.37 B C D

The bladder responds to increased pressure due to outflow obstruction by muscular hypertrophy. Causes of bladder outflow obstruction are abnormalities in the prostate gland and urethra. Abnormalities in the ureter and kidneys do not give rise to increased pressure in the bladder.

15.38 C D

Most bladder tumours are epithelial cell in origin, and the majority are transitional cell tumours. They frequently occur in multiples and are papillary in appearance. As they initially project into the bladder lumen before invading the bladder muscles, early diagnosis by cystoscopy is possible. A tumour near a ureteric orifice may cause urinary obstruction, and the back-pressure may result in hydronephrosis.

SYSTEM-BASED MEDICAL SCIENCES

The renal and urinary system

15.39   A D
Chemicals used in textile, printing, rubber and plastic industries are known to cause bladder tumours, and aniline compounds are thought to be responsible. Heavy smokers are also more prone to develop bladder tumours. Schistosomiasis infection is associated with squamous cell bladder tumour, but not transitional cell tumours. There is no evidence of association between either diabetes mellitus or excessive alcohol intake with transitional cell bladder tumours.

15.40   A B E
Bladder diverticuli are outpouchings from the bladder epithelium, and may be congenital or acquired. Congenital diverticuli are usually solitary, whilst acquired diverticuli are usually small and multiple. Acquired diverticuli are usually associated with bladder outflow obstruction, and occur between two ridges of hypertrophic muscles (trabeculae). As prostatic enlargement is a common cause of bladder outflow obstruction, bladder diverticuli occur more commonly in men than women.

15.41   C D
The prostate gland is shaped like an inverted cone, and lies below the neck of the bladder and above the urogenital diaphragm. Hence enlargement of the prostate gland may give rise to urinary obstruction. It lies just posterior to the symphysis pubis, and anterior to the rectum. Hence the gland can be palpated in a rectal examination. It surrounds the prostatic urethra, into which prostatic secretion is discharged. The prostatic secretion is alkaline and neutralises the acid in the vagina.

15.42   A D E
Benign enlargement of the prostate gland is due to hyperplasia of glandular tissue. It occurs in men over 50 years of age. The exact aetiology is unknown. However, it is thought that a reduction in androgen level and an increase in oestrogen level are important factors. There are often multiple circumscribed solid nodules and cysts. If the median lobe is involved, it often compresses the prostatic urethra and causes urinary obstruction. The bladder may respond by muscular hypertrophy and develop prominent bands of thickened smooth muscle (trabeculation).

15.43   B D
Although some drugs are effective in partially relieving symptoms of benign prostatic hypertrophy, surgery cannot be avoided once urinary retention has occurred. The prostatic stromal tissue is rich in α_1-adrenoceptors, whilst the glandular tissue is sensitive to androgens. α_1-adrenoceptor antagonists (e.g. prazosin) and 5 α-reductase inhibitors (e.g. finasteride) may reduce the prostatic volume, and are used to relieve the symptoms of benign prostatic hypertrophy. 5α-Reductase inhibitors inhibit the conversion of testosterone into the more active dihydrotestosterone.

15.44   D
Prostatic carcinoma may be clinical or latent. Latent carcinoma may be found incidentally at histological examination after prostatectomy. The latent carcinoma appears to have a different natural history from the clinical types, and may remain latent for a long time. Unlike benign prostatic hyperplasia which occurs most commonly in the peri-urethral areas, clinical prostatic carcinomas mostly arise from the posterior lobe of the gland. Hence, if the median grove is obliterated on rectal examination, a diagnosis of prostatic carcinoma is likely. The prostate gland produces both acid phosophatase and prostatic specific antigen, and the levels of these substances increase in the presence of prostatic carcinoma. This is useful for diagnostic purposes, although screening for prostatic carcinoma using these biochemical markers is not currently recommended. Bone is the most frequent site for prostatic cancer metastasis, which typically causes a sclerotic lesion.

15.45
A

i   The renal clearance of a substance is the volume of blood which would contain the same amount of the substance excreted in the urine per unit time. Hence, if the substance is X, the renal clearance is:

$$\frac{U_x V}{P_x}$$

where U_x and P_x are the urinary and plasma concentrations of the substance X respectively and V is the rate of urinary excretion.
From the question,

$$U_{In} = 10\,mg/ml$$
$$V = 1000\,ml \text{ in } 180\,min$$
$$= 5.5556\,ml/min$$
$$P_{In} = 0.46\,mg/ml$$

Hence, renal clearance
$$= (10 \times 5.5556)/0.46\,ml/min$$
$$= 120.8\,ml/min$$

ii   Since inulin is filtered in the glomeruli and neither reabsorbed nor secreted in the renal tubules, the amount of inulin in the urine per unit time must have come from the same volume of plasma which has been filtered. Hence, the renal clearance approximates the glomeular filtration rate. The other assumptions about the properties of inulin in approximating its renal clearance to the glomerular filtration rate are that:

- it is not metabolised
- it is not stored in the kidneys
- it is not toxic to the kidneys
- it does not affect the filtration rate.

B

i Using the same notation as above,

$$U_{PAH} = 25\,\text{mg/ml}$$
$$V = 1000\,\text{ml in } 120\,\text{min}$$
$$= 8.333\,\text{ml/min}$$
$$P_{In} = 0.35\,\text{mg/ml}$$

Hence, renal clearance
$$= (25 \times 8.333)/0.35\,\text{ml/min}$$
$$= 595.2\,\text{ml/min}$$

ii Since PAH is filtered by the glomeruli and the tubular cells actively secrete it into the lumen, the amount of inulin in the urine per unit of time must have come from the same volume of blood passing through the kidney. Hence, the renal clearance of PAH approximates the renal blood flow. If the renal venous concentration of PAH is not actually zero, the clearance of PAH underestimates the amount of blood passing through the kidneys. Hence, it underestimates the renal blood flow.

C

Filtration fraction is the proportion of renal blood flow which is filtered at the glomeruli (i.e. filtration rate = glomerular filtration rate/renal blood flow). From the question:

filtration fraction = 120.8/595.2 = 20.3%

D

The renal blood flow decreases with a sudden decrease in blood pressure, though to a lesser extent due to the autoregulation mechanism. The glomerular filtration rate in turn falls less than the renal plasma flow owing to efferent arteriolar constriction. These mechanisms ensure that the glomeular filtration rate is relatively constant. Hence, the filtration fraction increases with a sudden decrease in blood pressure.

15.46

A

In the normal young adult, glucose is present in the plasma and yet no glucose is detected in the urine. This is because the proximal tubule cells actively reabsorb glucose from the tubular lumen into the interstitial fluid. Glucose is transported from the tubular lumen into the proximal

tubule cells by secondary active transport with the Na^+-dependent glucose transporter (SGLT). Sodium is actively transported out into the interstitial fluid by an Na^+, K^+ pump, while glucose is transported into the interstitial fluid by GLUT. See Fig. 15.1.

B

The amount of glucose filtered is equal to the product of the glomerular filtration rate and the plasma concentration of glucose. Since the transport of glucose depends on secondary active transport, there is a maximum transport rate for glucose. In humans, the maximum is about 350 mg/min. The renal threshold for glucose is the plasma level at which the glucose first appears in the urine. Glucose appears in the urine of the diabetic young adult because the plasma concentration is so high that the transport maximum for glucose has been exceeded.

C

Glucose also appears in the urine of the non-diabetic elderly person in spite of a normal plasma glucose level. This is because the maximum transport rate for elderly person is lower than that for a young adult. Hence, the renal threshold in elderly persons is lower than for a younger person.

D

Diabetic patients with a high plasma glucose level often produce large volumes of urine in spite of dehydration. There are several reasons for this. First, the large quantities of glucose not reabsorbed in the proximal tubules increase the osmolarity of the proximal tubule fluid. This exerts considerable osmotic effects and prevents reabsorption of water. Second, less Na^+ is reabsorbed from

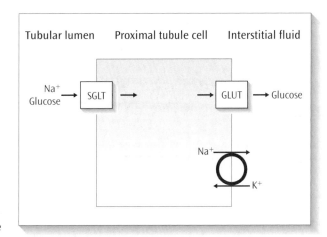

Fig. 15.1 Mechanism of glucose transport in the kidney.

227

The renal and urinary system

the proximal tubules as reabsorpton is against a higher concentration gradient. A larger volume of isotonic fluid enters the loop of Henle. As a result, hypertonicity in the medulla is reduced and less water is reabsorbed in the collecting ducts. Hence, the urine volume increases along with the excretion of Na⁺.

15.47

A

As the subject becomes dehydrated mainly through loss of water, the osmolality of the extracellular fluid increases. This stimulates the osmoreceptors in the anterior hypothalamus, causing an increased sensation of thirst and an increased intake of water.

B

See Table 15.3. The descending limb of the loop of Henle is permeable, whereas the ascending limb is not. Water is reabsorbed in the descending limb of Henle, which contributes to the hypertonicity at the turn of the loop. The ascending loop of Henle is impermeable to water but sodium and chloride ions are actively transported out, explaining the hypotonicity at the distal tubule. Finally, the collecting duct is highly permeable to water in the presence of ADH but relatively impermeable in its absence. This explains the central role of ADH in the control of the excretion of water by the kidneys.

C

In the subject with dehydration due to pure water loss, the hypertonicity in the extracellular fluid stimulates the osmoreceptors located in the anterior hypothalamus. This results in increased ADH (vasopressin) secretion from the posterior hypothalamus. From (B), reduced elimination of water from the kidneys results.

Table 15.3

Segment	ADH present	ADH absent
Loop of Henle		
Thin descending limb	+++	+++
Thin ascending limb	–	–
Thick ascending limb	–	–
Distal convoluted tubule	+	+
Collecting duct		
Cortical portion	+++	+
Medullary portion	+++	+

D

Free water clearance is a measure of the gain (or loss) of water by the excretion of urine which is more (or less) concentrated than plasma. It is calculated by the difference between the urine volume and the clearance in osmoles:

$$C_{water} = V - C_{osm} = V - (U_{osm}V/P_{osm})$$

where C is the free water clearance, C_{osm} is the clearance of osmoles, V is the urine volume, and P_{osm} and U_{osm} are the plasma and urine osmolality, respectively.

E

In order for the ADH to reduce renal elimination of water, the renal medulla must be hypertonic and there must be a gradient of increasing osmolality along the renal medullary pyramids so that water is extracted from the collecting ducts.

F

i The hypertonicity of the medulla is generated by the loops of Henle which act as 'countercurrent multipliers'. 'Countercurrent' refers to the inflow (the ascending limb) running parallel but in the opposite direction to the outflow (the descending limb). This countercurrent multiplier is mainly driven by the active transport of Na⁺ and Cl⁻ out of the thick ascending limbs and partly by the cotransport of Na⁺/Cl⁻ in the distal tubule. The thin descending limb is highly permeable to water. Hence, the continuous flow of hypotonic fluid into the descending limb generates an increasing gradient of hypertonicity in the medulla.

ii The countercurrent multipliers described above would not work if the Na⁺ and urea in the interstitial spaces in the medulla were removed by the circulation. This is prevented by the vasa recta which act as countercurrent exchangers. Solutes diffuse out of the vessels conducting blood towards the cortex and into the vessels conducting towards the pyramids. Similarly, water diffuses out of the descending vessels and into the ascending vessels. Hence, solutes tend to recirculate in the medulla and preserve the hypertonicity.

iii Urea is important in maintaining the osmotic gradient in the medulla. It diffuses passively out of the proximal tubule. The rest of the nephron is impermeable to urea, except the inner portion of the collecting duct. Hence, urea moves out into the inner medulla from this part of the collecting duct and adds to the hypertonicity of the medulla.

G

i Thiazide diuretics act by reducing the active reabsorption of sodium ions and accompanying chloride ions in the early portion of the distal convoluted tubule. Since the countercurrent multiplier system depends less on the transport of sodium from the distal convoluted tubule than from the thick ascending limbs of the loop of Henle, thiazides diuretics are less powerful than loop diuretics such as furosemide (frusemide).

ii Furosemide (frusemide) is a 'loop diuretic'. It acts by inhibiting Na^+ and K^+/Cl^- cotransport in the medullary thick ascending limb of the loop of Henle. Since the countercurrent multiplier system depends mainly on this sodium transport, furosemide (frusemide) is a powerful diuretic.

15.48
A
See Fig. 15.2.

B
i Respiratory acidosis.
ii The relevant Henderson–Hassalbalch equation is, for the reaction

$$CO_2 + H_2O \rightleftharpoons H_2CO_3 \rightleftharpoons H^+ + HCO_3^-$$

$$pH = pK + \log\left(\left[HCO_3^-\right]/CO_2\right)$$

It follows from this equation that as $[CO_2]$ increases, pH decreases.

iii From the diagram in (A), as $[CO_2]$ increases, H^+ and HCO_3^- are formed. H^+ is excreted in the urine and HCO_3^- diffuses into the interstitial fluid. Hence, this increase in $[HCO_3^-]$ partially compensates for the respiratory acidosis.

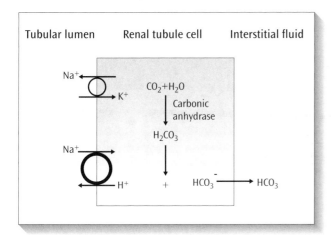

Fig. 15.2 Excretion of acid by a renal proximal tubule cell.

15.49
A
A high therapeutic dose of salicylates causes increased oxygen consumption and increased production of carbon dioxide. This occurs because salicylates uncouple oxidative phosphorylation, especially in skeletal muscle.

B
Before the overdose, the patient is likely to have had respiratory alkalosis due to direct stimulation of the respiratory centre by salicylates. This lowers the plasma carbon dioxide and causes an increase in pH.

C
The kidneys partially compensate for this respiratory alkalosis by increased bicarbonate excretion; a state of compensated respiratory alkalosis results.

D
The principal physiological buffers in the blood are bicarbonates, plasma proteins and haemoglobin.

$$H_2CO_3 \rightleftharpoons H^+ + HCO^-$$
$$Hprot \rightleftharpoons H^+ + Prot^-$$
$$HHb \rightleftharpoons H^+ + Hb^-$$

The main physiological buffer in the interstitial fluid is bicarbonate.

The main physiological buffers in the intracellular fluid are proteins and phosphate.

$$Hprot \rightleftharpoons H^+ + Prot^-$$
$$H_2PO_4 \rightleftharpoons H^+ + HPO_4^{2-}$$

E
Aspirin may cause fever in toxic overdose as a result of the increased metabolic rate due to uncoupled oxidative phosphorylation.

F
Possible reasons for severe acidosis on admission include:
- Metabolic acidosis caused by metabolites such as pyruvate, lactic acid and acetoacetic acid.
- Metabolic acidosis due to salicylate itself.
- Respiratory acidosis caused by respiratory depression. With therapeutic doses of aspirin, the patient usually had a low plasma bicarbonate due to respiratory alkalosis. Hence, when respiratory depression occurred with toxic overdose, the kidneys could not compensate by increasing the bicarbonate concentration.

G
Renal excretion of aspirin may be increased by correction of dehydration and forced alkaline diuresis with bicarbonate infusion. Bicarbonate increases urine pH and hence increases salicylate elimination.

The renal and urinary system

15.50

A

Primary glomerular diseases are renal diseases that affect the glomeruli but are not part of a systemic condition. Secondary glomerular diseases are renal damage occurring as part of a systemic condition. Examples of secondary glomerular diseases are:
- systemic lupus erythematosus
- Henoch–Schönlein purpura
- diabetes mellitus
- renal amyloidosis
- infective endocarditis.

B

i According to their aetiology, primary glomerular diseases might by classified into immunological and non-immunological injuries. Immunological injuries may be further classified into anti-glomerular basement membrane antibody or immune complex deposition.

ii According to their histology, primary glomerular diseases might be classified according to the reaction of the glomeruli to injury, such as proliferative, membranous thickening, membrano-proliferative or crescentic. The histological features sometimes help to identify the aetiology and to predict the prognosis of the diseases.

C

The glomerular capillary consists of endothelial cells, basement membrane and epithelial cells. The main function of the glomerular capillaries is to provide a filtration barrier based on charge and size. The functions of the capillary components are as follows:
- *Endothelial cell* polyanionic glycoproteins contribute to the charge-dependent filtration barrier.
- *Basement membrane* proteoglycans (e.g. heparan sulphate) are anionic and carry a negative charge. Hence, the basement membrane also contributes to the charge-dependent filtration barrier. In addition, it contains a network of type IV collagen which contributes to the size-dependent filtration.
- *Epithelial cell* slit diaphragms between foot processes contribute to the size-dependent filtration; the cells also synthesise the glomeular basement membrane and contribute to the charge-dependent filtration system.

D

i Excessive release of renin secondary to renal ischaemia in primary glomerular disease may have caused the patient to present with hypertension.

ii With severe glomeular injury, red blood cells may go through the damaged filters of the glomeuli (epithelial cells): blood may appear in the urine.

iii Increased permeability of the glomeular basement membrane to proteins may cause protein to appear in the urine.

15.51
See Table 15.4.

Table 15.4

	Renal cell tumour	Bladder tumour
Histological types	Clear or granular cell	Transitional cell (mostly) Squamous cell/ adenocarcinoma (rarely)
Unifocal/multifocal	Usually unifocal	Usually multiple
Smoking as risk factor	Yes	Yes
Chemicals as risk factors	No	Yes, e.g. dyes in textiles and printing
Other predisposing factors	Genetic predisposition such as von Hippel–Lindau disease	Analgesic abusers; schistosomiasis (for squamous cell carcinoma)
Association with hypercalcaemia	Yes, due to release of PTH	No
Association with polycythaemia	Yes, due to release of erythropoietin	No

The nervous system

16.1 The following structures of the brain develop from the embryological forebrain (proscencephalon):
- **A** Pons
- **B** Cerebellum
- **C** Cerebral cortex
- **D** Thalamus
- **E** Corpus striatum

16.2 The following structures contain fibres which link matching areas in the two hemispheres:
- **A** Corpus callosum
- **B** Anterior commissure
- **C** Superior longitudinal fasciculus
- **D** Posterior commissure
- **E** The uncinate fasciculus

16.3 The following cranial nerves emerge from the pons:
- **A** Oculomotor nerve
- **B** Trochlear nerve
- **C** Trigeminal nerve
- **D** Abducens nerve
- **E** Facial nerve

16.4 The following structures can be found in the midbrain:
- **A** Substantia nigra
- **B** Superior colliculus
- **C** Cerebral peduncle
- **D** Gracile and cuneate nuclei
- **E** Fourth ventricle

16.5 The following statements about the cranial meninges are correct:
- **A** The venous sinuses lie between the dura mater and the arachnoid mater
- **B** The falx cerebri is a fold of dura mater
- **C** The tentorium cerebelli is a fold of arachnoid mater
- **D** Cerebrospinal fluid can be found between the pia mater and the surface of the brain
- **E** The middle meningeal artery can be found between the inner surface of the temporal bones and the dura mater

16.6 Meningiomas:
- **A** Are the commonest type of CNS tumours
- **B** Occur more frequently in children
- **C** Frequently invade the brain
- **D** Frequently invade the dura and skull bones
- **E** Usually have irregular edges

16.7 Adult bacterial meningitis is commonly caused by:
- **A** *Staphylococcus aureus*
- **B** *Salmonella*
- **C** Anaerobic organisms
- **D** *Streptococcus pneumoniae*
- **E** *Pseudomonas*

16.8 A cerebral abscess may result from spread of infection from:
- **A** The paranasal sinuses
- **B** The bloodstream
- **C** The lymphatics
- **D** The mastoid cavity
- **E** The middle ear

16.9 Cerebrospinal fluid (CSF):
- **A** Is secreted by the choroid plexuses of the lateral ventricles
- **B** Enters the third ventricle through the interventricular foramen
- **C** Enters the fourth ventricle via the aqueduct of Sylvius
- **D** Enters the subarachnoid space via the central canal in the spinal cord
- **E** Is returned to the blood via the lymphatic system

16.10 Causes of hydrocephalus include:
- **A** Obstruction at the fourth ventricle into the subarachnoid space
- **B** Obstruction at the aqueduct
- **C** Obstruction at the central canal of the spinal cord
- **D** Meningitis
- **E** Tumour of the choroid plexus

16.11 In most people, branches of the internal carotid arteries include:
- **A** Ophthalmic arteries
- **B** Posterior cerebral arteries
- **C** Basilar artery
- **D** Anterior cerebral arteries
- **E** Middle cerebral arteries

16.12 The following areas of the brain are supplied by the middle cerebral arteries:
- **A** The pons
- **B** The parietal lobes
- **C** The anterior limb of the internal capsule
- **D** The posterior limb of the internal capsule
- **E** The optic radiation

16.13 Factors which relax the arteriolar smooth muscle of the cerebral vessels include:
- **A** Increased pH
- **B** Increased carbon dioxide
- **C** Increased systemic blood pressure

SYSTEM-BASED MEDICAL SCIENCES

The nervous system

D Hyperventilation
E Increased oxygen

16.14 Causes of a stroke include:
A Intracerebral haemorrhage
B Meningitis
C Encephalitis
D Cerebral infarction
E Subarachnoid haemorrhage

16.15 Causes of cerebral infarction include:
A Emboli from mural thrombus after a myocardial infarction
B Atheroma of the intracranial arteries
C Atheroma of the extracranial arteries
D Thrombosis of the intracranial arteries
E Cerebral hypotension following a cardiac arrest

16.16 Intracerebral haemorrhage:
A Occurs more commonly in hypertensive subjects
B May cause an increase in intracranial pressure
C May cause cerebral herniation
D Is commonly caused by rupture of arterial aneurysms at the circle of Willis
E Is commonly caused by rupture at the bifurcation of intracerebral arterioles

16.17 The following statements about the blood–brain barrier are true:
A The lining of the choroid plexus constitutes part of the blood–brain barrier
B It is bound by tight junctions
C Fenestrations occur frequently at the barrier
D It modulates the entry of glucose
E It prevents toxins from entering the CNS from the bloodstream

16.18 Significant quantities of the following drugs cross the blood–brain barrier:
A Lipid-insoluble drugs
B Lipid-soluble drugs
C Inhaled anaesthetics
D Alcohol
E Chloramphenicol in the presence of meningitis

16.19 The following statements about neurones are true:
A There are more neuroglial cells than neurones
B Nissl bodies contain endoplasmic reticulum
C Nerve impulses are conducted via the axon
D There is usually one dendrite per neurone
E Microtubules play an important role in neuronal transport

16.20 Retrograde neuronal transport:
A Includes transport of substances from the cell body to the dendrites
B Includes transport of substances from the axon to the cell body
C Is the principal means of transporting synthesised neurotransmitters
D Is the principal means of transporting neuronal waste products
E Plays an important role in target cell recognition

16.21 In an action potential, the firing level:
A Occurs when the membrane potential reaches 0 mV
B Is associated with a sudden increase in the openings of sodium channels
C Is associated with an increased K^+ influx into the cell
D Is associated with an increased Na^+ efflux out of the cell
E Is associated with a rapid increase in sodium conductance

16.22 Immediately after the spike potential of the action potential:
A The sodium channels become inactivated
B The potassium channels are gradually opened
C The sodium conductance increases
D The potassium conductance increases
E There is a net movement of potassium out of the cells

16.23 The excitation threshold of the neurone to stimulation is increased:
A When the membrane potential is made more negative
B During the rising phase of the spike potential
C In the initial falling phase of the spike potential
D During the after-depolarisation period
E During the after-repolarisation period

16.24 The following statements about the chemical synapse are true:
A Neurotransmitters are released from the pre-synaptic membrane by exocytosis
B Neurotransmitters are transported from the Golgi apparatus to the synaptic boutons in vesicles
C The neurotransmitter receptor is located on the membrane of the target neurone
D Most synapses are dendrito-axonic
E Pre-synaptic inhibition may be achieved by axo-axonic synapses

16.25 Known inhibitory neurotransmitters include:
  A Glycine
  B Serotonin (5-HT)
  C Noradrenaline (norepinephrine)
  D γ-Aminobutyric acid (GABA)
  E Glutaric acid

16.26 The following statements about the neuromuscular junction are true:
  A Acetylcholinesterase can be found on the post-synaptic membrane
  B Choline is transported from the synaptic cleft to the pre-synaptic neurone
  C Each nicotinic receptor binds to two molecules of acetylcholine
  D Binding of acetylcholine to its receptors results in the opening of sodium channels
  E Cyclic GMP acts as the second messenger

16.27 Known second messengers for synaptic transmission include:
  A Cyclic AMP
  B Substance P
  C Inositol triphosphate (IP$_3$)
  D Diacylglycerol (DAG)
  E Nitric oxide

16.28 Types of neuroglial cells in the brain include:
  A Astrocytes
  B Fibrocytes
  C Ependymal cells
  D Transitional epithelium
  E Oligodendrocytes

16.29 Myelination:
  A Is the function of microglial cells
  B Increases the speed of nerve conduction
  C Occurs in almost all nerve cells in the brain
  D Is usually accompanied by deletion of potassium channels
  E Never takes place in patients with multiple sclerosis

16.30 Multiple sclerosis:
  A Occurs more commonly in tropical than temperate countries
  B Is more common in males than females
  C Affects both the peripheral and central nervous system
  D Is characteristically associated with a loss of myelin in affected tissues
  E Characteristically gives an oligodendrocyte-predominant histological picture

16.31 The following sensory phenomenon and the type of nerve endings in the skin are correctly matched:
  A Sensation of heat – free nerve endings
  B Sensation of vibration – Pacinian corpuscles
  C Short-lasting touch sensation when clothes are put on – Ruffini endings
  D Differentiating between smooth and rough table surface – Meissner's corpuscles
  E Awareness of a fork held in the hand – Merkel cells

16.32 The following sites and their segmental innervation are correctly matched:
  A Around the nipple – T8
  B At the umbilicus – T10
  C Inguinal region – L3
  D Lateral side of the sole of the foot – S2
  E The thumb – C8

16.33 Symptoms due to S1 nerve root compression by a disc prolapse include:
  A Pain in the sole of the feet
  B Tingling sensation in the sole of the feet
  C Weakness of dorsiflexion of the ankle
  D Absent knee jerk
  E Exaggerated ankle jerk

16.34 Consequences of damage to the radial nerve at the radial groove of the humerus include:
  A Wrist drop
  B Inability to extend the elbow
  C Inability to extend the middle and distal phalangeal joints of the fingers
  D Diminished sensation over the ulnar side of the dorsum of the hand
  E Diminished sensation over the radial side of the palm

16.35 Consequences of damage to the ulnar nerve at the wrist include:
  A Inability to abduct the thumb
  B Inability to adduct the thumb
  C Clawed hand appearance of the fourth and fifth fingers
  D Loss of sensation on the ulnar side of the dorsum of the hand
  E Reduced sensation in the ulnar side of the palm

16.36 The following statements about the knee jerk elicited in a clinical examination are true:
  A Type Ia and type II muscle spindles in the quadriceps muscles discharge impulses to the spinal cord

16

Q

SYSTEM-BASED MEDICAL SCIENCES

The nervous system

B The nerve fibre from the muscle spindle synapses with the dendrites of α motoneurons supplying the quadriceps muscles

C Signals in the spinal cord are transmitted to the thalamus

D The nerve impulses must pass through two synapses before the knee jerk can occur

E Inhibitory impulses are sent to the α motor neurones supplying the hamstring muscles

16.37 The following statements about the posterior column–medial lemniscal pathway are true:

A The cell bodies of the first-order neurones lie in the anterior root ganglia in the spinal cord

B The first-order neurones cross the midline in the spinal cord a few spinal segments above

C The cell bodies of the second-order neurones lie in the nuclei gracilis and cuneatus in the posterior column

D The second-order neurone does not cross the midline

E The third-order neurone projects from the thalamus to the sensory cortex

16.38 The spinothalamic tract and the posterior column–medial lemniscal pathway show the following similarities:

A Both consist of three-order sets of neurones

B The second-order neurones cross over in both pathways

C Both pathways cross over in the spinal cord

D The third-order neurones project from the thalamus to the cerebral cortex

E The representations of different parts of the body in the cerebral cortex are similar

16.39 The following functions are lost in diseases affecting the posterior column – medial lemniscal pathway:

A Vibration sensation

B Temperature sensation

C Pain sensation

D Two-point discrimination

E Muscle power

16.40 The following lesions may cause loss in temperature whilst preserving joint position sensation:

A Peripheral neuropathy

B Diseases affecting spinal cord root ganglia

C Syringomyelia (cyst in and around the central canal of the spinal cord)

D Diseases affecting the thalamus

E A cerebral tumour affecting the sensory cortex

16.41 The following statements about neural transmission of pain are true:

A Sharp localised pain is transmitted by C fibres

B Dull diffuse chronic pain is transmitted by myelinated fibres

C Pain impulses for chronic pain travel slower than those for sharp pain

D Substance P is the neurotransmitter in the afferent pain fibres in the dorsal horn of the spinal cord

E Gating of pain impulses takes place at the dorsal horn cells of the spinal cord

16.42 Interventions for which the release of endogenous opioid neurotransmitters is a probable mechanism of pain relief include:

A Acupuncture

B Placebo

C Paracetamol

D Naloxone

E Transcutaneous nerve stimulation

16.43 The following drugs and their mechanisms of analgesic action are correctly matched:

A Diamorphine – μ-opioid receptor agonist

B Morpine – δ-opioid receptor agonist

C Non-steroidal anti-inflammatory drugs (NSAIDs) – cyclooxygenase inhibitor

D Corticosteroid – increased breakdown of prostaglandins

E Paracetamol – increased prostaglandin synthesis

16.44 Characteristic side effects of opiates include:

A Constipation

B Respiratory depression

C Dilated pupils

D Tachycardia

E Drowsiness

16.45 The following statements about the sympathetic nervous system are true:

A The pre-ganglionic fibres emerge from the cervical and thoracic segments of the spinal cord

B Most of the sympathetic ganglia lie in the sympathetic chain

C Some pre-ganglionic fibres synapse at the adrenal cortex

D Some post-ganglionic fibres synapse at the adrenal medulla

E The male genital tract receives sympathetic supply via the pelvic ganglion

16.46 Stimulation of the sympathetic nervous system causes an increase in:

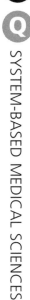
   A Heart rate
   B Blood flow to the skin
   C Blood flow to skeletal muscle
   D Gut motility
   E Sweating

16.47 Symptoms and signs of disruption of the sympathetic nerves immediately after their emergence from the superior cervical ganglion (i.e. Horner's syndrome) include:
   A Ptosis (drooping of eyelid)
   B Failure to abduct the eye
   C Increased tear secretion
   D A dilated pupil
   E Reduced sweating on that side of the face

16.48 Pre-ganglionic parasympathetic fibres emerge in the following cranial nerves:
   A Oculomotor nerve
   B Trochlear nerve
   C Trigeminal nerve
   D Facial nerve
   E Glossopharyngeal nerve

16.49 Actions of antimuscarinic drugs (e.g. atropine) include:
   A Small pupils
   B Dry mouth
   C Increased heart rate
   D Bronchoconstriction
   E Diarrhoea

16.50 The following statements about the left corticospinal tract are true:
   A It carries voluntary motor fibres
   B It passes through the left internal capsule between the thalamus and the basal ganglia
   C Most of its fibres cross over to the right side in the pons
   D Most of its fibres descend in the right side of the spinal cord as the anterior corticospinal tract
   E Less than 20% of its fibres descend in the right side of the spinal cord as the lateral corticospinal tract

16.51 Lesions at which of the following sites in the motor pathway usually result in a clinical 'upper motor neurone lesion'?
   A Corticospinal tract
   B Reticulospinal tract
   C Corticonuclear tract
   D Anterior horn cells of the spinal cord
   E Peripheral nerve

16.52 Characteristic signs of lower motor neurone lesions include:
   A Spasticity
   B Absent tendon reflex
   C Positive Babinski sign
   D Fasciculation
   E Pronounced muscle wasting

16.53 The basal ganglia include the following:
   A Caudate nucleus
   B Putamen
   C Hypothalamus
   D Substantia nigra
   E Subthalamic nucleus

16.54 Parkinson's disease is associated with:
   A A reduction in striatal activity
   B A reduction in nigrostrial neurones
   C Reduced activity of cholinergic neurones
   D A loss of GABA-ergic pathway
   E A reduction of MPTP (1-methly-4-phenyl-1,2,5,6-tetrahydropyridine)-like substance

16.55 Recognised drug treatments for Parkinson's disease include:
   A Monoamine oxidase B inhibitors (e.g. selegiline)
   B Phenothiazines (e.g. chlorpromazine)
   C Levodopa with peripheral decarboxylase inhibitor
   D Bromocriptine
   E Anticholinergic agents

16.56 The neocerebellum:
   A Constitutes over 50% of the whole cerebellum
   B Includes the vermis
   C Receives afferent fibres from the pontocerebellar tract
   D Sends efferent fibres from the dentate nucleus to the contralateral motor cortex via the thalamus
   E Coordinates the movements of the limbs

16.57 Characteristic features associated with lesions in the vestibulocerebellum include:
   A Inability to stand upright without support
   B Finger–nose incoordination
   C Impaired articulation
   D Increased muscle tone in the limbs
   E Nystagmus

16.58 Characteristic features of neocerebellar lesions include:
   A Tremor at rest
   B Impaired 'heel-to-toe' walking
   C Impaired ipsilateral 'heel-to-shin' test

D Uneven speech production
E Staggering gait

16.59 The following functions and their corresponding cranial nerves are appropriately matched:
A Sensation of the posterior third of the tongue – hypoglossal nerve
B Phonation – spinal accessory nerve
C Tongue protrusion – glossopharyngeal nerve
D Mastication – facial nerve
E Sensation to the forehead – ophthalmic branch of the trigeminal nerve

16.60 The mandibular division of the trigeminal nerve:
A Originates from the Gasserian ganglion in the petrous temporal bone
B Exits the skull base through the foramen rotundum
C Innervates the tip of the nose
D Mediates the jaw jerk
E Supplies the teeth and gums of the upper jaw

16.61 The following functions and their corresponding cranial nerves are appropriately matched:
A Taste in the posterior third of the tongue – glossopharyngeal nerve
B Taste in the anterior two-thirds of the tongue – trigeminal nerve
C Corneal reflex – maxillary branch of the trigeminal nerve
D Attenuation of loud sounds – facial nerve
E Parotid gland secretion – facial nerve

16.62 A unilateral upper motor neurone facial nerve palsy:
A May be caused by a vascular stroke
B May be caused by Bell's palsy
C May be caused by compression of the nerve in its bony canal
D Is associated with inability to close one eye
E Is associated with inability to retract the lip

16.63 A unilateral lower motor neurone facial nerve palsy:
A Is commoner than a corresponding lesion of any other cranial nerves
B Is associated with inability to raise the eyebrow
C Is associated with sensitivity to loud noise
D Is associated with the inability to smile
E Almost never recovers spontaneously

16.64 The oculomotor nerve supplies:
A The lateral rectus
B The superior rectus

C The sphincter pupillae
D The levator superioris
E The superior oblique

16.65 Clinical features of a complete oculomotor nerve palsy include:
A A constricted pupil
B Inability to abduct the eye
C Inability to close the eye
D Reduced sweating on that side of the face
E Inability to look upwards

16.66 The following statements about the medial longitudinal fasciculus (MLF) are true:
A It connects the oculomotor, trochlear and abducens nuclei
B It receives neural input from the vestibular nuclei
C It is essential for maintaining visual fixation on a moving target
D A lesion in the MLF may result in failure of abduction of the ipsilateral eye
E A lesion in the MLF may result in nystagmus of the contralateral eye

16.67 The following are neural pathways involved in the direct pupillary light reflex:
A The ganglion cells within the retina conduct impulses via the optic tracts to the lateral geniculate body
B The lateral geniculate body conducts impulses towards the superior cervical ganglion in the sympathetic chain
C The superior cervical ganglion conducts impulses towards the Edinger–Westphal nucleus
D The fibres from the Edinger–Westphal nucleus enter the oculomotor nerve and synapse in the ciliary ganglion
E Post-ganglionic fibres from the ciliary ganglion supply the sphincter pupillae in the iris

16.68 When a strong light is shone into the left eye, the right pupil constricts but the left pupil does not react. These clinical findings may be explained by a:
A Left optic nerve lesion
B Left oculomotor nerve lesion
C Right optic nerve lesion
D Right oculomotor nerve lesion
E Left sympathetic chain lesion

16.69 Cones and rods are the two types of photoreceptors in the retina. Compared to cones, rods:
A Are more numerous
B Are less sensitive to light
C Function less well in dim light

D Are mainly found in the fovea

E Are abnormal in patients with red – green colour-blindness

16.70 The following events occur in the photosensitive pigments of the retina in the presence of light:

A Conformal changes in the pigments occur

B Transducin (G_{t1}) is activated

C Phosphodiesterase is inhibited

D Intracellular cAMP is increased

E Sodium channels are opened

16.71 When an individual with normal vision moves from a very bright to a very dark room:

A The retina becomes less sensitive to light

B The changes in visual threshold occur more quickly than the reverse changes on moving from a very dark to a very bright room

C The initial changes in visual threshold are due to adaptation in the rods

D The later changes in visual threshold are due to adaptation of the cones

E The changes occur quicker if the individual had worn red-tinted glasses in the bright room

16.72 Myopia (short-sightedness):

A May be due to an abnormally short eyeball

B May be due to excessive curvature and convergence power of the cornea or lens

C Is associated with images formed in front of the retina

D May be corrected using concave lenses

E Is often genetic in aetiology

16.73 The following statements about the optic nerve are true:

A It develops from an outgrowth of the brain embryologically

B It is wrapped round by Schwann cells

C It can regenerate if damaged

D The cell bodies occupy the pretectal nucleus

E Almost all the fibres cross over to the lateral geniculate body on the opposite side

16.74 The following lesions in the visual pathway and their resulting visual field defects are correctly matched:

A Complete left optic nerve lesion – left homonymous hemianopia

B Optic chiasm – bitemporal hemianopia

C Left optic tract – right homonymous hemianopia

D Right optic radiation – right homonymous hemianopia

E Left occipital cortex – right homonymous hemianopia

16.75 Sound vibrations from outside the ear pass through the following to reach the acoustic nerve:

A Tympanic membrane

B Malleus

C Stapes

D The round window

E The inner hair cell of the cochlea

16.76 The auditory nerve impulses in the acoustic nerve pass through the following to reach the primary auditory cortex:

A Ipsilateral cochlear nuclei in the medulla

B Ipsilateral vestibular nuclei

C Ipsilateral lateral geniculate body

D Contralateral medial geniculate body

E Ipsilateral superior colliculus

16.77 The following features of sound waves and their associated qualities of sound are correctly matched

A Amplitude – loudness

B Frequency – pitch

C Wavelength – rhythm

D Harmonics – timbre

E Speed – duration

16.78 The differentiation between sound coming from:

A The left and the right side is partly due to the time difference between the arrival of stimulus in the two ears

B The left and the right side is partly due to the primary auditory cortex receiving signals produced by the stimuli only from the contralateral ear

C The left and the right side is partly due to the sound being louder on the side of the source

D The front and the back is partly due to the time difference between the arrival of stimulus in the two ears

E The front and the back is contributed to by the positioning of the pinna

16.79 The following statements about Wernicke's area are true:

A It is usually found in the right superior temporal gyrus

B Its main function is to understand speech

C Lesions in this area result in receptive aphasia

D It is connected to Broca's area by the arcuate fasciculus

16 Q

The nervous system

E It is usually damaged by vascular occlusion of the left anterior cerebral artery

16.80 Alzheimer's disease:
- A Is a metabolic disease
- B Occurs more commonly in older people
- C Is the second commonest cause of dementia
- D May occur in families
- E Is associated with the ApoE4 genotype on chromosome 19

16.81 Pathological features of Alzheimer's disease include:
- A Cortical hypertrophy
- B Small ventricles
- C Neurofibrillary tangles
- D Excessive cholinergic fibres
- E Predominant cerebellar involvement

16.82 Benzodiazepines are:
- A Antipsychotic
- B Sedative
- C Anxiolytic
- D Anticonvulsants
- E Muscle relaxants

16.83 Benzodiazepines:
- A Act on three different subtypes of receptors
- B Inhibit the effect of GABA
- C Result in opening of chloride ion channels in target cells
- D Act mainly on the reticular activating system
- E Are antagonists at the neuromuscular junction

16.84 Phenothiazines are:
- A Agonists of dopamine D_2 receptors
- B Agonists of serotonin receptors
- C Used to treat schizophrenia acutely
- D Used as long-term maintenance therapy for schizophrenia
- E Used as antidepressants

16.85 Characteristic side effects of phenothiazines include:
- A Parkinsonian symptoms
- B Akathisia
- C Involuntary movement of the face and tongue
- D Hypoprolactinaemia
- E Insomnia

16.86 Drugs effective in the treatment of depression include:
- A Lithium
- B Benzodiazepines
- C Barbiturates

D Butyrophenones
E Selective serotonin reuptake inhibitors (SSRIs)

16.87 Tricyclic antidepressants:
- A Are muscarinic receptor agonists
- B Act by increasing the synthesis of noradrenaline (norepinephrine) in the pre-synaptic neurone
- C Are cardiotoxic
- D Protect against convulsions
- E Inhibit bladder contraction

16.88 Lithium:
- A Increases the synthesis of phosphatidylinositol
- B Is poorly absorbed in the gastrointestinal tract
- C Is extensively metabolised by the liver
- D Has a shorter half-life in patients with renal impairment
- E Level increases when a diuretic is administered at the same time

16.89 Before embarking on a minor surgical procedure to remove a mole, a doctor injected local anaesthetic just below the skin. After a few minutes, the patient did not feel pain when pricked with a needle, although he could still perceive touch and pressure.
- A i What is the resting membrane potential of a nerve axon?
     ii Discuss how this resting membrane potential is generated and maintained.
     iii Give the events leading to the action potential in an axon.
     iv Sketch the relationship between the following variables and time during an action potential in a nerve axon:
        • membrane potential
        • sodium conductance
        • potassium conductance.
- B List the main differences between the peripheral nerves conveying pain and those conveying pressure or touch.
- C For the peripheral nerves conveying pain, describe how the action potential is propagated along the nerve.
- D For the peripheral nerves conveying pressure and touch, describe how the action potential is propagated along the nerve. What are the advantages of such nerves over those conveying pain?
- E What is the mechanism of action of the local anaesthetic? Briefly explain why it differentially affects nerves conveying pain but not those conveying touch.

16.90 A patient underwent an operation under general anaesthetic and paralysis was achieved using pancuronium. At the end of the operation, the anaesthetist administered neostigmine and the patient was able to move his limbs soon afterwards.
  A Draw a simple diagram of a neuromuscular junction.
  B Briefly describe the structure of the post-synaptic receptor.
  C Explain how pancuronium caused paralysis.
  D Explain how neostigmine reversed the paralysis.

16.91 Another patient underwent an operation under general anaesthetic and paralysis was achieved using suxamethonium. Unfortunately, the patient suffered from a congenital deficiency of an enzyme and had to be ventilated for several hours after the operation before he could breathe spontaneously.
  A Explain how suxamethonium achieved paralysis.
  B What clinical feature would you expect during paralysis with suxamethonium which you would not see with pancuronium?
  C Would you expect the paralysis to be reversed by neostigmine? Why?
  D Explain how suxamethonium causes prolonged paralysis in patients with certain enzyme deficiencies but not in other patients.

16.92 A young woman presented with easy fatigability and drooping eyelids. To determine whether she was suffering from myasthenia gravis, 5 mg edrophonium was given intravenously as a diagnostic test and her symptoms disappeared rapidly.
  A Explain the basic defects in myasthenia gravis.
  B Why might myasthenia gravis present with muscle fatigability?
  C What did the test show?
  D Why did the symptoms disappear rapidly?
  E What abnormal antibodies might be detectable in the patient's serum?

16.93
  A Explain the mechanism of action of atropine.
  B Illustrate the actions and uses of the group of drugs to which atropine belongs by completing Table 16.1.

16.94 A patient suffering from depression was prescribed imipramine; however, as he developed postural hypotension and was subsequently found to suffer from ischaemic heart disease, he was switched over to paroxetine.

Table 16.1

System	Actions	Possible clinical uses
Cardiovascular		
Eyes		
Respiratory		
Gastrointestinal		
Neurological		

  A Explain the mechanisms of action of imipramine and paroxetine.
  B Given that imipramine and paroxetine are effective in some patients with depression, what are the possible mechanisms for depression?
  C Why is paroxetine safer than imipramine if the patient suffers from ischaemic heart disease? What are other advantages of paroxetine over imipramine?

16.95 On neurological examination, the doctor taps on the patient's quadriceps femoris tendon with a tendon hammer and a knee jerk is elicited.
  A What structures in the muscle tendon are stimulated?
  B Give a concise account of the pathways and events responsible for the knee jerk.
  C It is well-known that the knee jerk response is exaggerated if the patient tries to pull the hands apart when the flexed fingers of each hand are hooked together. Give a possible mechanism for this.
  D What conclusion can you draw from the observation that the knee jerk is intact?

16.96 Give the spinal nerve roots responsible for the movements and reflexes listed in Table 16.2.

16.97 A child suffers from hydrocephalus (excessive accumulation of CSF in the ventricles leading to dilatation of the cerebral ventricles).
  A Where is CSF secreted? Trace the path of secreted CSF from its secretion to its return to the bloodstream.
  B What are the physiological functions of CSF?
  C What are the possible causes of hydrocephalus?

16.98 Alcohol is well known to have rapid effects on the central nervous system; gentamicin is regarded as unreliable in the treatment of meningitis.

239

16 **Q**

SYSTEM-BASED MEDICAL SCIENCES

The nervous system

Table 16.2

Movement or reflex	Spinal nerve root
Shoulder abduction	
Shoulder adduction	
Elbow flexion	
Elbow extension	
Wrist flexion	
Wrist extension	
Finger flexion	
Finger abduction	
Hip flexion	
Hip extension	
Knee flexion	
Knee extension	
Ankle dorsiflexion	
Ankle plantar flexion	
Biceps reflex	
Triceps reflex	
Knee reflex	
Ankle reflex	

A Briefly describe the structure of the blood–brain barrier.

B What are the main factors governing the permeability of the blood–brain barrier to drugs? Explain the higher permeability of the blood–brain barrier to alcohol compared with gentamicin.

C Could gentamicin be effective in treating bacterial meningitis? Explain.

16.99 A patient with recent head injury suffered from cerebral oedema. His blood pressure was abnormally high. Raised intracranial pressure was suspected as inspection of his optic discs revealed papilloedema. The physician attempted to lower the intracranial pressure temporarily by hyperventilating the patient so that the partial pressure of carbon dioxide fell below 3.5 kPa.

A Why does intracranial pressure increase with cerebral oedema?

B How do the optic nerves develop embryologically? Why might raised intracranial pressure cause the appearance of papilloedema in the optic disc?

C Why might raised intracranial pressure cause neurological injury?

D Why did the patient have a raised blood pressure?

E How might hyperventilation lower the intracranial pressure?

16.100 A strong light is shone onto the right eye. The left pupil constricts but the right pupil does not.

A Give a concise account of the neurological pathway for the direct pupillary reflex.

B Give a concise account of the neurological pathway for the consensual pupillary reflex.

C Where is the neurological lesion in this patient? Explain.

16.101 Two subjects, A and B, move from outdoors to a very dark room. Subject A has normal vision; subject B suffers from vitamin A deficiency. Subject A found that he could hardly see anything immediately; however, after 15 min, he could see the objects and find his way around in the room, although he could not identify the colour of the objects. Subject B still could not see any objects in the room.

A Sketch a graph showing the relationship between the log intensity of the threshold of effective stimulus of the retina and time after entering the dark room for subject A.

B Describe the mechanism that enables subject A to see the objects in the dark room after 15 min.

C What are the differences between rods and cones?

D Why was subject A not able to identify the colour of the objects in the dark room?

E If subject A had worn red goggles in the bright room, what would be the effect on the time for adaptation?

F Why could subject B still not see any objects 15 min after he entered the dark room?

16.102 Where is the likely site of lesion if a patient has the following?

A Complete visual defect in the right eye.

B Bitemporal hemianopia (defects of the temporal fields for both eyes).

C Left homonymous hemianopia without macular sparing.

D Left homonymous hemianopia with macular sparing.

16.103 For each of the neurological localising signs listed in Table 16.3 indicate the likely part of the brain involved and the likely artery involved if the symptom was caused by occlusion of arteries in the CNS territory.

16.104 A patient presented with double vision. Examination and investigation revealed that he had right oculomotor nerve palsy caused by compression by a posterior communicating aneurysm.
A What extraocular muscles do the oculomotor nerve supply?
B What other muscle does the oculomotor nerve supply?

Table 16.3

Localising signs	Site of lesion	Arteries in CNS territory involved
Reduced stereognosis		
Expressive dysphasia		
Receptive dysphasia		
Left hemianopia		
Ataxia		
Right hemiplegia		
Sensory loss in the right side of the face and arm		

C What abnormalities would you expect to find in right oculomotor nerve palsy regarding the following?
  i Eye movement.
  ii Eyelid position.
  iii Pupil size and reaction.

16.105 A patient diagnosed with an upper motor neurone facial nerve palsy secondary to a stroke was able to close his eyes. Another patient with a Bell's palsy was unable to close his eyes, and also became sensitive to loud noises.
A What group of muscles does the facial nerve supply?
B What is Bell's palsy?
C Explain why the patient with an upper motor neurone facial nerve palsy was able to close his eyes while the Bell's palsy sufferer was not.
D Why did the patient with Bell's palsy become sensitive to loud noises?

16.106 After an operation in the neck region, a patient was noted to have a droopy right eyelid and a small right pupil. He was diagnosed as having 'Horner's syndrome' resulting from interruption of the sympathetic nervous supply after its emergence from the superior cervical ganglion.
A Explain why interruption of the sympathetic nervous supply would result in a droopy eyelid and a small pupil.
B Give a brief account of the sympathetic nervous supply from the spinal cord to the superior cervical ganglion.
C At which other sites may lesions cause Horner's syndrome?

Table 16.4

	Upper motor neurone lesion	Lower motor neurone lesion
Nervous pathway affected		
Muscle weakness		
Muscle wasting		
Muscle tone		
Fasciculation		
Tendon reflex		
Babinski's sign		

241

16 **The nervous system**

Q

SYSTEM-BASED MEDICAL SCIENCES

16.107 **A** Compare a clinical 'upper motor neurone lesion' with a 'lower motor neurone lesion' by completing Table 16.4.
B If a patient suffers from cord compression at L4 level, deduce the clinical features from first principles.

16.108 A 70-year-old woman suffered a deterioration in intellect and reasoning abilities, and was diagnosed to suffer from Alzheimer's disease. She was treated initially with tacrine. This was found to have little effect and she was then treated with donepezil.

A What are the known risk factors for Alzheimer's disease?
B List the main gross pathological features of the disease.
C List the main histological features of the disease.
D What are the main hypotheses for the pathogenesis of Alzheimer's disease?
E Give one hypothesis for sufferers of Down's syndrome being more likely to develop Alzheimer's disease.
F What are the modes of action for tacrine and donepezil?

16.1   C D E
In its embryological development, the closed neural tube expands to form three brain vesicles:- the forebrain (prosencephalon), the midbrain (mesencephalon) and the hindbrain (rhombencephalon). The proscencephalon form the adult cerebral cortex and corpus striatum, and the diencephalon forms the adult thalamus and hypothalamus. The mesencephalon forms the adult midbrain. The rhomencephalon forms the adult pons, cerebellum and the medulla oblongata.

16.2   A B D
Fibres which link matching areas in the two hemispheres are called commissural fibres. The main commissure is the corpus callosum. It spans from the genu linking parts of the frontal lobe to the splenium linking the occipital lobes. The anterior commissure connects the anterior parts of the temporal lobe, and the posterior commissure lies in front of the pineal gland. The commissure of the fornix links the two hippocampi. Fibres which pass from one part of a hemisphere to another are association fibres. Examples are the superior longitudinal fasciculus, which links the frontal and the occipital lobes, and the uncinate fasciculus, which links the frontal lobe with the occipitotemporal cortex.

16.3   C D E
The third (oculomotor) and the fourth (trochlear) cranial nerves emerge from the midbrain. The fifth (trigeminal), sixth (abducens), seventh (facial) and eighth (vestibulocochlear) nerves emerge from the pons. The ninth to twelfth nerves emerge from the medulla oblongata.

16.4   A B C
The two large cerebral peduncles lie in the ventral part of the midbrain, and consist of the substantia nigra and the crus cerebri. The superior colliculus lies in the dorsal part of the midbrain, and is responsible for the orientation of the head and body towards visual stimuli. The aqueduct of Sylvius, the periaqueductal grey matter surrounding the aqueduct, and the red nuclei can be found in the central part of the midbrain.

16.5   B E
Three layers of meninges lie between the periosteum of the skull bones and the brain: the fibrous dura mater, the arachnoid mater and the pia mater. Between the periosteum of the skull bones and the dura mater is the extradural space. The middle meningeal artery can be found between the inner surface of the temporal bones and the dura mater. Skull fracture in the temporal bone may tear this artery, resulting in extradural haematoma. This often leads to initial concussion with loss of consciousness, a lucid interval of several hours, followed by acute deterioration due to cerebral compression. An emergency burr-hole is a life-saving procedure. The dura mater is made of strong fibrous tissue. The falx cerebri and the tentorium cerebelli are two large and strong dural folds which stabilise the brain. Between the dura mater and the arachnoid mater is the potential subdural space. Rupture of superficial veins in transit from the brain to a venous sinus may lead to a subdural haematoma (an accumulation of blood in the subdural space). This may present acutely following a head injury in children. On the other hand, it may present with gradual deterioration in personality changes without a history of head injury in the elderly. Between the subarachnoid mater and the pia mater is the subarachnoid space, where cerebrospinal fluid can be found.

16.6   –
Meningiomas are extrinsic CNS tumours. As a group, they occur less frequently than intrinsic CNS tumours (e.g. glioblastomas). Unlike CNS tumours in adults, those in children are usually intrinsic and below the tentorium. Meningiomas are usually lobulated with smooth edges. They seldom invade the dura, skull bones or the brain. Hence they have a better prognosis, as surgical removal is usually curative.

16.7   D
Bacterial meningitis is caused by different organisms at different ages. In neonates, *Streptococcus* and Gram-negative bacilli are common. In children, meningococcus is a common cause. *Haemophilus influenzae* type B commonly caused bacterial meningitis in children in the past, but the incidence has declined sharply since the introduction of universal vaccination against *Haemophilus* type B. Pneumococcus and meningococcus are the commonest organisms causing meningitis in adults.

16.8   A B D E
A cerebral abscess may result from spread of infection locally (e.g. paranasal sinus, middle ear), via the sigmoid cranial sinus (e.g. middle ear or the mastoid antrum) or from the bloodstream. There are no lymphatics in the CNS.

16.9   A B C
Most of the CSF is secreted by the choroid plexuses into the lateral ventricles, the remaining being secreted by the choroid plexus of the third ventricle. The CSF passes through the interventricular foramen into the third ventricle. It then passes through the aqueduct of Sylvius and reaches the fourth ventricle. From the fourth ventricle, it enters the subarachnoid space via the median and the lateral apertures. Only a very small proportion of the CSF enters the central canal of the spinal cord. The CSF is returned to the bloodstream directly via arachnoid mater

pouching through the dura of the superior sagittal sinus (arachnoid granulations).

16.10 A B D E

Hydrocephalus ('water in the head') is caused by the accumulation of CSF in the ventricles, which results in ventricular dilatation. The commonest cause is obstruction to the circulation of CSF. This may occur at the interventricular foramen, the third ventricle, the aqueduct, or the median and lateral apertures. Alternatively, obstruction may occur at the arachnoid granulations due to increased protein content of CSF (e.g. due to meningitis). A rare cause of hydrocephalus is excessive CSF production due to a tumour (papilloma) of the choroid plexus.

16.11 A D E

The internal carotid arteries enter the subarachnoid space in the roof of the cavernous sinus and give off ophthalmic, posterior communicating, and anterior choroidal arteries before dividing into their two terminal branches: the anterior and middle cerebral arteries. The basilar artery is formed from the two vertebral arteries, and divide into two posterior cerebral arteries at the upper part of the pons. The circle of Willis is completed by the posterior communicating arteries joining the posterior cerebral arteries, and the anterior communicating artery joining the two anterior cerebral arteries. In some people, the internal carotid arteries provide a significant proportion of blood to the posterior cerebral arteries via the posterior communicating arteries.

16.12 B D

The middle cerebral artery is the larger of the terminal branches of the internal carotid arteries. It gives off its central branches early on in its course. Deep to the lateral fissure, it divides into the upper and lower divisions. The upper division supplies the frontal and anterior parietal lobes. The lower division supplies the posterior parietal lobe, the temporal lobe and the middle of the optic radiation. It supplies about two-thirds of the lateral surface of the cerebral hemispheres. The central branches are important, and supply the corpus striatum, the thalamus and the posterior limb of the internal capsule. Hence blockage of this artery may cause paralysis of the opposite arm, leg and lower part of the face. The anterior limb of the internal capsule is supplied by the anterior cerebral artery. Blockage of the artery results in weakness of the opposite arm and face. The pons is supplied by branches of the basilar artery. The optic radiation is supplied by branches of the posterior cerebral arteries.

16.13 B

Cerebral blood flow is tightly regulated to maintain steady perfusion of the brain. Hence the perfusion of the brain remains relatively constant in spite of wide fluctuations in systolic blood pressure. An increase in acidity (a reduction in pH or an increase in carbon dioxide) leads to relaxation of the arteriolar smooth muscle of the cerebral vessels, and hence increases the cerebral blood flow. Increased systemic pressure leads to contraction of the arteriolar smooth muscle, so that blood flow to the brain can remain constant. Hyperventilation reduces carbon dioxide and hence reduces cerebral blood flow. Mechanical hyperventilation is sometimes used in treating patients with cerebral oedema. Oxygen concentration has relatively little effect on cerebral blood flow.

16.14 A D E

A stroke is a sudden disturbance of the functions of the CNS due to a vascular disease. Over 80% of strokes are due to cerebral infarction. Other causes include intracerebral haemorrhage and subarachnoid haemorrhage.

16.15 A B C D E

Cerebral infarction is due to a reduction of cerebral blood flow or cerebral oxygenation. Reduction in cerebral oxygenation may follow a respiratory arrest. Reduction in cerebral blood flow may be due to cerebral hypotension following cardiac arrest, occlusion of extracranial or intracranial arteries due to atheroma, thrombi or emboli. Other less common causes include head injury and venous thrombosis.

16.16 A B C E

Intracerebral haemorrhage occurs much more commonly in hypertensive subjects. It is caused by rupture at the bifurcation of intracerebral arterioles, and most commonly occurs in the basal ganglia, the brainstem, the cerebellum and the cerebral cortex. The resulting cerebral haematoma acts as an intracranial space-occupying lesion, and may therefore cause an increase in intracranial pressure or cerebral herniation. Rupture of arterial aneurysms at the circle of Willis causes subarachnoid haemorrhage.

16.17 A B D E

The blood–brain barrier exists to provide a chemically appropriate environment for the neurones to function optimally. It has two components: the ependymal lining of the choroid plexuses and the CNS capillary bed. In order to control substances entering and leaving the CNS, the cells lining the barrier are bounded by tight junctions, and fenestrations are absent. Functions of the blood–brain barrier include control of important metabolic substrate such as glucose, to prevent toxins and peripheral neurotransmitters from entering into the CNS, and to control ion movements.

роοен

16.18   B C D E
In general, lipid-insoluble drugs do not cross the blood–brain barrier easily, and their effect on the CNS is attenuated and delayed. Lipid-soluble drugs cross the blood–brain barrier easily, and their effect on the CNS is rapid. Inhaled anaesthetics and alcohol cross the blood–brain barrier, and produce CNS effects very rapidly. In the presence of meningitis, the blood–brain barrier is less effective. This can be made use of, as even drugs which usually do not cross the blood–brain barrier (e.g. gentamicin) can do so in the presence of meningitis. Chloramphenicol crosses the blood–brain barrier even in the absence of meningitis.

16.19   A B C E
Neurones are nerve cells whereas neuroglial cells are connective tissue supporting the nervous system. There are about 10 neuroglial cells to every neurone. Each neurone usually has many short dendrites which receive synaptic contacts from other neurones. However, each neurone only has one axon which conducts nerve impulses away from the neurone, although the axon may give rise to collaterals. Nissl bodies can be seen within the cytoplasm, and contain clumps of granular endoplasmic reticulum. Microtubules are intracellular organelles which can be seen in all parts of the neurone. They are involved in neuronal transport, and microtubule-associated proteins transport molecules along the outer surface of microtubules.

16.20   B D E
There are two types of neuronal transport: anterograde and retrograde. In anterograde transport, substances synthesised by the cell body move up the dendrites and axon. In retrograde transport, waste products from the axon and dendrites move to the lysosomes in the cell bodies to be destroyed. Retrograde transport is also important for target cell recognition. Axons constantly take up fragments of the plasma membrane of the target neurone and transport them back to the cell body. Retrograde transport may also be important for the transport of viruses to the CNS from the peripheral nervous system.

16.21   B E
At the resting membrane potential (−70 mV), there is continuous K⁺ efflux and Cl⁻ influx to maintain the negative membrane potential. In an action potential, the firing level is reached when the membrane is depolarised by about 15 mV (i.e. membrane potential is depolarised from −70 mV to about −55 mV). The voltage-gated sodium channels are suddenly opened at an increased rate as a result of positive feedback, and the sodium conductance increases. As the sodium concentration is usually higher

outside than inside the cell due to Na⁺, K⁺-ATPase, sodium ions readily enter the cell. The membrane potential moves towards though does not reach the equilibrium potential for Na⁺. This effect is much larger than the normal repolarising effect of the K⁺ efflux and Cl⁻ influx.

16.22   A B D E
Immediately after the spike potential of the action potential, the sodium channels rapidly enter the inactivated state, and the sodium conductance rapidly decreases. The K⁺ channels are gradually opened for a prolonged period of time, and the potassium conductance increases. There is a net movement of K⁺ out of the cells, as the concentration of K⁺ inside the cell is normally higher than that outside the cell. The prolonged opening of the K⁺ channels also explains the after-hyperpolarisation phase.

16.23   A B C E
Before the firing level is reached, the excitation threshold of the neurone to stimulation is higher (i.e. less excitable) the more negative the membrane potential. The absolute refractory period lasts from the time when the firing level is reached until after the first third of the repolarisation. During this period, the neurone cannot be excited irrespective of the strength of the stimulus. The relative refractory period occupies the rest of the repolarisation. During this period, the neurone can be excited, although a stronger stimulus is required. The threshold for excitation is increased during both the absolute and relative refractory periods. During the brief after-depolarisation period which comes immediately after the repolarisation, the neurone is slightly more excitable. However, during the prolonged after-repolarisation period, the neurone becomes less excitable than in its normal resting state.

16.24   A B C E
A synapse is where one neurone meets another. In humans, most synapses are chemically mediated, although electronic synapses do exist. Neurotransmitters are manufactured and loaded into vesicles within the Golgi apparatus of the sending neurone. Neurotransmitters are released from the pre-synaptic membrane by exocytosis. The neurotransmitters diffuse across the synaptic cleft, and act on receptors located on the membrane of the target neurone. Most synapses are axo-dendritic. However, axo-axonic synapses may achieve pre-synaptic inhibition either by preventing the generation of impulses in the target axon or by preventing the release of neurotransmitters.

16.25   A D
GABA and glycine are the two main inhibitory amino acid neurotransmitters. GABA is found mainly in the cerebellum and the cerebral cortex, and glycine is found mainly in the

The nervous system

spinal cord and brainstem. Most amines (e.g. dopamine, noradrenaline (norepinephrine), adrenaline (epinephrine), 5-HT) are excitatory neurotransmitters. Glutaric acid is an excitatory amino acid neurotransmitter.

16.26   A B C D
At the neuromuscular junction, acetylcholine is synthesised in the cholinergic neurone from acetyl-CoA and choline catalysed by the enzyme choline acetyltransferase. It is then taken into vesicles and is ready to be released into the synaptic cleft on the arrival of an action potential. After the acetylcholine vesicles are released, a proportion of the acetylcholine molecules bind to their receptors on the post-synaptic membrane. The nicotinic receptor is made up of five subunits: two identical α, one β, one γ and one δ subunits. Each α subunit binds to an acetylcholine molecule. When both α subunits are bound to an acetylcholine molecule, the sodium channel opens and depolarisation occurs. A second messenger is not required. To allow repolarisation to occur, the remaining acetylcholine molecules in the synaptic cleft are broken down into choline and acetic acid by acetylcholinesterase found on the post synaptic membrane. The choline is recycled and transported back to the pre synaptic neurone.

16.27   A C D
Most neurotransmitters exert their effects via a second messenger. Cyclic AMP is the commonest second messenger, followed by IP$_3$ and DAG. Nitric oxide is a neurotransmitter, and employs cGMP as the second messenger. Substance P is a neurotransmitter.

16.28   A C E
The types of neuroglial cells in the brain include astrocytes, oligodendrocytes, microglia and ependymal cells. Astrocytes maintain the structure of the capillary endothelium in the brain. Oligodendrocytes are responsible for myelination. Microglia are phagocytes in the brain. Ependymal cells line the ventricles and their cilia help the circulation of the CSF within the ventricular system.

16.29   B D
Myelination is the process of wrapping myelin sheaths around the axons of the neurones in the white matter of the brain, and is the main function of oligodendrocytes in the brain. Not all nerves are myelinated. For example, less than half of all peripheral nerves are myelinated. The axon is exposed at intervals between the myelin wrappings, and these are known as nodes. Myelination significantly increases the conduction of nerve impulses along the axon, as the impulses jump from node to node. During myelination, the potassium ion channels are deleted as

they are no longer necessary. Multiple sclerosis is a disease characterised by patches of demyelination in the white matter, and usually occurs in young adults in the temperate latitudes. Since the potassium ion channels have already been deleted, nerve conduction is compromised. Multiple sclerosis causes a variety of neurological symptoms depending on the anatomical site involved.

16.30   D
Multiple sclerosis is the commonest demyelinating disorder of the CNS. It does not usually affect the peripheral nervous system. It occurs more commonly in temperate than tropical countries, and in women than in men. The aetiology of the disease is not entirely clear, although it has been hypothesised that it may be an autoimmune disorder triggered by viral infection in genetically susceptible individuals. Histologically, the chronic plaque characteristically shows a loss of myelin, scarcity of oligodendrocytes (which make myelin) and a predominance of fibrillary astrocytes.

16.31   A B D E
There are many types of receptors in the skin. As they have different speeds of adaptation and they are located in different areas, they detect different stimuli and perform different functions. Free nerve endings respond to variations in temperature and painful stimuli. Pacinian corpuscles are found especially on the fingers and the palms, and are particularly effective in detecting vibration. Follicular nerve endings detect touch, and are rapidly adapting. This explains the short-lived touch sensation when clothes are put on. Meissner's corpuscles are mainly found on the pulp of the fingers, and are rapidly adapting. They are responsible for the detection of the texture of objects. Merkel cells adapt slowly, and discharge continuously in response to constant pressure. This explains the continued awareness of an object (e.g. knife and fork) held in the hand.

16.32   B
Knowledge of the segmental nerve supply is sometimes important in making a diagnosis in neurological examinations. The correct answers are:
- Around the nipple – T5
- At the umbilicus – T10
- Inguinal region – L1
- Lateral side of the sole of the foot – S1
- The thumb – C6

16.33   A B
Nerve root compression in the vertebral canal commonly affects the cervical roots (e.g. due to cervical spondylosis) or the lumbosacral roots (e.g. due to intervertebral disc

prolapse). It generally causes a feeling of numbness or tingling within that dermatome, referred pain in the muscles supplied by the relevant spinal nerves, weakness of muscles supplied by the spinal nerve and a loss of tendon reflex supplied by the spinal nerve. Hence compression of the S1 nerve root would cause pain in the sole of the feet, tingling or numbness in the area supplied by S1, weakness of the plantar flexion of the ankle and an absent ankle jerk. The knee jerk is unaffected, as its segmental level is L3/4.

16.34 A
Damage to the radial nerve at the radial groove of the humerus results in damage to the posterior interosseous nerve. Hence the long digital and carpal extensors are paralysed. The branch to the triceps is given off in the axilla. Hence extension of the elbow is unaffected. The middle and distal phalangeal joints of the fingers are extended by the interossei and lumbricals, and are therefore preserved. There may be diminished sensation over the radial side of the dorsum of the hand.

16.35 B C E
Damage to the ulnar nerve at the wrist results in paralysis of the adductor pollicis, the hypothenar muscles, and the third and fourth lumbricals. This results in inability of the thumb to adduct, and a clawed hand appearance. Sensation is diminished over the ulnar side of the palm, and over the palmar side of the little finger and the ulnar side of the fourth finger. However, sensation of the ulnar side of the dorsum of the hand is preserved, as the dorsal cutaneous branch is given off in the forearm.

16.36 A B E
When the hammer strikes the tendon of the quadriceps muscles, the muscle spindles in the muscle belly are passively stretched, and the type Ia and type II fibres discharge impulses to the posterior horn of the spinal cord. They then synapse with the dendrites of α motorneurones supplying the quadriceps muscles, and elicit contraction of the extrafusal muscle fibres. Most tendon reflexes involve only one synapse, and only occur at the spinal cord level. The muscle spindles also send inhibitory impulses simultaneously to the α motor neurones supplying the antagonist muscles (i.e. hamstrings). This is called reciprocal inhibition.

16.37 C E
The posterior column–medial lemniscal pathway is the larger of the two sensory pathways, and carries sensory fibres for joint position sense, vibration sense and discriminative touch. Like the spinothalamic pathway, it consists of three sets of neurones. The cell body of the first-order neurone lies in the posterior root ganglia. The

fibres are projected from the sensory receptors to the nuclei gracilis and cuneatus, and the fibres are collected in the gracilis and cuneate fasciculi. Unlike the spinothalamic tract, the first-order neurone does not cross over. The cell bodies of the second-order neurones lie in the nuclei gracilis and cuneatus, and project to the ventral posterior nucleus of the thalamus. The fibres cross over at the level of the medulla oblongata, and the fibres form the medial lemniscus after crossing over. The cell bodies of the third-order neurones lie in the ventral posterior nucleus of the thalamus, and project to the sensory cortex.

16.38 A B D E
There are great similarities between the spinothalamic tract and the posterior column–medial lemniscal pathway. Both have three-order sets of neurones. The cell bodies of the first-order neurones lie in the posterior root ganglia. The second-order neurones cross over to the opposite side for both pathways. One major difference is that whilst the spinothalamic tract crosses over in the spinal cord, the posterior column–medial lemniscal pathway crosses over in the medulla oblongata. The cell bodies of the third-order neurones lie in the thalamus for both pathways, and the third-order neurones project from the thalamus to the sensory cortex. Moreover, the representation of different parts of the body on the cortex is similar for both pathways.

16.39 A D
The two sensory pathways are the posterior column–medial lemniscal pathway and the spinothalamic pathway. The posterior column–medial lemniscal pathway mediates joint position and vibration senses, as well as two-point discrimination. The spinothalamic pathway mediates pain and temperature sensation.

16.40 C
Dissociated sensory loss affecting temperature but not joint position sensation can only occur if the anatomical pathways for the two sensory functions are separate. As the nerves or their cell bodies relaying messages for these two functions run close to each other in the peripheral nerves, posterior root ganglia, thalamus and cerebral cortex, lesions at these sites are likely to produce abnormalities in both sensory modalities. However, as the posterior column and lateral spinothalamic tract run separately in the spinal cord, a cyst in the central canal (syringomyelia) may initially affect the spinothalamic tract whilst leaving the posterior column intact.

16.41 C D E
Sharp localised pain is transmitted by the larger and faster myelinated Aδ fibres, whilst dull diffuse chronic pain is transmitted by smaller and slower unmyelinated C fibres.

16

A

SYSTEM-BASED MEDICAL SCIENCES

The nervous system

This accounts for the delay between the feeling of a localised sharp pain and the diffuse dull pain which follows it.

Substance P is the neurotransmitter in the afferent pain fibres in the dorsal horn of the spinal cord. The dorsal horn cells act as 'gates' to the pain pathway: the synapse between the peripheral pain fibres and the dorsal horn cells can be modified by drugs, or by other fibres (e.g. collaterals from touch fibres) via pre-synaptic inhibition.

16.42   A B E

Endogenous opioid neurotransmitters (e.g. endorphins, enkephalins) in the spinal cord and the brain form the natural pain inhibitory system. The mechanism of action for acupuncture and transcutaneous nerve stimulation is thought to be the release of these endogenous opioid neurotransmitters, and placebo may also work in this way. The analgesic action of paracetamol is peripheral by inhibiting the synthesis of prostaglandin. Naloxone is an opioid antagonist.

16.43   A C

The correct mechanisms of analgesic actions for the drugs are:

- Opiates – μ-opioid receptor agonist
- NSAIDs – cyclooxygenase inhibitor, reduction of prostaglandin synthesis both centrally and peripherally
- Corticosteroids – prevention of prostaglandin synthesis by reduction of arachidonic acid release
- Paracetamol – same as NSAIDs, but, peripheral action predominant

16.44   A B E

Stimulation of μ_2-opioid receptors causes respiratory depression and reduced gastrointestinal motility. Opioids also stimulate vagal tone and reduce sympathetic drive, and bradycardia may result. This effect is useful in the treatment of acute left ventricular failure with excessive sympathetic drive. The increased predominance of parasympathetic over sympathetic drive may cause pupil constriction, and may help in the clinical diagnosis of opiate overdose.

16.45   B E

The pre-ganglionic fibres of the sympathetic nervous system emerge from the anterior nerve root of the thoracic and lumbar segments of the spinal cord, and enter the sympathetic chain. They may ascend or descend to supply various parts of the body. Most of the sympathetic ganglia are in the sympathetic chain (e.g. superior cervical ganglion, stellate ganglion, thoracic ganglion, lumbar and sacral ganglia), although some lie outside (e.g. adrenal medulla, coeliac ganglion, pelvic ganglion). The adrenal medulla develops from the neural

crest embryologically, and acts as a sympathetic ganglion. The adrenal cortex does not receive innervation from pre-ganglionic sympathetic fibres, although it might receive post-ganglionic fibres from the renal ganglion. The male genitalia receive post-ganglionic fibres from the pelvic ganglion.

16.46   A C E

The sympathetic nervous system prepares the body for 'fright, flight and fight'. Effects include dilated pupils, increased heart rate, sweating, blood diverted from the skin and intestines to the skeletal muscles, reduced gut motility, and closure of sphincters for defecation and micturition. Hence, in patients with Raynaud's phenomenon with intermittent cold and painful fingers due to restriction of blood supply, interruption of the sympathetic nervous supply (sympathectomy) may be carried out. Similarly, the procedure might be considered in patients with serious excessive sweating of the hands.

16.47   A E

As the sympathetic nervous system normally dilates the pupils and increases sweating, interruption of the sympathetic nervous system after its emergence from the superior cervical ganglion would result in a small pupil and reduced sweating on that side of the face. Since the sympathetic nervous system also supplies the levator muscle of the upper eyelid, drooping of the eyelid (ptosis) may be seen in Horner's syndrome. Enophthalmos (sunken eye) may be seen in very severe cases. Eye movements are not affected, as the extraocular muscles are supplied by the third, fourth and sixth cranial nerves. Tear secretion is not affected. The lacrimal glands receive parasympathetic nervous supply from the pterygopalatine ganglion.

16.48   A D E

The pre-ganglionic parasympathetic fibres emerge from the cranial nerves and the sacral segments of the spinal cord. The cranial nerves carrying parasympathetic nerves include the oculomotor nerve (the post-ganglionic fibres from the ciliary ganglion supply the eye), the facial nerve (the post-ganglionic fibres from the pterygopalatine ganglion supply the lacrimal, submandibular and sublingual glands), the glossopharyngeal nerve (the post-ganglionic fibres from the otic ganglion supply the parotid gland) and the vagus nerve (the post-ganglionic fibres supply the heart and intestine).

16.49   B C

Acetylcholine is the neurotransmitter for the post-ganglionic parasympathetic fibres. Most of the post-ganglionic receptors are muscarinic, but different subtypes of muscarinic receptors have been found. Antimuscarinic drugs tend to block the parasympathetic effects, and cause dilated pupils, dry mouth, increased heart rate, bronchodilation, reduced gut motility and retention of urine.

16.50 A B
The corticospinal tract is the main voluntary motor pathway. Most of its fibres originate from the primary motor cortex in the pre-central gyrus, with contributions from the sensory cortex. It descends through the corona radiata and the internal capsule to reach the brainstem. It passes through the midbrain cerebral peduncles and the pons to form the pyramid in the medulla oblongata. About four-fifths of the fibres then cross over to the opposite side at the medullary decussation, and continue as the lateral corticospinal tract in the spinal cord. About one-fifth of the fibres remain uncrossed. Amongst these uncrossed fibres, half continue as anterior corticospinal fibres in the spinal cord, and half continue as uncrossed lateral corticospinal fibres. These uncrossed fibres may be important in the partial recovery of power in the affected limbs after hemiplegia caused by cerebrovascular accident.

16.51 A C
A clinical 'upper motor neurone lesion' is characteristically associated with weakness, increased muscle tone, spasticity, clasp-knife rigidity, exaggerated tendon reflexes and positive Babinski sign. It occurs when the upper motor neurone of the primary voluntary motor pathway is affected. These are the corticonuclear tract (for facial and lingual muscles) and the corticospinal tract. The anterior horn cells are the cell bodies of the 'lower motor neurones'. Periphery nerve lesions cause lower motor neurone lesions. The reticulospinal tract forms part of the extrapyramidal pathway responsible for posture and coordination of the limbs.

16.52 B D E
The distinction between upper and lower motor neurone lesions is important clinically, as it may give valuable clues about the aetiology of a neurological disease. The characteristic signs of a lower motor neurone lesion are weakness, wasting, reduced muscle tone, fasciculations and loss of tendon reflexes. Wasting occurs probably as a result of the loss of a factor produced by motorneurones. Fasciculations result from spontaneous discharge of motorneurones.

16.53 A B D E
The basal ganglia are concerned with the control of movement, and consist of a number of nuclei and nerve fibres at the level between the thalamus and the midbrain. They include the striatum (which include the caudate nucleus and the putamen of the lentiform nucleus), the globus pallidus, the substantia nigra and the subthalamic nucleus.

16.54 B
The main lesion in Parkinson's disease is a loss of dopaminergic neurones in the nigrostriatal pathway. The exact functions for each component of the basal ganglia are not yet entirely understood. However, it is generally accepted that there is a balance between the output of cholinergic and dopaminergic neurones in the striatum, and that the cholinergic output becomes unopposed in Parkinson's disease. The GABA-ergic neurones are reduced in Huntingdon's disease but not in Parkinson's disease. It was found that injection of the drug MPTP causes an acute clinical picture very similar to Parkinson's disease. MPTP is metabolised by monoamine oxidase B. Since monoamine oxidase B inhibitors (e.g. selegiline) appear to slow the progress of Parkinson's disease, it has been hypothesised that Parkinson's disease may be partly caused by the presence of a natural substance resembling MPTP.

16.55 A C D E
See question 16.54 above. Phenothiazines are dopamine antagonists, and tend to worsen Parkinsonian symptoms. Bromocriptine has dopaminergic agonist activity, and is sometimes useful in the treatment of Parkinson's disease.

16.56 A C D E
The cerebellum can be functionally divided into vestibulocerebellum, spinocerebellum and neocerebellum. The vestibulocerebellum consists of nuclei in the midline, and includes the vermis and fastigial nuclei. It communicates with the vestibular nucleus, and is important in maintaining balance. The spinocerebellum includes the anterior lobe. It receives fibres from the spinocerebellar tract, and is important in controlling gait and posture. The neocerebellum is the largest of all, and consists of the lateral parts of the cerebellum. It receives fibres from the pontocerebellar tract, and sends efferent fibres to the opposite cerebral cortex via the thalamus. Its main functions include coordination of the movements of the ipsilateral limbs and maintaining smooth contraction of the diaphragm and other speech muscles.

16.57 A E
The function of the vestibulocerebellum is most often impaired by midline cerebellar tumours. As the vestibulocerebellum communicates with the vestibular nuclei, vestibulocerebellar lesions usually result in the inability to stand upright without support (truncal ataxia) and nystagmus. Finger–nose incoordination and impaired articulation are characteristic features of neocerebellar lesions.

The nervous system

16.58   C D
See question 16.56 above. As the function of the neocerebellum is the coordination of ipsilateral limb movements and the maintenance of smooth contraction of speech muscles, characteristic features of neocerebellar lesions include impaired ipsilateral 'heel-to-shin' and 'finger-to-nose' tests and impaired articulation and phonation.

16.59   E
The correct cranial nerves responsible for the functions are:
- Sensation of the posterior third of the tongue – glossopharyngeal nerve
- Phonation – cranial accessory and vagus nerves
- Tongue protrusion – hypoglossal nerve
- Mastication – trigeminal nerve (motor root)
- Sensation to the forehead – ophthalmic branch of the trigeminal nerve

16.60   A D
The trigeminal nerve emerges from anterolateral surface of the pons, and enters the Gasserian ganglion in the petrous temporal bone. The three divisions emerge from the Gasserian ganglion and leave the skull through different foramina (the ophthalmic branch through the superior orbital fissure; the maxillary branch through the foramen rotundum; the mandibular branch through the foramen ovale). It has both sensory and motor functions. The motor branch innervates the muscle of mastication. The sensory branch supplies the dura mater of the middle and anterior cranial fossa, teeth and gums of the lower jaw, and the anterior two-thirds of the tongue. The mandibular division of the trigeminal nerve mediates the jaw jerk. The tip of the nose is innervated by the maxillary division.

16.61   A D
The correct cranial nerves responsible for the functions are:
- Taste in the posterior third of the tongue – glossopharyngeal nerve
- Taste in the anterior two-thirds of the tongue – facial nerve (via chorda tympani)
- Corneal reflex – (afferent limb) ophthalmic division of the trigeminal nerve; (efferent limb) facial nerve
- Attenuation of loud sound – facial nerve (branch to stapedius muscle)
- Parotid gland secretion – glossopharyngeal nerve (via otic ganglion)

16.62   A E
The nuclei of the facial nerve lie in the caudal part of the pons. Upper motor neurone lesion of the facial nerve is supranuclear, and is commonly caused by a vascular stroke which affects the corticonuclear fibres either in the cerebral cortex or the internal capsule. As the nuclei for the upper part of the face are bilaterally represented, a unilateral upper motor neurone facial nerve palsy affects only the lower part of the face, but spares the upper part of the face.

16.63   A B C D
The commonest cause of a unilateral lower motor neurone facial nerve palsy is Bell's palsy. It is caused by compression resulting from inflammation of the nerve inside the bony canal above the labyrinth between the geniculate ganglion and the stylomastoid foramen. This affects both the lower and upper parts of the face. As a result of loss of the stapedius function, the patient may complain of increased sensitivity to loud noise. Most cases resolve within a few weeks, although recovery in a few patients is incomplete.

16.64   B C D
All the extraocular muscles are supplied by the oculomotor nerve, apart from the lateral rectus (supplied by the abducens nerve) and the superior oblique (supplied by the trochlear nerve). In addition, the upper division of the oculomotor nerve also supplies the levator palpebrae. The oculomotor nerve also carries parasympathetic fibres to the eye to supply the sphincter pupillae (which constricts the pupil) and the ciliary muscle (for accommodation). The parasympathetic fibres originate from the Edinger–Westphal nucleus and synapse in the ciliary ganglion.

16.65   E
All extaocular muscles apart from the lateral rectus and superior oblique are paralysed in oculomotor nerve palsy. Hence the position of the eye is 'down and out'. Paralysis of the levator superioris results in complete ptosis due to the action of unopposed orbicularis oculi. Paralysis of the sphincter pupillae results in a fully dilated pupil due to unopposed action of dilator pupillae. Sweating is controlled by the sympathetic nervous system, which is unaffected in oculomotor nerve palsy.

16.66   A B C E
The MLF is a central brainstem nerve tract which connects the oculomotor, trochlear and abducens nuclei. It also receives neural input from the vestibular nuclei and the cerebellum. It is important for conjugate eye movement to ensure that the visual axes of both eyes are parallel, and to maintain visual fixation on a moving target. The MLF is often affected by multiple sclerosis. This results in internuclear ophthalmoplegia. The ipsilateral eye is unable

to adduct, and nystagmus appears in the contralateral abducting eye.

16.67 D E
Direct pupillary light reflex describes the constriction of the pupil when light is shone onto the same eye, whilst consensual light reflex describes the constriction of the pupil when light is shone onto the opposite eye. Only the first-order neurone of the visual tract is involved. In direct pupillary light reflex, the ganglion cells within the retina conduct impulses along the optic nerve and the optic tracts to the pretectal nucleus near the superior colliculus in the midbrain. The pretectal nucleus is linked by internuncial neurones to the parasympathetic (Edinger–Westphal) nucleus. The pre-ganglionic fibres from the Edinger – Westphal nucleus enters the oculomotor nerve and synapses in the ciliary ganglion, and the post-ganglionic fibres supply the sphincter pupillae in the iris. Stimulation of the sphincter pupillae causes papillary constriction. For consensual light reflex, impulses are conducted from the pretectal nucleus to the opposite Edinger–Westphal nucleus via the posterior commissure.

16.68 B
The fact that the right pupil constricts in response to light shone onto the left eye indicates the pathway along the left optic nerve and the right oculomotor nerve are intact. A lesion in either the pathway along the left optic nerve or the left oculomotor nerve may explain why the left pupil fails to react in response to light shone on the left eye. Other explanations may include a lesion in the left Edinger–Westphal nucleus or paralysis of the sphincter pupillae (e.g. due to drugs). From these two deductions, the only given option which may explain the clinical findings is a left oculomotor nerve lesion.

16.69 A
The are two types of photoreceptor cells: the rods and the cones. The photosensitive compounds are contained in the outer segments, which contain regular stacks of membrane. In the rods, the outer segments are thin and rod-like, whilst those of the cones are more pointed. There are about 6 million cones in each eye, and they are mainly found in the fovea. On the other hand, there are about 120 million rods in each eye, and they are found outside the fovea. The rods are more sensitive to light than cones, and function in dim light. Hence they are important for night vision. However, they are not able to differentiate between different colours. The cones are important for vision in daylight. They are capable of distinguishing between different colours, and can achieve a higher level of visual acuity than rods.

16.70 A B
When the photosensitive pigments (opsin and $retinene_1$) are exposed to light, structural changes in the $retinene_1$ occur. This results in a conformation change of the photopigment, and activates an associated G protein-transducin (G_{t1}). This in turn activates a cGMP-associated phosphodiesterase, and hence causes a reduction in intracellular cGMP. This leads to a closure of the sodium channel, and hyperpolarisation of the photoreceptor occurs. This hyperpolarisation leads to an action potential in the ganglion cells in the retina.

16.71 E
When an individual with normal vision moves from a very bright to a very dark room, the visual threshold declines due to dark adaptation. The initial decline in visual threshold is mainly due to adaptation of the cones as the changes are tested at relatively high intensity of light when cones are active. The later changes in visual threshold are due to rod adaptation at a much lower intensity of light. The dark adaptation is due to the regeneration of the photopigments from their 'bleached' configuration. On the other hand, when a person moves from a very dark to a very bright room, the visual threshold increases due to the conversion of the photopigments into their 'bleached' configuration. This is a much faster process. If the individual had worn red-tinted glasses in the bright light, the rods would only be minimally stimulated as its peak sensitivity to light is at a lower wavelength of 505 mm. Hence the dark adaptation process would be quicker.

16.72 B C D E
Myopia is often genetic in origin, and is commoner amongst Chinese and Japanese than the Caucasians. It is due to an abnormally long eyeball, excessive convergence power of the cornea or lens, or a combination of the two factors. As a result, the images formed lie in front of the retina, and they appear blurred to the subject. It may be corrected by concave lenses, which tend to diverge the light rays and move the images further back onto the retina.

16.73 A
Both the retina and the optic nerve develop embryologically from an outgrowth of the brain (the optic vesicle). Hence the optic nerve is wrapped round by neuroglial cells (i.e. astrocytes and oligodendrocytes) and not Schwann cells as in peripheral nerves. The optic nerve is also surrounded by meninges. Whilst peripheral nerves can regenerate if damaged, the optic nerve cannot. The cell bodies of the optic nerve are in the ganglion layer of the retina. It synapses at the lateral geniculate bodies of the thalamus. The optic nerve is therefore homologous

16

A

SYSTEM-BASED MEDICAL SCIENCES

The nervous system

with the second-order neurone in the sensory pathway (e.g. spinothalamic tract). Whilst the fibres from the nasal side of the retina at the optic chiasma cross over to the opposite lateral geniculate body, those from the temporal side of the retina do not cross over, and join the ipsilateral lateral geniculate body.

16.74   B C E
Lesions before the optic chiasma will only affect vision in that eye. As the other eye is unaffected, the visual field with both eyes open is full. A lesion at the optic chiasma (e.g. due to a pituitary gland) may result in the fibres from the nasal side of the retina from both eyes being interrupted. This gives rise to bitemporal hemianopia. Lesions beyond the optic chiasma result in fibres of the temporal side of the retina from the ipsilateral eye and the nasal side of the retina from the opposite eye being interrupted. This gives rise to homonymous hemianopia in the visual field on the side opposite to the lesion. The correct matches between the lesions and the resulting visual field defects are:
- Complete left optic nerve lesion – blindness in left eye
- Optic chiasm – bitemporal hemianopia
- Left optic tract – right homonymous hemianopia
- Right optic radiation – left homonymous hemianopia
- Left occipital cortex – right homonymous hemianopia

16.75   A B C E
Sound vibrations from outside the ear must enter the outer ear to set up vibrations in the tympanic membrane. The handle of the first ossicle (malleus) is attached to the back of the tympanic membrane, and the sound vibrations must pass through all three ossicles in the middle ear (malleus, incus, stapes) to reach the oval window. The foot plate of the stapes closes the scala vestibuli at the oval window, which separates the middle and the inner ear. The sound vibrations from the stapes stimulate the inner hair cells of the cochlea, which are the auditory sense organs.

16.76   A D
The axons of the neurones that innervate the inner hair cells form the auditory nerve, which synapse at the dorsal and ventral cochlear nuclei in the medulla. This is the first-order neurone. The second-order neurone runs from these nuclei to the contralateral medial geniculate body at the thalamus. It also sends fibres to the ipsilateral medial geniculate body through different pathways. The third-order neurone runs from the medial geniculate body to the primary auditory cortex in the superior temporal gyrus. Lateral geniculate bodies and superior colliculi are part of pathways for vision and visual reflexes.

16.77   A B D
The amplitude and frequency of sound waves determine the loudness and pitch of the sound respectively. The harmonics of the sound waves (i.e. the proportion of sound with harmonic vibrations) determine the timbre of the sound (e.g. the difference in sound quality of notes between different musical instruments of the same pitch). The speed of the sound is determined by the medium in which the sound is transmitted (e.g. faster in water than in air), but the sound appears the same. The wavelength can be calculated by the equation
Wavelength = Speed/Frequency
For a given speed of sound, the higher the wavelength, the lower the pitch.

16.78   A C E
Two factors contribute to the lateral localisation of sound. Firstly, there is a slight time difference in the arrival of stimulus in the two ears. This results in a phase difference in the sound waves on the two sides. Secondly, the sound is louder on the side of the source. These differences are interpreted by the auditory cortex. However, there is no time difference in the arrival of the sound from in front and behind in the two ears. Localisation is achieved by the shape and position of the pinna. The pinna also explains the localisation of sound coming from directly above or directly below the subject.

16.79   B C D
About 90% of the population are left hemisphere/right hand dominant. Amongst these people, Wernicke's area is found in the left superior temporal gyrus. Its main function is to understand speech. Hence lesions in the area result in receptive aphasia, and patients have difficulty in understanding the speech of others, retrieving the appropriate names of objects, and monitoring their own speech, although they might appear to speak fluently and they may not be aware of the gross errors in their speech.

Broca's area is usually found in the left inferior frontal gyrus. Its main function is to express what the subject wishes to say. Hence a patient with a lesion in Broca's area understands other people's speech. However, their own speech is slow, hesitant and telegraphic. Patients are well aware of their speech problem. The two speech areas are supplied by branches of the left middle cerebral artery. Broca's and Wernicke's areas are connected by the arcuate fasciculus.

16.80   B D E
Alzheimer's disease is the commonest cause of dementia. It is a degenerative condition, and therefore occurs more commonly amongst older people. Most cases of Alzheimer's disease are sporadic, and occur more

commonly in individuals with the ApoE4 genotype on chromosome 19. However, a small proportion of cases run in families and appear to have an autosomal dominant inheritance. A gene on chromosome 21 appears to be involved in these cases.

16.81   C
Alzheimer's disease characteristically causes a severe loss of both white and grey matter. Marked cortical atrophy is characteristic, with consequent ventricular dilatation. The hippocampus, frontal and temporal lobes are most affected. This explains the clinical features of deterioration in personality, memory and cognition. Histologically, senile plaques and neurofibrillary tangles are characteristic, although the nature of these structures is not entirely known. Senile plaques are neuritic processes surrounding a central amyloid core. Neurofibrillary tangles are long corkscrew-like structures consisting of thickened fibrils within the neuronal cytoplasm. There is a reduction of cholinergic neurones in Alzheimer's disease. The effectiveness of drugs which enhance cholinergic activities in the CNS is currently being evaluated.

16.82   B C D E
Benzodiazepines have sedative, hypnotic, anxiolytic, anticonvulsant and muscle relaxant properties, and are used clinically for each of these properties. There are three different subtypes of benzodiazepine receptors. The traditional benzodiazepines act at all three subtypes. However, newer types of benzodiazepines might act selectively on one or two of these subtypes, and actions can be more specific.

16.83   A C D
Benzodiazepines act mainly on the reticular activating system (causing sedation and hypnosis), but also act on the limbic system. They act by attaching to a specific site on the GABA receptor/chloride channel complex. Their action is to potentiate the effect of GABA, which is an important inhibitory neurotransmitter. GABA acts by opening chloride ion channels in cells. The muscle relaxant properties of benzodiazepines are central and not peripheral.

16.84   C D
Neuroleptics are anti-schizophrenic agents. Schizophrenia is associated with excess dopaminergic D_2 receptors in the limbic system of the brain. Phenothiazines (e.g. chlorpromazine) belong to one of the traditional groups of neuroleptic drugs. Other neuroleptic drugs include butyrophenones (e.g. haloperidol) and thioxanthenes. They act mainly by competitively antagonising the dopaminergic D_2 receptors. However, phenothiazines also have other significant pharmacological actions, such as

antagonists at serotonin, cholinergic, and α-adrenergic receptors. They are used to treat schizophrenia both in acute treatment and for maintenance therapy. Neuroleptics are not antidepressants.

16.85   A B C
As phenothiazines are antagonists of dopamine receptors, they may antagonise the dopamine receptors in the nigrostriatal tract and cause Parkinsonian symptoms. As dopamine inhibits the release of prolactin from the anterior pituitary gland, phenothiazines may cause hyperprolactinaemia. Tardive dyskinesia is a disorder characterised by involuntary movements of lips, tongue and face, and may occur after neuroleptics have been used for a few years. Akathisia (extreme restlessness of legs) may occur in about a fifth of the patients, but the exact mechanism of action is unclear. Phenothiazines are generally sedative. The newer types of neuroleptics (e.g. clozapine, risperidone) generally have fewer neurological side effects.

16.86   A E
The major types of antidepressants include tricyclic (e.g. amitriptyline), SSRIs (e.g. fluoxetine, paroxetine), monoamine oxidase inhibitors (e.g. phenelzine), and reversible selective MAO-A inhibitors (e.g. moclobemide). Lithium and carbamazepine are used in the treatment of manic-depressive illnesses, as well as mood stabilisers in unipolar depression. Benzodiazepines, barbiturates and neuroleptics have no place in the treatment of depression.

16.87   C E
Tricyclic antidepressants act by inhibiting the reuptake of noradrenaline (norepinephrine) into the neuronal stores. Hence, the sympathomimetic actions of adrenergic agonists (e.g. adrenaline (epinephrine) and noradrenaline (norepinephrine)) are potentiated by tricyclic antidepressants. The cardiotoxic effects are also potentiated. Tricyclic antidepressants are antimuscarinics, and may cause blurred vision, urinary retention, dry mouth and raised intraocular pressure. The bladder inhibitory action is used clinically in the treatment of childhood enuresis. Tricyclics may also precipitate seizures as they lower the seizure threshold.

16.88   E
Lithium acts by reducing the recycling of free myoinositol for the synthesis of phosphatidylinositol, which is an important intracellular signalling molecule for regulating intracellular calcium concentration. As lithium has a narrow therapeutic window, a good understanding of the pharmacokinetics is important. Lithium is a small ion, and is therefore normally easily absorbed throughout the gastrointestinal tract. However, a sustained-release preparation may delay the absorption. It is not bound to

The nervous system

plasma proteins, and it is not significantly metabolised by the liver. It is mainly eliminated by the kidneys, and the rate of elimination is proportional to the plasma sodium concentration. Hence the half-life increases in patients with renal impairment, and lithium clearance is inversely proportion to sodium clearance. Thus lithium clearance decreases when a diuretic is administered at the same time.

16.89

A

i The resting potential of a nerve axon is about −70 mV.
ii In the resting condition, the membrane is relatively impermeable to Na^+; thus, the resting membrane potential originates mainly from K^+ and Cl^-. It is generated and maintained by the following factors:
1. There are non-diffusible negatively charged proteins inside the cell.
2. Cl^- moves inside the cell down its concentration gradient.
3. K^+ moves inside the cell to preserve electroneutrality outside the cell.
4. Hence, $[K^+]$ is higher inside than outside the cell.
5. There are more osmotically active particles inside than outside the cell.
6. To restore the balance of osmotically active particles, the Na^+, K^+-ATPase pumps Na^+ out of the cells in exchange for K^+ into the cells.
7. Hence, the higher $[K^+]$ inside than outside the cell and the higher $[Cl^-]$ outside than inside the cell are maintained.
8. The resting membrane potential results from a combination of the equilibrium membrane potentials for $[K^+]$ and $[Cl^-]$.
iii When a stimulus is applied, the voltage-gated Na^+ channels begin to open after a latent period of about 2 ms. This causes depolarisation of the axon as the resting membrane potential for $[Na^+]$ is +60 mV. When the membrane potential reaches about −55 mV, the voltage Na^+ channels open at an increasing rate. This is the firing level and the membrane potential increases to a peak of about +35 mV very rapidly, within about 0.5 ms. The Na^+ channels are then rapidly inactivated and enter a closed state. At the same time, voltage-gated K^+ channels open and the axon enters into repolarisation.
iv See Figs 16.1 and 16.2.

B

The peripheral nerves conveying pain are:
• C fibres
• smaller fibre diameter (about 1 μm)
• lower conduction velocity (about 1 m/s)
• unmyelinated.

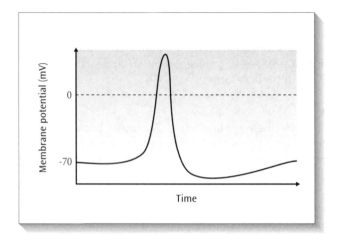

Fig. 16.1 Action potential.

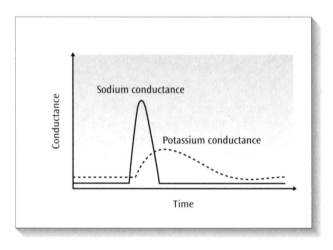

Fig. 16.2 Changes in soidum and potassum conductance during an action potential.

The peripheral nerves conveying pressure and touch are:
• A fibres
• larger fibre diameter (about 10 μm)
• higher conduction velocity (about 50 m/s)
• myelinated.

C

For unmyelinated fibres, the propagation of nerve impulses depends on local circular current flow. When a portion of nerve axon is depolarised, the positive charges from the membrane move forward into an area of negativity until the firing level is reached. The action potential fails to depolarise the area behind it, which has entered into a refractory state. In this way, action potential is propagated forward along the nerve axon.

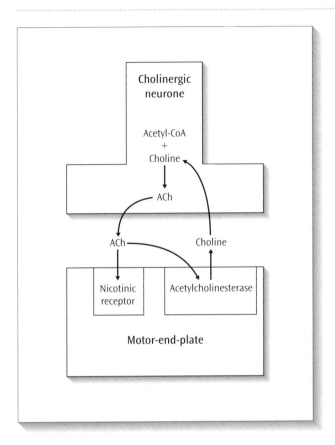

Fig. 16.3 The neuromuscular junction.

D

For myelinated fibres, current flow through the myelin is negligible because myelin does not conduct current well. Propagation of nerve impulses results from depolarisation jumps from one node of Ranvier to the next. Hence, it is a faster process.

E

Local anaesthetics block Na⁺ channels by plugging the transmembrane pore. They preferentially bind to the inactivated stage of the channels, blocking the initiation and propagation of action potentials and preventing the voltage-dependent increase in Na⁺ conductance in the axon. Local anaesthetics block conduction in small-diameter nerve fibres more readily than in large fibres. Hence, peripheral nerves conveying pain are more easily blocked than those conveying touch.

16.90
A
See Fig. 16.3.

B

The post-synaptic receptor in the motor end-plate is the nicotinic receptor. It is made up of five subunits: two

identical α subunits, one β, one γ, and one δ subunit. There is a binding site for acetylcholine for each α subunit. When acetylcholine binds to the α subunit, a configurational change is induced so that the sodium channels open and increase the sodium conductance.

C

Pancuronium is a non-depolarising neuromuscular blocking drug with an intermediate duration of action. It acts by blocking the nicotinic acetylcholine receptors in the motor end-plate.

D

Neostigmine is a medium-duration anticholinesterase. It acts by inhibiting peripheral acetycholinesterase. This prevents the breakdown of acetylcholine in the synaptic cleft and increases the local acetylcholine concentration to compete with any neuromuscular blocking agent in binding to the nicotinic receptors.

16.91
A
Suxamethonium is a depolarising neuromuscular blocking agent. It acts by causing a maintained depolarisation at the motor end-plates, so that they are no longer electrically excitable.

B

As suxamethonium acts by maintained depolarisation of the motor end-plates, brief fasciculation usually occurs when the drug is given.

C

Suxamethonium is not reversed by anticholinesterase. As the motor end-plates become electrically non-excitable, an increase in the local concentration of acetylcholine would have no effect.

D

Normally, suxamethonium only acts for a short time because it is hydrolysed by a plasma cholinesterase such as pseudocholinesterase (butyrocholinesterase); however, in a small group of subjects with a congenital deficiency of this enzyme, the paralysing effect of suxamethonium may last a long time.

16.92
A
Myasthenia gravis is an autoimmune condition caused by circulating antibodies to the nicotinic acetylcholine receptors. These antibodies destroy some of the receptors and the destroyed receptors are removed by endocytosis.

The nervous system

Table 16.5

System	Actions	Possible clinical uses
Cardiovascular	Increase heart rate	Treatment of sinus bradycardia
Eyes	Pupillary dilatation and paralysis of accommodation	Dilatation of eye and paralysis of accommodation (e.g. in fundus examination, treatment of iritis)
Respiratory	Prevent reflex bronchoconstriction Dry secretions	Use during general anaesthetia to prevent aspiration of secretions Treatment of asthma (ipratropium)
Gastrointestinal	Inhibit gastrointestinal motility	Treatment of abdominal colic
Neurological	Reduce Parkinsonian extrapyramidal effects	Treatment of Parkinsonian symptoms

B

As there is a relative lack of functioning nicotinic receptors in the motor end-plates, the few functioning receptors present are rapidly used up by initial stimulation. Hence, patients present with muscle fatigability.

C

The symptoms disappear rapidly after an intravenous injection of edrophonium. This confirms the diagnosis that she suffers from myasthenia gravis.

D

Edrophonium is a short-acting anticholinesterase. It inhibits the breakdown of acetylcholine in the neuromuscular junction and temporarily increases the acetylcholine concentration. Hence, it leads to temporary disappearance of symptoms.

E

Anti-acetylcholine receptor antibodies are present in about 90% of patients with myasthenia gravis.

16.93
A

Atropine is a long-acting muscarinic receptor competitive antagonist. Since muscarinic receptors are present in a wide variety of peripheral tissues, it has widespread clinical effects.

B
See Table 16.5.

16.94
A

Imipramine is a tricyclic antidepressant. Its main action in the central nervous system is to block the reuptake of

noradrenaline (epinephrine) in noradrenergic neurones. It thus increases the availability of noradrenaline (epinephrine) and facilitates neuronal transmission; it also has some action in inhibiting neuronal 5-HT uptake. Paroxetine is a selective 5-HT uptake inhibitor. Its main action is to inhibit the reuptake of 5-HT in serotonin neurones but with little effect on noradrenergic neurones.

B

Both imipramine and paroxetine are effective in treating depression in some patients, suggesting that depression is caused by a deficiency of monoamine neuronal transmission in the brain (the monoamine hypothesis of depression). However, this hypothesis cannot explain all observations (e.g. it fails to predict the effectiveness of some newer antidepressants).

C

Paroxetine has much less risk of cardiotoxicity than imipramine because paroxetine has little effect on peripheral noradrenergic neurones. The other advantages of paroxetine over imipramine are:
- fewer cholinergic side effects (e.g. dry mouth, blurred vision, frequency of urine)
- less risk of postural hypotension
- safer in overdose.

16.95
A

Muscle spindles are stimulated when the muscle tendon is struck.

B

1. Impulses travel in the Ia fibre from the muscle spindle of the quadriceps femoris to the afferent sensory neurone to enter the dorsal root of the spinal cord.

2. Excitatory neurotransmitters are released from the sensory neurone into the synapse with the motor neurone.
3. Impulses travel in the motor neurone from the ventral root of the spinal cord to the motor end-plate of the quadriceps femoris.

C

This phenomenon is known as 'reinforcement'. It may be due to increased efferent discharge to the muscle spindle of the quadriceps tendon from the afferent γ discharge from the hands. Increased efferent γ discharge may also explain an exaggerated tendon reflex in anxious patients.

D

From the observation that the knee jerk is intact, we can conclude that:
• the afferent Ia fibres to the spinal cord are intact
• the spinal cord at the segment of the tendon is intact
• the motor neurone at the segment is intact.
However, we cannot draw any conclusions about other levels of the spinal cord.

16.96
See Table 16.6.

16.97
A
CSF is mainly secreted by the choroid plexuses into the lateral ventricles. A small amount is secreted in the third ventricle. The CSF from the lateral ventricles passes through the interventricular foramina (of Magendie and Luschka) to the third ventricle, via the aqueduct of Sylvius, and reaches the fourth ventricle. It then enters the subarachnoid spaces via the median and lateral apertures. A small proportion of the CSF enters the spinal cord. Most of the CSF is returned directly to the bloodstream via arachnoid mater pouching through the dura of the superior sagittal sinus (arachnoid granulations).

B
The physiological functions of CSF include:
• mechanical protection of the brain, reducing the weight of the brain by acting as a 'water bath' and as a cushion against trauma
• provision of the ideal biochemical environment for the neuronal tissues (e.g. pH, K^+, Ca^{2+}, Mg^{2+}).

C
Hydrocephalus is caused by the abnormal accumulation of CSF in the ventricles, resulting in ventricular dilatation. Possible causes for hydrocephalus are:
• Increased production of CSF, e.g. tumour of the choroid plexus.

Table 16.6

Movement or reflex	Spinal nerve root
Shoulder abduction	C5
Shoulder adduction	C5–C7
Elbow flexion	C5–C6
Elbow extension	C7
Wrist flexion	C7–C8
Wrist extension	C7
Finger flexion	C7–C8
Finger abduction	T1
Hip flexion	L1–L2
Hip extension	L5–S1
Knee flexion	S1
Knee extension	L3–L4
Ankle dorsiflexion	L4
Ankle plantar flexion	S1–S2
Biceps reflex	C5–C6
Triceps reflex	C7–C8
Knee reflex	L3–L4
Ankle reflex	S1–S2

• Obstruction. This may occur at the interventricular foramen, the third ventricle, the aqueduct of Sylvius, or the median and lateral apertures.
• Prevention of return of CSF into the bloodstream, e.g. blockage at the arachnoid granulations due to increased protein content of CSF in meningitis.

16.98
A
The blood–brain barrier is formed by the tight junctions between capillary endothelial cells in the brain and between epithelial cells in the choroid plexus.

B
The permeability of the blood–brain barrier to drugs increases with:
• higher lipid solubility of the drug
• smaller drug size

- disruption of the integrity of the blood–brain barrier (e.g. in meningitis).

Alcohol crosses the blood–brain barrier more effectively than gentamicin mainly because alcohol has a higher lipid solubility.

C

Gentamicin may be effective in the treatment of bacterial meningitis because the integrity of the blood–brain barrier is usually breached in this disorder. However, it is too unreliable to be of value in clinical practice.

16.99
A

The brain is enclosed in a rigid cranial cavity and the brain tissue and CSF are not compressible. Hence, any brain swelling is likely to lead to an increase in intracranial pressure.

B

The optic nerves develop embryologically from the forebrain; hence, the optic nerves are part of the brain. The optic disc occurs where the optic nerves leave the eye. The appearance of papilloedema in the optic disc is due to the accumulation of axoplasm in the optic nerve when axonal flow is impeded by pressure on the nerve.

C

Increased intracranial pressure might cause neurological injury if it results in:

- compression of the cerebral vessels and a reduction in cerebral blood flow
- intracranial shift of the brain (if the cause for the increased intracranial pressure is an intracranial space-occupying lesion)
- intracranial herniation (through the tentorium or foramen magnum).

D

The blood pressure rises with increased intracranial pressure (the Cushing reflex). This is a physiological protective mechanism to protect the brain from reduced cerebral perfusion. The increased intracranial pressure causes a reduction in blood supply to the vasomotor area of the brain. The resultant local hypoxia increases discharges from the vasomotor area and the arterial blood pressure rises.

E

Hyperventilation lowers the arterial [CO_2]. The reduction in arterial [CO_2] induces cerebral vasoconstriction, which rapidly reduces the intracranial pressure.

16.100
A

The direct pupillary light reflex describes the constriction of the pupil when light is shone on to the same eye. The ganglion cells within the retina conduct impulses along the optic nerve and the optic tracts to the pretectal nucleus near the superior colliculus in the midbrain. The pretectal nucleus is linked by internuncial neurones to the parasympathetic (Edinger–Westphal) nucleus. The pre-ganglionic fibres from the Edinger–Westphal nucleus enter the oculomotor nerve and synapse in the ciliary ganglion, and the post-ganglionic fibres supply the sphincter pupillae in the iris, which constricts the pupil.

B

The consensual pupillary light reflex describes the constriction of the pupil when light is shone on to the opposite eye. The neurological pathway is similar to that for the direct pupillary light reflex except that impulses are conducted from the pretectal nucleus to the opposite Edinger–Westphal nucleus via the posterior commissure.

C

In this patient, the left pupil constricts when light is shone on to the right eye. We can conclude that the right optic nerve and the right optic tract are intact. However, the right pupil does not constrict; therefore, the lesion must be in the pathway between the right pretectal nucleus and the right sphincter pupillae. The most likely site of the lesion is in the right oculomotor nerve. Alternatively, it may be due to lesions in the Edinger–Westphal nucleus or paralysis of the sphincter pupillae.

16.101
A
See Fig. 16.4.

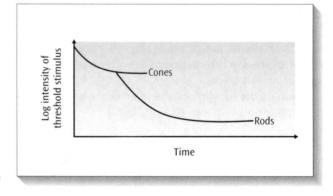

Fig. 16.4 Dark adaptation.

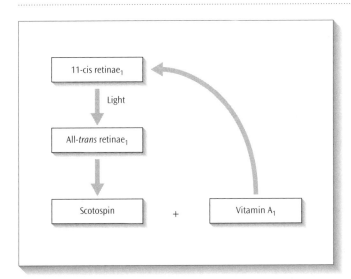

Fig. 16.5 Synthesis of retinae in rods.

D
Cones are not functional under low light intensity. Hence, when A was in the dark room, only the rods were functional. Since cones are essential for colour perception, A could not identify any colours in the dark room.

E
As rods are maximally responsive at a lower wavelength of about 505 mm, red light would cause little bleaching of rhodopsin. Hence, the time for adaptation would be greatly reduced if subject A had worn red goggles in the bright room.

F
Vitamin A is essential in the regeneration of 11-*cis* retinae$_1$. Hence, the ability to regenerate is greatly reduced in vitamin A deficiency. The explains why subject B could not see any objects in the room 15 min after entering it.

16.102
A
Right eye or right optic nerve.

B
Optic chiasm (e.g. pituitary tumour).

C
Right optic tract.

D
Right geniculocalcarine tract or right occipital cortex.

16.103
See Table 16.7.

16.104
A
The oculomotor nerve supplies all extraocular muscles except lateral rectus (supplied by abducens VI nerve) and superior oblique (supplied by trochlear IV nerve).

B
Levator palpebrae.

C
The oculomotor nerve also transmits parasympathetic innervation for pupil constriction. The abnormalities in a complete oculomotor nerve palsy are as follows:
i In the resting position, the eye position is 'down and out'. This is because the only functioning extraocular muscles are lateral rectus (abductor) and superior oblique (depressor and abductor).

B
Subject A was able to see the objects in the dark room by dark adaptation. From the sketch in (A), the initial decrease in visual threshold was due to the dark adaptation of the cones, whereas the later larger decrease in visual threshold was due to the dark adaptation of the rods. The photosensitive pigment in the rods is called rhodopsin. Light converts the retinae$_1$ of the rhodopsin to the all-*trans* isomer (Fig. 16.5). Other than the conversion from 11-*cis* retinae$_1$ to all-*trans* retinae$_1$, all reactions take place continuously irrespective of the presence of light. Hence, in the bright room, all the retinae$_1$ is in all-*trans* form. When subject A enters the dark room, 11-*cis* retinae is gradually synthesised. This explains why subject A was able to see the objects in the dark room after a period of adaptation.

C
1. Rods are more sensitive than cones. Hence, rods are mainly functional in the dark (e.g. at night), whereas cones are mainly functional when it is relatively bright.
2. Cones are mostly found in the fovea and are important for central vision. Rods are found in the periphery of the retina and are important for peripheral vision.
3. There are three different types of cones maximally responsible to light of different wavelengths, and they are essential for colour vision.
4. A higher level of visual acuity can be achieved with cones compared with rods.
5. There are more rods (120 million) than cones (6 million) in each eye.

The nervous system

Table 16.7

Localising signs	Site of lesion	Arteries in CNS territory involved[a]
Reduced stereognosis	Parietal lobe	Middle cerebral
Expressive dysphasia	Broca's area (left parietal frontal)	Left middle cerebral
Receptive dysphasia	Wernicke's area (posterior end of superior temporal gyrus)	Left middle cerebral
Left hemianopia	Right occipital lobe	Right posterior cerebral
Ataxia	Cerebellum	Vertebral or posterior inferior cerebellar
Right hemiplegia	Left motor cortex (temporal lobe)	Left middle cerebral
Sensory loss in the right side of the face and arm	Left sensory cortex (temporal lobe)	Left middle cerebral

[a] The cerebral arterial supply varies between individuals.

ii There will be complete ptosis due to paralysis of the levator palpebrae.

iii As the oculomotor nerve carries the parasympathetic innervation, oculomotor nerve palsy results in widely dilated non-reactive pupil.

16.105

A

The facial nerve generally supplies the muscles of facial expression.

B

Bell's palsy is a palsy of the facial nerve. Patients present with unilateral facial weakness. The cause is unknown, although a viral aetiology has been suspected.

C

The muscles around the forehead and the eyes are bilaterally innervated by the upper motor neurone of the facial nerve. Hence, a unilateral upper motor neurone facial nerve palsy does not result in weakness in facial muscles around the forehead or the eyes. Bell's palsy is a lower motor neurone lesion of the facial nerve.

D

Patients with Bell's palsy may become sensitive to loud noises because the facial nerve supplies stapedius muscle. Stapedius muscle is in the middle ear. In response to loud noises, it pulls the footplate of the stapes out of the oval window and helps to protect the ear against such noises.

16.106

A

The sympathetic nervous system supplies both the sphincter muscle of the iris and partly the levator muscle of the upper eyelid: interruption of the sympathetic nervous system may cause a droopy eyelid and a constricted pupil.

B

The pre-ganglionic fibres of the sympathetic nervous system originate from the anterior nerve root of the thoracic and lumbar segments of the spinal cord and enter the sympathetic chain. They ascend or descend to supply various parts of the body via ganglia (including the superior cervical ganglion) or the adrenal medulla.

C

Horner's syndrome may also occur in lesions:
- of the brainstem (e.g. in multiple sclerosis or stroke)
- of the spinal cord (e.g. in syringomyelia)
- of the thoracic outlet (e.g. Pancoast tumour of lung)
- in the skull (e.g. carotid aneurysm).

16.107

A

See Table 16.8.

B

The general symptoms and signs of nerve root compression at the vertebral column are:
- numbness or tingling sensation in that dermatome

Table 16.8

	Upper motor neurone lesion	Lower motor neurone lesion
Nervous pathway affected	Corticonuclear or corticospinal tracts	Anterior horn cell and peripheral nerves
Muscle weakness	Some	Marked
Muscle wasting	Minimal	Marked
Muscle tone	Increased	Decreased
Fasciculation	Absent	Present
Tendon reflex	Increased	Decreased or absent
Babinski's sign	Positive	Negative

- weakness of muscle supplied by the spinal nerve
- lower motor neurone signs for that dermatome
- upper motor neurone sings for the levels below.

Hence, nerve root compression at L4 level may cause:

- pain or numbness in the dermatome supplied by L4
- weakness of ankle dorsiflexion and knee extension
- reduced or absent knee jerk
- exaggerated ankle jerk
- positive Babinski's sign.

16.108

A

There are both familial and sporadic forms of Alzheimer's disease. Known risk factors for Alzheimer's disease include:

- old age
- female sex
- family history of the disease, especially those with amyloid precursor protein (APP) gene on chromosome 21 (familial form)
- individuals with ApoEe-4 genotype on chromosome 19 (sporadic form).

B

Gross pathological features of Alzheimer's disease include:

- shrinkage of brain tissue
- cortical atrophy, especially in the frontal and temporal lobes
- loss of both cortical grey and white matter
- dilatation of ventricles.

C

The main histological features of Alzheimer's disease include:

- Aβ amyloid plaques
- neurofibrillary tangles – tortuous and elongated corkscrew-like structures formed from thickening of fibrils within neuronal cytoplasm
- reduction in cholinergic activity.

D

The main hypotheses for the pathogenesis of Alzheimer's disease are:

- altered processing of amyloid protein from its precursor APP: abnormal processing of the cell surface glycoprotein APP coded by a gene on chromosome 21 leads to the formation of Aβ plaque and neuronal death
- selective loss of cholinergic neurones in the cerebral cortex, especially in the hippocampus.

E

This may be explained by the hypothesis for altered processing of amyloid protein from its precursor APP. There are three copies of chromosome 21 in Down's syndrome and their APP gene load is higher.

F

Both tacrine and donepezil are cholinesterase inhibitors and act by increasing the availability of acetylcholine in the cortex. Tacrine may produce peripheral cholinergic side effects (e.g. nausea, abdominal cramps) and hepatotoxicity. Donepezil seems to be free of these side effects.

The musculoskeletal system

SYSTEM-BASED MEDICAL SCIENCES

17.1 The following statements about a typical long bone are true:
A It is covered by a tough membrane made up of mainly fibrous tissue
B Collagen makes up over 50% of its organic matrix
C It is formed by ossification of membranes
D When the rate of bone growth decreases, the epiphyseal plate widens
E The linear growth rate increases sharply when the epiphyseal plate fuses with the shaft

17.2 Osteoblasts:
A Make collagen
B May differentiate into osteoclasts
C Reabsorb bone
D Are stimulated by parathyroid hormone
E Are stimulated by corticosteroids

17.3 Predisposing factors for pathological fractures include:
A Bone metastasis
B Osteomalacia
C Osteoporosis
D Paget's disease
E Myeloma

17.4 The clavicle:
A Articulates with the first costal cartilage medially
B Articulates with the coracoid process of the scapula laterally
C Is essential for the abduction of the upper limb
D Very rarely fractures
E Fractures more commonly in its lateral than its middle third

17.5 The following statements about the shoulder joint are true:
A The glenoid cavity is deep
B It has a wider range of movement than the hip joint
C Abduction is initiated by the supraspinatus
D The axillary nerve runs anterior to the joint
E Anterior dislocation is commoner than posterior dislocation

17.6 The rotator cuff muscles include:
A Supraspinatus
B Deltoid
C Latissimus dorsi
D Subscapularis
E Pectoralis major

17.7 The following muscles extend the elbow:
A Biceps

B Triceps
C Pronator teres
D Brachioradialis
E Extensor carpi radialis longus

17.8 The following statements about the scaphoid are true:
A It is a carpal bone in the distal row
B It is attached by the flexor retinaculum
C Most of the blood supply enters at the proximal end
D Fracture usually results from a fall on the outstretched hand
E Non-union is more likely after fracture of the tuberosity (distal part) rather than the waist of the scaphoid

17.9 The flexor retinaculum:
A Is a thickening of the palmar deep fascia
B Is attached to the hamate and the pisiform
C Gives origin to the muscles of the thenar eminence
D Forms the carpal tunnel
E Covers the median nerve

17.10 The following muscles of the hand and their actions are correctly matched:
A Abductor pollicis brevis – abduction of the thumb
B Opponens pollicis – extension of the thumb
C Dorsal interosei – adduct the fingers
D Palmar interosei – abduct the fingers
E Lumbricals – flex the proximal phalanx; extend the middle and distal phalanxes

17.11 The following statements about the hip joint are true:
A It has a deep acetabulum cup
B The associated ligaments are stronger than those of the shoulder joint
C Dislocation of the adult hip is common
D The sciatic nerve runs posterior to the joint
E It is commonly affected by osteoarthritis in older people

17.12 The following statements about the ligaments of the knee joint are correct:
A The anterior cruciate ligament passes from the front of the intercondylar area to the medial surface of the lateral femoral condyle
B The posterior cruciate ligament passes from the front of the intercondylar area to the lateral surface of the lateral femoral condyle

C The lateral collateral ligament passes from the lateral epicondyle of the femur to the head of the fibula

D The medial collateral ligament passes from the medial epicondyle of the femur to the head of the fibula

E The patellar ligament passes from the apex of the patella to the tibial tuberosity

17.13 The following statements about testing the stability of the knee joint are true:

A The knee should be fully flexed when the lateral collateral ligament is tested

B Excessive movement of the knee on varus testing indicates medial collateral ligament weakness

C The knee should be in half-flexed position when the medial collateral ligament is tested

D Anterior and posterior cruciate ligaments should be tested with the knee in full extension

E The patella should be tested by assessing the up-and-down movement when the knee is fully flexed

17.14 The following regions of the vertebral column and their corresponding number of vertebrae (before fusion occurs) are correctly matched:

A Cervical – 8

B Thoracic – 12

C Lumbar – 4

D Sacral – 4

E Coccygeal – 4

17.15 The following regions of the vertebral column are convex anteriorly (i.e. secondary curvature):

A Cervical

B Thoracic

C Lumbar

D Sacral

E Coccygeal

17.16 Osteoporosis is associated with:

A A reduction of total bone mass

B Gross histological abnormalities

C Gross biochemical abnormalities

D Increased susceptibility to fracture

E An excess of bone formation over resorption

17.17 Osteoporosis occurs more commonly in:

A Men than women

B Older than younger people

C Negroes than Caucasians

D After a period of bed rest

E Those on corticosteroid therapy

17.18 The following statements about the arrangements of filaments in the muscle fibre are correct:

A The overlapping patterns of the thick and thin filaments account for the characteristic striations seen on electron microscopy

B The thick filaments are made of actin

C The thin filaments are made of myosin

D Troponin binds to myosin

E Tropomyosin are located between filaments of actin

17.19 Which of the following events occur when an action potential in the skeletal muscle fibre leads to its contraction?

A The action potential is transmitted to different sarcomeres via the T tubules

B Calcium ions diffuse from the extracellular space to the thick and thin filaments

C Calcium ions increase the concentration of tropomyosin

D There is increased availability of troponin in the sarcomere

E There is increased formation of cross-linkages between actin and myosin

17.20 When the muscle fibre contacts:

A The length of the thick filaments decrease

B The length of the thin filaments decrease

C The length of the sarcomere decreases

D The overlap between the thick and the thin filaments increases

E Energy released from ATP is utilised

17.21 Compared to the red (type I) muscle fibres, the white (type II) muscle fibres:

A Contract less rapidly

B Have a longer latent period

C Are smaller

D Contain more mitochondria

E Are richer in glycogen

17.22 The following substances which relax muscles and their mechanisms of action are correctly matched:

A *Clostridium botulinum* toxin – irreversible antagonist at the neuromuscular junction

B Tubocurarine – irreversible antagonist at the neuromuscular junction

C Suxamethonium – depolarisation of the motor end-plate

D Organophosphorus compounds – prevention of release of acetylcholine from pre-synaptic neurone

E Baclofen – glycine agonist in the spinal cord

The musculoskeletal system

17.23 Anticholinesterase drugs (e.g. neostigmine):
  A Increase the synthesis of acetylcholine in the pre-synaptic neurone
  B Increase the acetylcholine concentrationin the neuromuscular junction
  C May be used to reverse the paralytic effects of tubocurarine
  D May be used to reverse the paralytic effects of suxamethonium
  E Are effective in the treatment of myasthenia gravis

17.24 Suxamethonium:
  A Characteristically produces fasciculation before paralysis
  B Normally has a half-life of less than 1 h

  C Is usually metabolised by the enzyme acetylcholinesterase
  D Is mainly excreted by the kidneys
  E May have unusually prolonged effects in several members of the same family

17.25 The following statements about myasthenia gravis are true:
  A It is an autoimmune disorder
  B It is caused by a reduction of acetylcholine synthesis in the pre-synaptic neurone
  C Edrophonium improves the symptoms for many months
  D It is often associated with thymic abnormalities
  E Corticosteroid is an effective treatment

The musculoskeletal system

17.1 A B
The bones are covered by periosteum, which is a tough membrane made up of fibrous tissue. Bone is mainly made up of a matrix of collagen, with microscopic crystals of hydroxyapatites (phosphates of calcium). Whilst the skull bones (other than the base of the skull) ossifies in membranes, the long bones are initially modelled in cartilage, and ossification starts in the shaft of the bone. In childhood, the ends of the long bones (the epiphyses) are separated from the shaft by a plate of actively proliferating cartilage (the epiphyseal growth plate). Linear bone growth is dependent on the formation of new bone laid down by this plate, and the rate of linear growth is proportional to the width of the epiphyseal plate. When the epiphyseal plate fuses with the shaft in adulthood, linear bone growth ceases.

17.2 A D
There are three types of bone cells: osteoblasts, osteocytes and osteoclasts. Osteoblasts are specialised fibroblasts which make collagen. They may differentiate into osteocytes. Osteoblasts are involved in the formation of new bones, and are stimulated by parathyroid hormones. On the other hand, osteoclasts are involved in breaking down bones. However, corticosteroids inhibit osteoblasts. Hence, if corticosteroids are given to children, growth may be stunted.

17.3 A B C D E
Any bone abnormalities which reduce the strength of the bones are predisposing factors for pathological fractures. They include primary or secondary malignancies, metabolic bone disease (e.g. osteoporosis, osteomalacia, Paget's disease), congenital bone disease (e.g. osteogenesis imperfecta) and infection of the bone (oeteomyelitis).

17.4 A C
The clavicle is a long bone which articulates with the manubrium of the sternum medially, and the acromion of the scapula laterally. It is convex anteriorily in its medial two-thirds, and concave anteriorly in its lateral third. It allows the upper limb to move away from the trunk, and it also transmits part of the weight of the upper limb to the trunk. It is very commonly fractured, especially in children and young adults. This usually occurs at the middle third of the bone.

17.5 B C E
The shoulder joint is a ball-and-socket joint. It has a wider range of movement than any other joint in the body. Hence the glenoid cavity is shallow, and the capsule is generally lax, especially inferiorly. The relative lack of muscles inferiorly also contributes to the frequency of downward dislocation of the shoulder after a fall on the hands with the arm abducted. As the head of the humerus which is forced out almost always moves up anteriorly due to the internal rotation – abduction force of the rotator cuff muscles, anterior dislocation is much commoner than posterior dislocation. The abduction of the shoulder is initiated by the supraspinatus and continued by the deltoid muscle. The supraspinatus is subject to the greatest mechanical strain compared to other rotator cuff muscles. Hence pain on active abduction of the shoulder is a common feature in the 'frozen shoulder' syndrome, especially between 90° and 135° abduction (the painful arc).

17.6 A D
The rotator cuff muscles are the short articular muscles of the shoulder joint which insert into the tuberosities of the humerus, and help to stabilise the shoulder joint. These muscles are affected in the 'frozen shoulder'. The rotator cuff muscles are the supraspinatus, infraspinatus, subscapularis and teres minor.

17.7 B
The triceps muscle is the only extensor of the elbow joint. The biceps and brachioradialis flex the elbow. The pronator teres pronates the forearm. The extensor carpi radialis longus extends and abducts the wrist.

17.8 B D
The scaphoid is a carpal bone at the lateral end of the proximal row. The flexor retinaculum (thickening of the deep fascia of the palmar aponeurosis) attaches to the tubercle of the scaphoid and the ridge of the trapezium laterally, and the pisiform and hook of the hamate medially. Fracture of the scaphoid often results in younger people from a fall on the outstretched hand. As most of the blood supply enters the scaphoid at the distal end, ischaemia may occur to the proximal end of the scaphoid after fracture of the waist of the scaphoid. This may lead to non-union or avascular necrosis. However, the blood supply to the scaphoid is preserved after fracture of the tuberosity.

17.9 A B C D E
See question 17.8 above. The flexor retinaculum is a thickening of the palmar deep fascia over the carpal bones. It is attached to the scaphoid and trapezium laterally, and the pisiform and the hamate medially. It gives rise to the origin of the muscles of the thenar and hypothenar eminence, and forms the carpal tunnel for the long flexor tendons. It also covers the median nerve. In the carpal tunnel syndrome, the median nerve is compressed by the flexor retinaculum, and pain and numbness in the distribution of the median nerve may occur. This may occur without any obvious cause, or may

The musculoskeletal system

be associated with osteoarthritis of the wrist, hypothyroidism, pregnancy or rheumatoid arthritis. It may be treated initially by corticosteroid injection, but surgical decompression may be necessary.

17.10 A E
The correct responses are:
- Abductor pollicis brevis – abduction of the thumb (supplied by median nerve)
- Opponens pollicis – opposition of the thumbs to tips of fingers (supplied by median nerve)
- Dorsal interrossei – abduct the fingers (mnemonic: Dorsal ABduct, DAB) (supplied by the ulnar nerve)
- Palmar interrosei – abduct the fingers (mnemonic: Palmar ADduct, PAD) (supplied by the ulnar nerve)
- Lumbricals – flex the proximal phalanges, extend the middle and distal phalanges (lateral two supplied by median nerve, medial two by the ulnar nerve). This explains the 'clawed hand' abnormality of the fourth and fifth fingers in ulnar nerve palsy

17.11 A B D E
The hip joint has a deep acetabulum cup, and the associated ligaments are strong. Hence grossly excess force (e.g. in a road traffic accident) is necessary to dislocate the hips, and hip dislocations are rare. As the sciatic nerve runs posterior to the hips, it may be damaged by posterior dislocation of the hip. Osteoarthritis of the hips commonly affects older people due to excessive cumulative wear and tear, and total hip replacement may be necessary.

17.12 A C E
The correct attachments of the important ligaments of the knee joint are:
- Anterior cruciate ligament – from front of intercondylar area to medial surface of the lateral femoral condyle
- Posterior cruciate ligament – from back of intercondylar area to lateral surface of the medial femoral condyle
- Lateral collateral ligament – from lateral epicondyle of femur to head of fibula
- Medial collateral ligament – from medial epicondyle of femur to upper medial surface of tibial shaft
- Patellar ligament – from apex of patella to tibial tuberosity

17.13 –
To test the collateral ligaments, the knee should be very slightly flexed whilst varus or valgus stress is applied. Excessive movement of the knee on varus testing may indicate lateral collateral ligament weakness. The cruciate ligaments should be tested with the knee flexed at 90°. The stability of the patella can be tested by assessing side-to-side movement when the knee is fully extended.

17.14 B E
The correct number of vertebrae in each region are as follows:
- Cervical – 7
- Thoracic – 12
- Lumbar – 5
- Sacral – 5
- Coccygeal – 4

The sacral and coccygeal vertebrae are fused in adults to form the sacrum and the coccyx.

17.15 A C
In the fetus, the vertebral column is flexed throughout its length (primary curvature). After birth, extension of the cervical region allows the head to be raised, and extension of the lumbar region allows the adoption of an upright posture.

17.16 A D
Osteoporosis is caused by an excess of bone resorption over bone formation, the result being a reduction of total bone mass. However, the bones are otherwise quite normal both histologically and biochemically. The main risk of osteoporosis is that it predisposes to fractures, especially of the femur and the wrist.

17.17 B D E
Men generally have greater bone mass than women. Hence women are more susceptible than men to osteoporosis. As the bone mass generally decreases with age, osteoporosis is commoner in the elderly. Negroes generally have greater bone mass than Caucasians. Hence osteoporosis is commoner in Caucasians than Negroes. Bone mass decreases with immobility. Other aetiology factors of osteoporosis include smoking, excess corticosteroids (either Cushing's syndrome or corticosteroid therapy), diabetes and excess alcohol.

17.18 A E
There are two types of filaments in the muscle fibre: the thick and the thin filaments. The overlapping patterns of the thick and thin filaments account for the characteristic striations seen on histology sections and electron microscopy. The thick filaments are made up of myosin. The thin filaments are made up of two long helical chains of actin. Tropomyosin molecules are located in the groove between the two chains of actin. Troponin molecules are located at intervals along the tropomyosin molecules.

17.19 A E
The correct version of events is:
- Depolarisation of the action potential spreads to other muscle fibrils through the T tubules, so that all

sarcomeres in the muscle fibres contract at the same time
- Calcium ions are released from the terminal cisterns of the sarcoplasmic reticulum and diffuse to the thick and thin filaments in the sarcomere
- Calcium ions bind to troponin C, a subunit of troponin
- This causes movement of tropomyosin, and uncovers sites on actin which myosin can bind to
- Increased cross-linkages between actin and myosin occur, leading to shortening of the sarcomere

17.20   C D E
When the muscle fibre contracts, the thick and thin filaments slide over one another, and the overlap between the thick and thin filaments increases. However, the lengths of the individual filaments remain constant. Energy released from ATP is required for muscle contraction. The breakdown of ATP is catalysed by ATPase activity in the heads of the myosin molecules.

17.21   E
There are two types of muscle fibres: type I (red) and type II (white) muscle fibres. Type I fibres can contract for a prolonged period of time. Hence they are found mainly in the large muscles responsible for maintaining posture. They are mainly aerobic. Thus they contain more mitochondria and myoglobin and less glycogen store and glycolytic capacity. The high myoglobin content accounts for their red colour. They are smaller, contract slower, and have a longer latent period than type II fibres. On the other hand, type II fibres contract faster and are more suitable for fine, accurate movements. Hence they are found in the extraocular muscles and in the muscles of hands and arms.

17.22   C
The correct answers are:
- *Clostridium botulinum* toxin – prevention of release of acetylcholine from pre-synaptic neurone
- Tubocurarine – competitive antagonist at the neuromuscular junction
- Suxamethonium – depolarisation of the motor end-plate
- Organophosphorus compounds – irreversible antagonist at the neuromuscular junction

- Baclofen – agonist at GABA receptors in the spinal cord

17.23   B C E
Acetylcholinesterase (true cholinesterase) is an enzyme which normally destroys acetylcholine at the neuromuscular junction. Anticholinesterase increases the concentration of acetylcholine in the synapse by reducing its breakdown by inhibiting acetylcholinesterase. Hence it may be used to antagonise the paralytic effects of tubocurarine. It is also used in the treatment of myasthenia gravis caused by autoantibodies to acetylcholine receptors. However, as suxamethonim acts by depolarisation, anticholinesterase would, if anything, increase the effect of suxamethonium.

17.24   A B E
As suxamethonium acts by depolarisation, it causes stimulation to the motor end-plate before depolarisation block occurs. Hence fasciculation often precedes paralysis after suxamethonium is administered. Suxamethonium is destroyed by plasma pseudocholinesterases, and thus the half-life of the effect of suxamethonium is short (about 10 min). Therefore, suxamethonium is often used for short procedures (e.g. electroconvulsion therapy). However, pseudocholinesterase deficiency occurs as a hereditary disorder in about one in every 2500 individuals in the population. As they are unable to inactivate suxamethonium, the effect of suxamethonium may last for many hours. They often require artificial ventilation during this period.

17.25   A D E
Myasthenia gravis is caused by the presence of circulating antibodies to the nicotinic acetylcholine receptors. This prevents synaptic transmission at the neuromuscular junction. It is typical of autoimmune disease: it is commoner in women than men, it may be associated with thymic abnormalities, it is sometimes associated with other autoimmune disorders, and treatment with corticosteorid or other immunosuppressive drugs is often effective. Edrophonium is a very short-acting anticholinesterase, and is used as a diagnostic test for myasthenia gravis. The symptoms of myasthenia gravis improve dramatically following an intravenous injection of edrophonium, but the effect usually only lasts for minutes.

INDEX

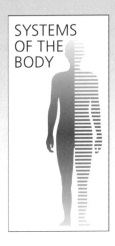

SYSTEMS
OF THE
BODY

The page numbers in **bold** denote illustrations.

A
ABO blood group, 77, 84
Acetazolamide, 27, 216, 223
Acetylcholine, 13, 25, 212, 248, 255, 261
Acetylcholinesterase, 264, 267
Acid-fast bacilli, 54, 60
Acidic drugs, 19, 27
Acids, 50
Acquired immunological memory, 41, 46
Acromegaly, 182, 195
Acute inflammation, 42–3, 48–9, 53
Adenosine, 125
ADH secretion, 175, 184
Adhesion pili, 50
Adrenal steroids, 179–80, 190–1
Adrenaline, 25, 179, 190, 214
Afterload, 111, 126, 128
Aggressins, 50
Agonists, 15, 17, 18, 21, 23, 24, 26, 214
Alcohol, 20, 29, 50, 170, 173, 239, 258
Alkalization, of urine, 216–17, 224
Alkalosis, respiratory, 135, 144, 151
Alleles, 77–8, 85
Allergy, drugs, 17, 23, 50
Allosteric enzymes, 5, 11, 14
Alzheimer's disease, 238, 242, 252–3, 261
Amenorrhoea, 182, 194–5
Amino acids, 165
Amiodarone, 124
Amniocentesis, 200, 209
Amniotic fluid, 200, 209
Amphotericin B, 65
Amylase, 155, 161
Anaemias, 90, 92–3, 97, 101–2
Anaesthesia, 238–9, 254–5
Analgesics, 234, 248
Androgens, 198, 202, 212
Angina, 112
Antacids, 164
Antagonism, between drugs, 15, 21–2
Antagonists, 15, 18, **19**, 21, 23, 26, 27
Antianginal drugs, 108, 119
Antiasthmatics, 134, 143, 151
Antibacterial agents/defences, 54, 57, 59, 65
Antibiotics, 55, 56–7, 61, 65
Anticoagulants, 153
Antidepressants, 15, 238, 239, 253, 256
Antiemetics, 155, 160–1
Antifungal agents, 57, 65
Antihypertensives, 107, 118, 128
Antimicrobial agents, 57
Antimuscarinic agents, 225, 235, 248–9
Antiplatelet agents, 91, 98
Antiviral agents/defences, 54, 55, 59, 61
Aorta, arch of, 106, 117–18
Apex beat, 109, 121
Apoptosis, 42, 48, 51, **52**
Appendicitis, 158, 169
Arrector pili muscles, 70, 72
Arterial pressure, 107, 118
Arterioles, 106–7, 118

Aspirin, 27, 98, 164, 219, 229
Asthma, 134, 139, 143, 151
Atenolol, 113, 129
Atherosclerosis, 107, 118–19, 128
ATP, conversion to ADP, 30, 34
Atrial fibrillation, 105, 111, 115, 124
Atropine, 123, 256
Auditory nerve impulses, 237, 252
Auscultatory method, 112, 127
Autosomal disorders, 74, 75, 79–80, 81

B
Bacteria, and disease, 43, 50, 54, 56, 57, 59, 63–4
Bacterial cell walls, 56, 63
Bacteriophages, 55, 61
Bacteroides, 55, 60–1
Basal ganglia, 235, 249
Basement membrane, epithelial, 70, 72
Bell's palsy, 241, 260
Benzodiazepines, 23–4, 238, 253
Bicarbonate, 27
Biguanides, 178–9, 188
Bile, 171, 173
Bilirubin, 171, 173–4
Biological response, drugs, 18–19, 25–7
Bismuth, 164
Bisphosphonates, 178, 187
Bladder, 217, 218, 220, 225, 226, **230**
Blood and bone marrow, 89–104, 108–9, 120, 134, 142
Blood cells, 89, 90, 92, 95, 97, 100, 102, 134
Blood flow, 107, 119, 126, 215, 222, 244
Blood pressure, 107, 112, 127, 182, 196, 218, 227, 258
Blood-brain barrier, 232, 240, 244, 245, 257–8
Body temperature, 70, 72, 175, 183
Body volume, 92, 99–100
Brain, 32, 38, 231, 243
Breasts, female, 199, 207
Bromocriptine, 195, 207, 249
Bronchial breath sounds, 137, 140, 146–7, 152
Bronchial carcinoma, 136, 139, 146, 152
Bronchioles, respiratory, 133, 141
Bronchus, right main, 133, 141
Brown fat, 31, 36

C
Calcitonin, 177, 187
Calcium, 177, 186
Calcium channel blockers, 105, 115–16
Calculi, urinary, 217, 225
Calorimetry, 37
Capillary circulation, 108, 120
Carbimazole, 176, 185
Carbohydrate digestion, 155, 157, 161
Carbon dioxide, 5, 11, 134, 142–3, 144
Carcinomas, 136, 139, 146, 152, 154, 160, 171, 173, 176, 185, 198–9, 207, 217, 218,

225, 226
Cardiac failure, 106, 109, 117, 121
Cardiac glycosides, 105, 116
Cardiac murmurs, 110, 113, 122, 130
Cardiac muscle, 105, 115
Cardiac output, 106, 110, 111, 116–17, 122, 125
Cardiac thrills, 109, 122
Cardiovascular system, 105–32
Carotid arteries, 231, 244
Carotid sinus message, 125
Catecholamines, 176, 184, 189
Cell-mediated immune responses, 50
Cells, 3–14, 89, 95
Cellular injury, 42, 47–8
Cellulitis, 44–5, 53
Cerebellum, 235–6, 249–50
Cerebral abscesses, 231, 243
Cerebral arteries, 231, 244
Cerebral infarction, 232, 244
Cerebral oedema, 240
Cerebrospinal fluid, 231, 239, 243, 257
Cervical carcinomas, 199, 207
Chemical control, respiration, 143
Chemical messengers, 3–4, 7, 9
Chemical reactions, 4, 7, 9–10
Chlamydia, 56, 63
Chloride ions, 3, 5, 6, 8
Cholecystokinin, 171, 174
Chronic bronchitis, 148–9
Chronic inflammation, 43, 49
Cigarette smoke, 50, 103, 148, 152
Cirrhosis, 170–1, 173
Citric acid cycle, 30, 34–5, 38–9
Clavicle, 262, 265
Clomifene, 202, 214
Clostridia, 54, 60, 263, 267
Coagulation, 91, 94, 99
Codon, 10
Coeliac disease, 156, 157, 161–2, 167–8
Colchicine, 12
Colon, 155, 161
Communicating junctions, 70, 73
Congenital infection, 57, 66, 67
Contraceptives, 198, 202–3, 206, 214
Contractility, 111, **126**
Coronary arteries, 112, 128
Corticospinal tract, 235, 249
Cortisol, 180, 190, **194**
Cough, 135, 138, 144–5, 148
Cranial meninges, 231, 243
Cranial nerves, 231, 236, 243, 250
Crohn's disease, 156, 157, **158**, 162, **168**
Cromoglycate, 151
Culture mediums, 56, 62
Cushing's syndrome, 181–2, 194
Cyanosis, 121
Cyclizine, 166
Cyproterone acetate, 199, 208, 212
Cytochrome P_{450}, 16, 23
Cytoplasmic membrane, 63
Cytoskeleton, 3, 8

D
Dead spaces, respiratory, 133, 141, 148
Dehydration, 216, 219, 223, 227, 228
Deoxygenated blood, 108, 120, 142
Dermis, 70, 72
Diabetes insipidus, 175, 183–4
Diabetes mellitus, 178, 179, 180, 181, 188, 189
Diagnostic tests, 56, 61
Diffusion, 9
Digoxin, 105, 111, 122, 124, 207
Diltiazem, 113, 129
Diphtheria, 54, 60
Dipyridamole, 98
Disinfection, 56, 62
Disopyramide, 98
Dissacharides, 155, 161
Dizygotic twins, 71, 73, 208
DNA, 3, 6, 8, 49, 61, 74, 79
Donepezil, 261
Dopamine, 207
Dose-response curve, 15, 18, 21, 25, 26
Down's syndrome, 75, 80, 97
Ductus arteriosus, 113, 130
Duodenal ulcers, 154, 159–60
Dysplasia, 41, 47, **52**

E
Ectoderm, 70, 73
Edrophonium, 256
Elderly, effects of drugs, 17, 23
Elimination, 6, 12, 16, 22, 23, 28, 29
Embryology, 70–3, 201, 210
Emphysema, 136, 145–6, 148
Endocrine system, 175–96
Endoderm, 70–1, 73
Endometrial carcinomas, 198–9, 207
Endotoxins, 50, 57, 68
Energy, 3, 5, 30–40
Enzyme inhibitors, 5, 11, 15, 21, 24–5
Enzymes, 4–5, 7, 9–11, 32, 38, 155–6, 161
Epidermis, 70, 72
Epithelia, 70, 72
Epstein-Barr virus, 55, 61, 68
Exercise, 37, 106, 111, 117, 126
Exotoxins, 50, 57, 68
Extracellular microorganisms, 41, 46

F
Facial nerve palsy, 236, 241, 250, 260
Fats, 155, 161
Femoral canal, 168
Fertilisation, 200, 208
Fetal circulation, 113–14, 131
Fetal development, 71, 73
Fibrinolytic system, 92, 94, 99
Fibrinolytics, 99, 153
Fick principle, 125
Filaments, muscle fibre, 263, 266
Filtration fraction, 218, 227
Flexor retinaculum, 262, 265–6
Fluconazole, 65
Flucytosine, 65–6

Food poisoning, 58, 69
Fractional occupancy, 18, 25
Fragile X syndrome, 75, 81
Furosemide, 216, 223

G
GABA, 245, 253
Gallbladder, 171, 174
Gap junctions, 4, 9
Gas exchange, 133, 141
Gastric secretions, 154, 159
Gastro-oesophageal reflux, 155, 161
Gastroenteritis, 156, 162
Gastrointestinal epithelium, 43, 50
Gastrointestinal infection, 69
Gastrointestinal system, 154–69
Genetics, 4, 10, 54, 56, 59, 64, 74–86
Gentamicin, 239, 258
Gestation, structural defects, 71, 73
GFR, 215, 222
Glomerular disease, 217, 220, 224, 230
Glucagon, 179, 189, 192
Glucocorticoids, 151, 152, 179, 190, 191, 194
Glucose, 5, 11, 32, 33, 35, 38, 165, 178, 181, 188, 192, 195, 219, 221, 222, 227
Glycine, 245–6
Glycogen, 30–1, 35
Glycolysis, 30, 35, 38
Glycopeptides, 65
GnRH, 198, 205–6
Goitre, 180, 191
Gonads, 197, 204
Graft rejection, after transplantation, 41, 47
Gram-negative bacteria, 54, 59–60
Gram-positive bacteria, 54, 59–60
Granulomatous disease, 45, 53
Grave's disease, 176, 185
Growth hormone, 179, 189, 195, 196
Growth mechanisms, 44, 51

H
HAART, 58, 69
Haemoglobin, 89, 92, 93, 95–6, 100–1, 102–3, 133–4, 138–9, 142, 149–50
Haemolysis, 90, 97
Haemolytic anaemia, 90, 97, 102
Haemophilia A, 92, 99
Haemophilus influenzae, 55, 60, 243
Half life, of drugs, 17, 24, 28
Heart block, 111, 125
Heart rate, 105, 111, 116, 125, 126
Heart sound, 109–10, 122
Heparin, 92, 99, 104
Hepatitis, 57, 68, 173
Hernias, 156, 158, 162, 168–9
Hexokinase, 38
Hip joint, 262, 266
Histology, 70–3
Hodgkin's disease, 91, 98
Homozygotes, 74–5, 80
Hormones, 38, 155, 160, 175, 176, 177,

179, 183, 184–5, 186, 189, 190, 195, 196
Horner's syndrome, 241, 260
Horseshoe kidneys, 215, 221–2
Hot flushes, 202, 211
Human chorionic gonadotrophin (hCG), 200, 209
Human immunodeficiency virus (HIV), 55, 58, 61, 69
Hydrocephalus, 231, 239, 244, 257
Hydrochloric acid, 163–4
Hydrogen ions, 216, 223
Hyoscine, 166
Hyperbilirubinaemia, 171, 174
Hypercalcaemia, 177–8, 187
Hyperparathyroidism, 178, 187, 192–3
Hyperplasia, 41, 47, 51
Hyperprolactinaemia, 207
Hypersensitivity, 41, 46–7
Hypertension, 107, 112, 118, 128
Hyperthyroidism, 176, 185
Hypertonicity, 228
Hypertrophy, 47, 51
Hyperventilation, 258
Hypoglycaemia, 179, 189, 191
Hypoparathyroidism, 177, 186
Hypothalamic maturation, 197, 205, 210
Hypothalamus, 175, 183
Hypothyroidism, 176, 185
Hypovolaemic shock, 114, 131–2
Hypoxia, 135, 144, 150, 151

I
Imipramine, 239, 256
Immune system, maternal, 200, 209
Immunoglubulins, 41, 46
Impotence, 200, 202, 208, 212
Incontinence, 217, 225
Infection, external barriers, 41, 46
Infectious diseases, 54–69
Infectious mononucleosis, 58, 68
Infertility, 202, 212–13, 214
Inguinal canal, 168
Inhibin, 198, 206
Inspiratory muscles, 136, 145
Insulin, 178, 180, 187–8, 191
Interactions, of drugs, 17–18, 24–5
Interferon, 54, 56, 59, 64–5
Intestines, 154, 155, 157, 160, 167
Intracellular junctions, 70, 72–3
Intracerebral haemorrhage, 232, 244
Inulin, 218, 226–7
Inverse agonists, 17, 23–4
Iodine, 191
Ionising radiation, 42, 47
Ipratropium, 151
Iron, 89–90, 93, 96, 101–2
Irradiation, therapeutic, 44, 51–2
Ischaemic symptoms, 107–8, 119
Islets of Langerhans, 178, 187
Isoenzymes, 4, 10
Isoprenaline, 111, 125
Isosorbide mononitrate, 113, 129

Index

J
Jugular vein, internal, 109, 121
Jugular venous pulse, 109, 121

K
Karotypes, 76, 82–3
Ketoacidosis, diabetic, 178, 188
Ketone bodies, 31, 35, 36
Kidneys, 22, 215, 221
Kilocalories, 32, 37
Knee jerk, 233–4, 239, 247, 256–7
Knee joint, 262–3, 266

L
Labour, 201, 203, 210, 214
Laxatives, 156, 162, 167
Left atrium, 106, 116
Legionella pneumophila, 55, 60
Leptin, 175, 183
Lesions, visual pathway, 237, 252
Leukaemia, 90, 93–4, 97, 103
Levothyroxine, 13
LH surge, 198, 206, 213
Lidocaine, 110, 124
Lipids, 155, 161
Listeria monocytogenes, 55, 57, 60, 67
Lithium, 238, 253–4
Liver and biliary system, 170–4
Lobar pneumonia, 140, 152
Lobules, liver, 170, 172
Long-acting thyroid stimulator (LATs), 176, 185
Loops of Henle, 216, 221, 222–3, 228
Lung disease, 141–2
Lung resonance, 136, 146
Lung volume, 133, 137, 141, 147
Luteal phase, 198, 206
Lymph nodes, 91, 97–8
Lymphatic circulation, 91, 98

M
Malabsorption, 155, 160, 161, 165
Mannitol, 222
Mastication, 154, 159, 162, 163
Medial longitudinal fasciculus (MLF), 236, 250–1
Megakaryocytes, 104
Meiosis, 74, 79
Membrane, human cell, 3, 8
Menarche, 211
Mendelian inheritance, 76, 77, 83, 84
Meningiomas, 231, 243
Meningism, 58, 69
Meningitis, 58, 69, 243
Meningococci, 55, 60, 243
Menopause, 212
Mesoderm, 73
Metabolic rate, 31, 32, 35, 37
Metastases, blood-borne, 43, 49
Metformin, 188, 191
Metoclopramide, 166
Michaelis-Menten equation, 4–5, 10–11, 14
Microcytes, 89, 96

Microtubules, 8, 12, 245
Micturition, 217, 225
Milk production, 199, 207–8
Minerals, dietary, 31, 36
Mitochondria, 8, 39
Mitosis, 4, 10
Mitral valve, 105–6, 114, 116, 131
Modified release capsules, 15, 22
Monosaccharides, 30, 34
Monozygotic twins, 73, 80, 208
Mosaics, 74, 79
Motor neurone lesions, 235, 236, **241**, 242, 249, 250, **261**
MRNA, 3, 8–9
Mucus, 164
Mullerian ducts, 197, 204
Multifactorial disorders, 75, 80
Multiple sclerosis, 233, 246
Muscle cells, 5, 11
Muscle fibre, 263, 266–7
Muscle relaxants, 263, 267
Musculoskeletal system, 111, 126, 262–7
Mutation, 54, 59, 76, 81–2
Myasthenia gravis, 239, 255–6, 264, 267
Mycobacterium spp., 60
Mycoplasma, 63, 65
Myelination, 233, 246
Myelomas, multiple, 90, 94, 97, 103
Myocardial infarction, 107, 108, 119–20, 129
Myoglobin, 134, 142, 150
Myopia, 237, 251

N
Na+,K+-ATPase, 3, 8, 9
Necrosis, 42, 47, 48, **52**
Neisseria spp., 60
Neostigmine, 255
Nephrons, 215, 216, 221
Nephropathy, obstructive, 217, 224
Nerve endings, 233, 246
Nerve root compression, 233, 246–7, 260–1
Nervous system, 231–61
Neural control, respiration, 134, 143
Neuroglial cells, 233, 246
Neuromuscular junction, 233, 246
Neurones, 43, 50–1, 232, 245
Neurotransmitters, 212, 233, 234, 245–6, 248
Neutrophils, 53
Nicotinic receptor, 255
Nitrogen balance, negative, 33, 40
Non-penetrance, 74, 80
Non-steroidal anti-inflammatory drugs, 19
Noradrenaline, 13, 25, 179, 189, 190, 214
Nucleus, 8, 89, 95
Nutrition, 30–40

O
Oculomotor nerve, 236, 250, 258, 259
Oestrogen, 206, 207
Omeprazole, 164
Oncogenes, 43, 49

Oncoproteins, 43, 49
Ondansetron, 166
Opiates, 234, 248
Optic nerve, 236, 237, 251, 258
Organelles, 3, 6
Organic nitrates, 129
Osmotic diuresis, 216, 223
Osteoblasts, 262, 265
Osteoporosis, 263, 266
Ovarian germ cells, 198, 205
Ovarian tumours, 199, 207
Ovulation, 213
Oxidative phosphorylation, 30, 34, 39
Oxygen, 5, 11, 107, 111, 119, 126, 133–4, 135, 139, 142, 144, 150
Oxygen-haemoglobin dissociation curve, 134, 142
Oxygenated blood, 108, 120
Oxytocin, 175, 184

P
P-Aminohippuric acid (PAH), 218, 227
Pancuronium, 255
Papaverine, 212
Parathyroid gland, 43, 51, 177, 186
Parkinson's disease, 235, 249
Parotid gland, 163
Paroxetine, 239, 256
Partial agonists, 17, 21, 24
Parturition, 201, 210
Passive immunisation, 56, 61, 66
Pathological processes, 41–53
Penile erection, 199–200, 208, 212
Peptic ulcers, 154, 157, 159, 164
Peptidoglycan, 63
Perfusion, 133, 141
Pericardium, 106, 118
Peripheral nerves, 254
Peristalsis, 167
Permeability, of drugs, 15, 21
Phagocytic cells, 41, 46
Pharmacology, 15–29
Phenothiazines, 207, 238, 249, 253
Phosphates, high energy, 30, 34, 39
Phosphofructokinase, 38
Photoreceptors, 236–7, 251
Pituitary gland, 175, 184
Placenta, 200, 209
Plasma concentration, of drugs, 16, 23
Plasma membrane, 15, 21
Plasma proteins, drug binding, 16, 22
Plasmodia, 55, 61
Platelets, 91, 94, 98, 103–4
Pneumothorax, 136, 146
Polycythaemia, 102, 103
Polyploidy, 74, 79
Polysaccharides, 66
Portal hypertension, 170, 172
Portal venous system, 170, 172
Posterior column-medial lemniscal pathway, 234, 247
Potassium ions, 3, 5, 6, 8
Pre-ganglionic fibres, 248, 260

Prenatal diagnosis, 75, 81
Progesterone, 206, 207
Prolactin, 195, 199, 207
Prostaglandins, 214
Prostate gland, 218, 226
Protein synthesis, 3, 6, 8–9, **13**
Proteins, 3, 4, 8, 9, 31, 36, 39, 40, 155–6, 157, 161, 165
Proton pump, 164
Proximal renal tubules, 215–16, 219, 222, **229**
Puberty, 197, 204–5, 210, 211
Pulmonary arterial hypertension, 136, 145
Pulmonary emboli, 48, 135–6, 140, 145
Pulmonary oedema, 136, 145
Pulse character, 109, 121
Pupillary light reflex, 236, 240, 251, 258
Pyelonephritis, 217, 224–5
Pyruvate, 30, 35

R
Radial nerve, 233, 247
Ranitidine, 164
Rashes, 57, 68
Rebound phenomenon, 17, 24
Reinforcement, 257
Renal and urinary system, 16, 22–3, 215–30
Renin-angiotensin-aldosterone system, 128, **196**
Reproductive system, 197–214
Respiratory chain, 30, 34
Respiratory failure, 135, 144
Respiratory quotient, 32, 37
Respiratory system, 133–53
Reticulocytes, 102
Retina, 237, 251
Retrograde neuronal transport, 232, 245
Rickets, 181, 192
Rickettsiae, 56, 63
Rotator cuff muscles, 262, 265

S
Salbutamol, 151
Saliva, 154, 159, 163
Scaphoid, 262, 265
Second messengers, 4, 9, 233, 246
Selectivity, of drugs, 15, 21
Seminiferous tubules, 198, 205
Sensitivity, to drugs, 15, 21
Sex-linked disorders, 74, 78, 79, 80, 85–6
Shoulder joint, 262, 265
Sildenafil, 200, 208, 212
Sino-atrial node, 105, 115, 123
Sinus rhythm, 110, 123
Sodium, 3, 5, 6, 8, 11, 128, 216, 222, 223
Somatomedins, 179, 189

Sound, 237, 252
Sounds of Korotkoff, 112, 127
Spermatozoa, 198, 199, 202, 208, 212, 213–14
Spherocytosis, 93, 102
Spinothalamic tract, 234, 247
Spirometers, 37
Spironolactone, 196, 216, 223
Squamous cell bronchial carcinomas, 136, 146, 152
Staining methods, 56, 62
Staphylococci, 54, 60
Starch, 157, 161, 164–5
Starling's law, 111, 126
Starvation, 31, 35
Steady state concentration, of drugs, 16, 23
Sterilisation, 54, 56, 59, 62
Streptokinase, 104
Stroke, 232, 244
Stroke volume, 111, 125–6
Submandibular/sublingual glands, 163
Sulphonylureas, 178, 188
Supraventricular tachycardia, 111, 124
Surfactant, 133, 141, 147
Suxamethonium, 255, 263, 264, 267
Swallowing, 156, 163
Sympathetic nervous system, 128, 208, 234–5, 241, 248, 260
Synapse, 232, 245
Systemic availability, drugs, 15, 17, 22, 24
Systemic emboli, 42, 48
Systolic pressures, 109, 120–1, 127

T
T-cells, 41, 46
Tacrine, 261
Temporomandibular joints, 162
Teratogenic agents, 71, 73
Terbinafine, 65
Testes, 197, 198, 204, 205
Testicular feminisation syndrome, 197, 204
Testosterone, 198, 205, 212
Thalassaemias, 93, 102
Theophylline, 151
Therapeutic index, 19, 27
Thiazide diuretics, 217, 224, 228–9
Thirst, 175, 181, 183, 193
Thrombosis, 42, 44, 48, 92, 99
Thymus gland, 91, 98
Thyroid gland, 176–7, 180, 185, 190
Thyroid hormones, 38, 175, 176, 184–5, 190
Ticlopidine, 98
Tissues, adult, 15, 21, 42, 47
Tolbutamide, 191

Toxoids, 56, 61
Trachea, 136, 146
Tranexemic acid, 104
Transitional epithelium, 70, 72
Translation, protein synthesis, 3, 8
Transmission, infectious agents, 57, 66
Transsexuals, 197, 201, 204, 210
TRH stimulation test, 191
Tricyclic antidepressants, 238, 253
Trigeminal nerve, 236, 250
Triglycerides, 157, 165
Trinucleotide repeat amplification, 74, 79
Trisomy, 74, 75, 79, 80
Trophoblasts, 70, 73
Tumours, 43, 49, 199, 207, 218, 220, 225, 226, **230**

U
Ulcerative colitis, 157, **158, 168**
Ulnar nerve, 233, 247
Ureters, 215, 221
Uterine muscle contraction, 201, 210

V
Vaccines, 56, 57, 61–2, 66
Vasopressin, 175, 183, 216, 222
Ventilation, 133, 135, 138, 141, 143–4, 149
Ventricular fibrillation, 110, 124
Ventricular septal defects, 113, 129
Ventricular systole, 105, 116
Ventricular tachycardia, 110, 124, 125
Vertebral column, 263, 266
Viral cell entry, 56, 63
Virulence, 56, 64
Viruses, 49, 54, 55, 56, 58, 59, 61, 62, 64, 68, 69
Visual threshold, 237, 240–1, 251, 258–9
Vitamins, 31, 36, 90, 91, 96–7, 99, 177, 186, 192, 259
Vocal folds, 136, 140, 146, 152
Volume of distribution, drugs, 16, 20, 22, 28
Vomiting, 155, 157, 160, 165–6

W
Warfarin, 91–2, 98, 99, 104
Water, 5, 11
Wernicke's area, 237–8, 252
Wolffian system, 197, 204

X
X chromosomes, 83, 84
X-linked dominant conditions, 75, 80

Z
Zero-order kinetics, 16, 20, 29